VASCULAR ENDOTHELIUM IN HEALTH AND DISEASE

ADVANCES IN EXPERIMENTAL MEDICINE AND BIOLOGY

Recent Volumes in this Series

VASCULAR ENDOTHELIUM IN HEALTH AND DISEASE

Edited by

Shu Chien

Institute of Biomedical Sciences
Academia Sinica
Taipei, Taiwan
Republic of China

PLENUM PRESS • NEW YORK AND LONDON

Library of Congress Cataloging in Publication Data

Vascular endothelium in health and disease / edited by Shu Chien.
    (Advances in experimental medicine and biology; v. 242)
        p.   cm.
    "Proceedings of the satellite symposium to the Fourth World Congress for Micro-
circulation on vascular endothelium in health and disease, held August 5–6, 1987, in
Taipei, Taiwan, Republic of China"—T.p. verso.
    Proceedings of the Symposium on "Vascular Endothelium in Health and Disease,"
held at the Institute of Biomedical Sciences, Academia Sinica.
    Includes bibliographies and index.

    DOI 10.1007/978-1-4684-8935-4
    1. Vascular endothelium—Pathophysiology—Congresses. 2. Vascular endothelium—
Physiology—Congresses. I. Chien, Shu. II. Symposium on "Vascular Endothelium in
Health and Disease" (1987: Institute of Biomedical Sciences, Academia Sinica) III.
World Congress for Microcirculation (4th: 1987: Tokyo, Japan) IV. Series.
    [DNLM: 1. Endothelium, Vascular—physiology—congresses. WI AD559 v. 242 /
QS 532.5.E7 V3314 1987]
RC691.4.V37   1988
616.1′3—dc19
DNLM/DLC   88-26583
for Library of Congress   CIP

Proceedings of the Satellite Symposium to the Fourth World Congress for
Microcirculation on Vascular Endothelium in Health and Disease,
held August 5-6, 1987, in Taipei, Taiwan, Republic of China

© 1988 Plenum Press, New York
MyCopy version of the original edition 1988
A Division of Plenum Publishing Corporation
233 Spring Street, New York, N.Y. 10013

Dedicated to my wife,

Kuang-Chung Hu Chien,M.D.,

and my colleagues at

Institute of Biomedical Sciences, Academia Sinica,

and

Division of Circulatory Physiology and Biophysics,
Department of Physiology and Cellular Biophysics,
Columbia University College of Physicians and Surgeons

PREFACE

In recent years there has been rapid progress in research on vascular endothelium. This has led to significant advances in our understanding of the structure and function of vascular endothelium in health and disease, including such aspects as the permeability of endothelium in relation to its ultrastructural correlates, theoretical basis, regulatory factors, and role in atherogenesis; the interaction between endothelium and blood cells; the endothelial release and processing of a number of important physiological agents, such as eicosanoids, hemostatic factors, and histamine; the cell biology of endothelium with respect to the cytoskeletal apparatus, cell activation, and cell locomotion; and the role of endothelium in microcirculatory regulation in normal and pathophysiological circumstances.

A Symposium on "Vascular Endothelium in Health and Disease" was held on August 5-6, 1987, at the Institute of Biomedical Sciences, Academia Sinica, Taipei, Taiwan, Republic of China, following the 4th World Congress for Microcirculation in Japan. Experts working on various aspects of vascular endothelium came from all over the world to participate in this two-day Symposium and gave excellent presentations. This volume, embodying the proceedings of that Symposium, is a collection of the papers given by the speakers with, in many cases, further updating and new information added subsequent to the Symposium.

The Institute of Biomedical Sciences (IBMS), the site of this Symposium, is a newly established research institution, which has vascular endothelium as one of its areas of research emphasis. Its parent organization, Academia Sinica, celebrates its 60th Anniversary on June 9, 1988. The Republic of China, with its remarkable economic advances, is now making a major effort in upgrading its biomedical research. Therefore, the holding of this Symposium was timely and valuable. It provided an opportunity for local scientists to learn state-of-the-art research from leading workers on vascular endothelium. The publication of this volume will ensure the dissemination of important information to a wide audience and the promotion of interest in endothelial research everywhere in the world.

This book consists of 25 manuscripts grouped under seven topics, viz. Microvascular Permeability, Role of Endothelium in Atherogenesis, Leukocyte-Endothelium Interactions, Prostaglandins and Hemostatic Functions of Vascular Endothelium, Histamine and Endothelium, Cell Biology of Endothelium, and Tumor Microcirculation. Thus, it encompasses the major developments in endothelial research outlined above. On the one hand, the book covers the current advances in basic science research on vascular endothelium in breadth and depth, elucidating many important biological processes such as macromolecular permeability, fluid transfer, interstitial transport, cell-cell interaction, chemotaxis, cell locomotion, receptor binding, eicosanoid biosynthesis, thrombosis and hemostasis, and angiogenesis. On the other hand, it contains important information relevant to a variety of clinical conditions, e.g., atherosclerosis, inflammation, edema formation, coagulationopathies, peripheral vascular disorders, peptic ulcer, and cancer. Therefore, this book presents a collection of important information on vascular endothelium in health and disease, and should be valuable to scientists, clinicians, and students in many different disciplines, including angiologists, biochemists, bioengineers, biophysicists, cell biologists, electron microscopists, hematologists, internists, oncologists, pharmacologists, physiologists, surgeons, and others.

Shu Chien
Institute of Biomedical Sciences
Academia Sinica
May 1988

ACKNOWLEDGMENTS

The successful holding of this Symposium on Vascular Endothelium in Health and Disease and the publication of this proceedings volume have been made possible by the support and efforts of many organizations and individuals. I would like to thank Professor M. Tsuchiya and the organizers of the 4th World Congress for Microcirculation for making this a satellite symposium of the Congress, thus facilitating the participation of many world leaders in the field. The participants from abroad included the Present and Past Presidents, and Present and Past Secretaries General of several international learned societies, e.g. the Bioengineering Society (U.S.A.), the European Society for Microcirculation, the International Society of Biorheology, the Microcirculatory Society (North America), and the 4th World Congress for Microcirculation. The speakers and chairpersons are outstanding scientists from ten nations on four continents; their wonderful contributions to the Symposium and to this book are gratefully appreciated.

I wish to acknowledge with gratitude the support and encouragement of Academia Sinica (President: Dr. Ta You Wu), the Advisory Committee of the Institute of Biomedical Sciences (Chairman: Dr. Paul N. Yu), and the National Science Council (Chairman: Dr. Li An Chen) in sponsoring this Symposium, and the co-sponsorship by the Foundation for Biomedical Sciences (Chairman: Mr. S.K. Huang) and the China Committee for Scientific and Scholarly Cooperation with U.S.A. (Chairman: Mr. K.T. Li), as well as the generous support of several government agencies and private sector.

I wish to thank Drs. C. Y. Chai and Kung-ming Jan and other members of the Organizing Committee, the Local Executive Committee, and the Program Committee for their excellent work and to express my appreciation to the International and Local Honorary Advisors for their valuable advice and counsel. I am most grateful to Mr. Ching Tung Chen for his marvelous editorial assistance and I would like to thank Ms. Grace Han for her excellent cooperation during the preparation of this book.

Shu Chien
Institute of Biomedical Sciences
Academia Sinica
May 1988

CONTENTS

PROSTAGLANDINS AND HEMOSTATIC FUNCTIONS OF VASCULAR ENDOTHELIUM

HISTAMINE AND ENDOTHELIUM

CELL BIOLOGY OF ENDOTHELIUM

TUMOR MICROCIRCULATION

MICROVASCULAR PERMEABILITY

THE PARACELLULAR PATHWAY IN CAPILLARY ENDOTHELIA

Magnus Bundgaard

Department of General Physiology & Biophysics
The Panum Institute, Blegdamsvej 3
DK- 2200 Copenhagen N, Denmark

INTRODUCTION

The main function of the circulation is exchange of gases and solutes between blood and tissue occurring across the walls of microvessels. In the days before electron microscopy the water-filled clefts between the endothelial cells were considered the obvious pathway for exchange of hydrophilic solutes.[1] The introduction of electron microscopy in studies of capillary wall structure somewhat confused this simple picture. The electron micrographs indicated that the clefts between the endothelial cells are closed by cell contacts;[2,3] and thus they could not serve as hydrophilic diffusion pathway. Consequently, an extensive search for transcellular pathways for hydrophilic solutes was initiated. Starling's original concept has now been revived. Recent data, both physiological and ultrastructural, strongly indicate that solutes - at least up to the size of small proteins - may permeate the microvascular endothelium via the paracellular pathway.[4,5] It remains unclear how macromolecules and particles (diameter larger than 5 nm) permeate the endothelium.

The intercellular tight junctions seem to be a dynamic system. Many autacoids, released by cells in the tissues, rapidly induce formation of large intercellular leaks (0.1-1.0 μm) in venular endothelium.[6] This phenomenon is reversible and dose-dependent. More subtle modulations of the endothelial tight junctions - leading to increased permeability - probably also occur.[7]

This report gives a brief overview of electron microscopical data on the organization of the paracellular pathway in microvascular endothelia. In addition, recent results on the organization of structures, potentially involved in modulation of junctional permeability, will be presented and discussed.

DIMENSIONS OF THE INTERCELLULAR CLEFTS

The dimensions of the intercellular clefts and the organization of the endothelial tight junctions are the structural parameters which define the significance of exchange of solutes via the clefts. Thus, permeability varies in direct proportion to the length of the clefts per unit area and to the average width of the clefts, and in inverse proportion to the depth of the clefts - the diffusion path length (Fig. 1).

Estimates of the average cleft length per unit area capillary wall (L) and of the cleft depth (ΔX) can be obtained using stereological principles. Cleft lengths have been determined for a series of capillaries. The average cleft length for capillaries is about 20 m/cm^2.[8] Cleft depths, (ΔX), measured along the tortuous clefts from the luminal to the abluminal openings vary among different types of capillaries - the average is about 0.7 μm.[8,9] The width of the clefts is about 20 nm outside the junctional region (i.e. in the larger part of the clefts).

The fractional area of the capillary wall occupied by the clefts can thus be calculated: L $\times$ W = 20 m/cm^2 $\times$ 20 nm = 0.004 (0.4%). The fractional area, accessible to free diffusion of small hydrophilic solutes, has been determined by physiological techniques to be

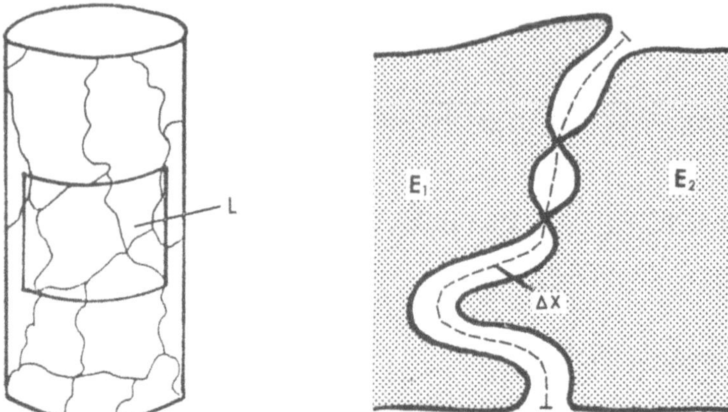

Fig. 1. Exchange of hydrophilic solutes via the interendothelial clefts of the capillary wall is defined by the following equation: $P = D \times (L \times W/\Delta X)$. P is permeability, D the diffusion coefficient of the solute and L the average length of the clefts per unit area capillary wall (illustrated by the left Figure). W is the average effective width of the clefts and ΔX is the length of the diffusion pathway. The right Figure illustrates how ΔX is measured, from the luminal to the abluminal openings of the tortuous intercellular clefts.

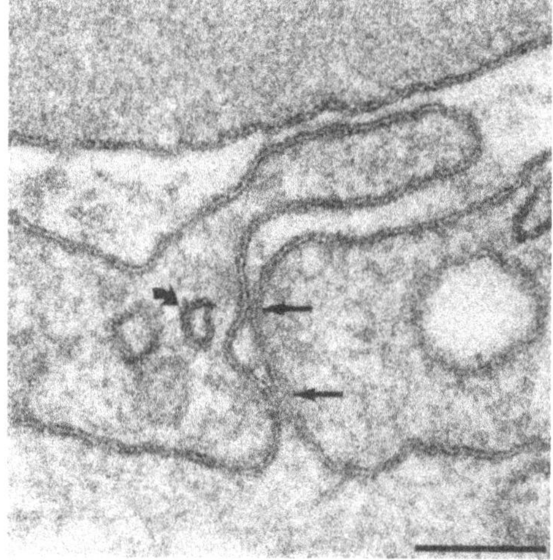

Fig. 2. High magnification electron micrograph of an intercellular cleft from rat heart capillary endothelium. Straight arrows mark the junctional appositions and/or contacts between adjacent cell membranes. Notice the irregular membrane profile (curved arrow), closely related to the junction. This profile represents a long projection – orientated in parallel to the tight junction – from a smooth surfaced cisterna. Lumen (dominated by a segment of an erythrocyte) at the top. Bar, 0.1 μm.

0.01-0.1%.[10] This means that, if the clefts are the main pathway for exchange of hydrophilic solutes, the tight junctions must be organized in such a way that they are permeable in only about 2.5% to 25% of their outline, i.e. neither completely open nor completely closed.

THE ORGANIZATION OF ENDOTHELIAL TIGHT JUNCTIONS

Most electron microscopical studies on endothelial tight junctions have been based on random, individual thin sections of the capillaries. In projections of such sections the tight junctions appear as 1-4 punctate contacts or appositions between neighbouring cell membranes (Fig. 2). The crucial question in this context is: do the punctate contacts represent a circumferential belt?

Some studies, with electron microscopical tracers, have indicated that the junctions are discontinuous and permeable structures. Wissig (1979)[10] observed a step-wise decline in the concentration of microperoxidase (MW:2000; diameter : 2 nm) in the clefts of mouse diaphragm capillary endothelium after i.v. injection of the tracer. This observation indicated that the punctate contacts do not represent a continuous barrier. Wissig proposed that the punctate contacts represent a labyrinthic network of discontinuous lines of contact. I decided to test this hypothesis by means of serial section electron microscopy, allowing reconstruction of the organization of the punctate junctional contacts in three dimensions.

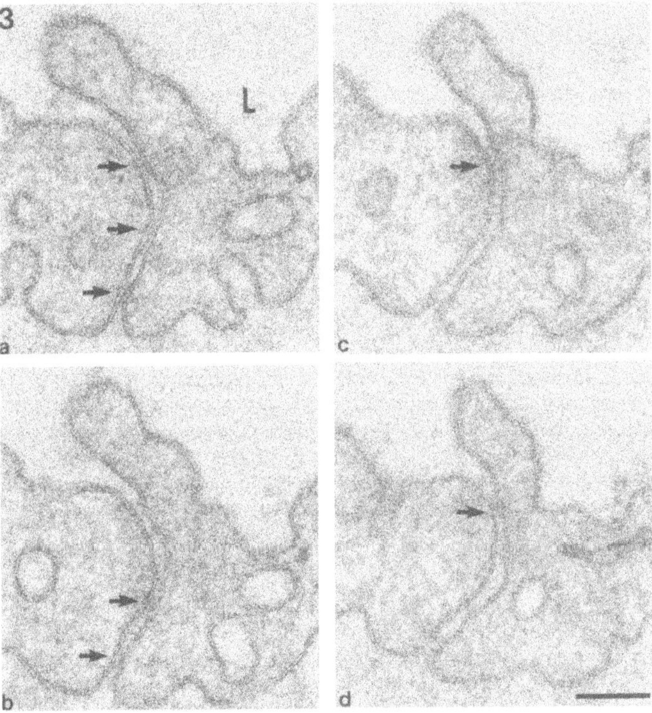

Fig. 3. Consecutive sections (average thickness: 35 nm) of an intercellular cleft from rat heart capillary endothelium. A tortuous pathway through the junctional region is included in these sections. In a, arrows mark three punctate junctional contacts. Section b contains an interruption in the luminal contact line. This pore closes in c; and in d there is a typical luminal punctate junction again. The abluminal part of the cleft is apparently devoid of junctional hindrance to diffusion in sections c and d. The interruption in the luminal contact line creates a pathway, which circumvent the abluminal junctional contacts in a and b. L, lumen, Bar, 0.1 μm.

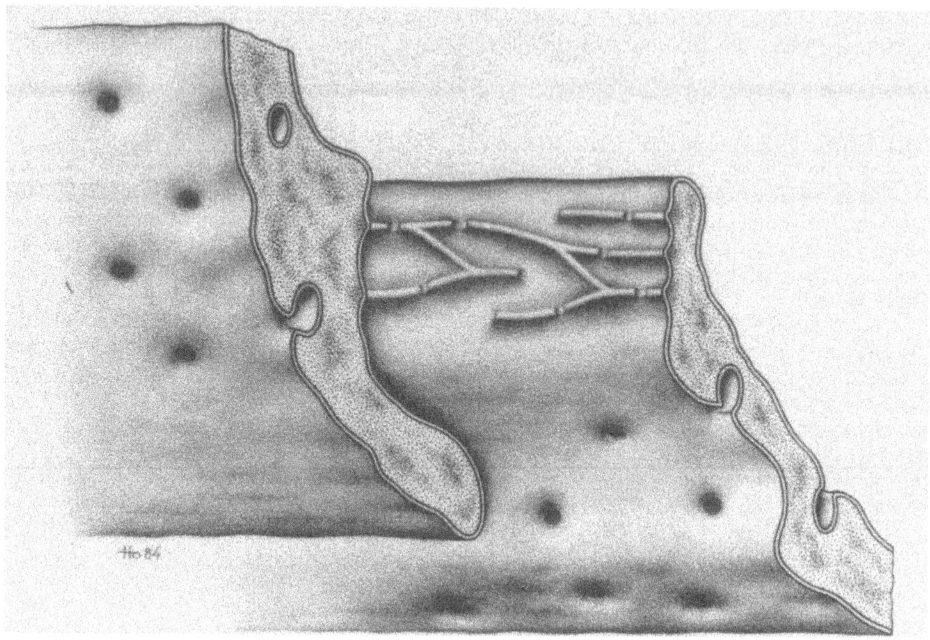

Fig. 4. Schematic drawing summarizing three-dimensional reconstructions of endothelial tight junctions. Lumen at the top. The lateral surface of an endothelial cell is exposed to the right. The tight junctions is organized as an irregular network of contact lines between adjacent cells. Passage of hydrophilic solutes through the junctional region probably occurs by circumvention of contact lines and via discrete discontinuities in the lines.

The freeze-fracture technique may seem useful for this purpose. However, the fracture plane does not follow the plane of interest – the intercellular clefts –, but the interior of membranes delimiting the clefts. Further, there is a poor correlation between junctional tightness and the appearance of junctional strands in the metal-replicas of the cleaved membranes.

Reconstructions of junctional segments, based on consecutive sections of rat heart and diaphragm capillaries, have shown that the punctate contacts, observed in projections of individual thin sections, represent contact lines.[4] The lines are organized as an irregular network. The important finding is the presence of discrete discontinuities (width:4-10 nm; length 10-20 nm) in the lines. A discontinuity is illustrated in Fig. 3 and the results of the reconstructions are summarized in Fig. 4. The interruptions obviously define a continuous – albeit tortuous – pathway from blood to interstitium. It is more than likely that the morphological substrate for the capillary pores[11] is these interruptions.

There are some technical limitations that reduce the resolving power; thus, it has not been possible to determine exactly the quantitative aspects of this diffusion pathway through the endothelial tight junctions. Section thickness is larger than the dimensions of the discrete discontinuities, implying that a substantial fraction of these are not being detected, due to overlapping electron dense material. Further, the tortuous pathways, circumventing the contact lines, may only rarely be wholly contained in the relatively small reconstructed series of segments (in average, each reconstructed segment was based on 15 consecutive thin sections).

The width of the paracellular pathway in chemically fixed and sectioned epithelia and endothelia is probably influenced by the preparative procedures. Consequently, estimates of the in vivo dimensions of diffusion pathways in the clefts have to be based on accessibility to electron microscopical tracers of known dimensions, administered in vivo. The discrete discontinuities in the junctional contact lines are accessible to horseradish peroxidase (MW: 40,000; diameter 5 nm).[12] In electron micrographs the intermembrane distance of the clefts is about 15-20 nm outside the junctional region, as mentioned above. Probably this figure comes close to the in vivo dimensions in most situations. Thus, it is known that horseradish peroxidase readily diffuses into the clefts,[13] whereas ferritin (MW: 450,000; diameter 11 nm) rarely or never is observed between the cells. The access to the clefts is clearly easier for large cationic than

6

for anionic molecules of identical dimensions, indicating that charge of the glycocalyx is an accessory perameter, determining permeability of large molecules.[14] Occasional observations of lipoproteins (diameter: 20-50 nm) in the clefts indicate that their width may fluctuate in vivo.

At this stage it seems clear that the intercellular clefts of microvascular endothelia are permeable to hydrophilic solutes. The quantitative aspects of junctional pathways remains to be further elucidated.

MODULATION OF ENDOTHELIAL TIGHT JUNCTIONS

The large inflammatory leaks between venular endothelial cells probably represent an extreme of a graded ability to modulate the paracellular pathway. Recently, it has been demonstrated with electrophysiological techniques on venous microvessels of the frog brain that a transient increase in permeability to small solutes, can be induced by a number of mediators, including some of the compounds involved in formation of inflammatory leaks.[7,15,16,17] It has been demonstrated that inflammatory mediators increase cytosolic free Ca^{2+} in endothelial cells[18] and that this calcium transient plays a central role in the permeability increase,[19] as it does when junctional permeability of epithelia is changed.[20] The mechanisms behind the modulation of junction permeability are unknown. However, recent studies have given some important hints.

The endothelial cells are provided with numerous vesicular profiles. Originally, these characteristic structures were considered plasmalemmal vesicles and their function was assumed to be transcellular transport of macromolecules. However, three-dimensional reconstructions, based on consecutive ultra-thin sections, have clearly demonstrated that the profiles represent invaginations of the cell membrane.[21,22,23,24] They may be considered as analogous to the invaginations involved in activation of contractile material in skeletal and smooth muscle cells.[25] This analogy has been further extended to the endothelial cells with the implication that the physiological significance of the invaginations is regulation of free cytosolic calcium concentration.[17] In this picture, an intracellular source and sink for free Ca^{2+}, comparable to the sarcoplasmic reticulum (SR) of smooth muscle cells, is needed. This led me to take a closer look at the profiles of smooth surfaced cisternae within the endothelial cytoplasm.

Three-dimensional reconstructions of these profiles, based on consecutive thin sections, have shown that endothelial cells contain a system of irregular cisternae, indistinguishable from the SR in smooth muscle cells.[23,26] The cisternae are often closely associated with the plasmalemmal invaginations. Some of the cisternae give off long slender processes, running parallel to the tight junctions at a distance of about 100 nm (Fig. 2). These long structures are present in about 50% of the outline of the junctions. Our working hypothesis is now that the reconstructed intraendothelial cisternae are functionally similar to SR in contractile cells. It is conceivable that the junction-related processes make it possible to deliver a localized Ca^{2+}-signal, only influencing the junctions.

The link between a rise in cytosolic Ca^{2+} and modulation of junctional organization is unknown. A modification of the cytoskeleton – either contraction or degradation of filaments – is a possibility. Application of available experimental techniques to cultured endothelial cells will probably help to clarify these fundamental aspects of the function of the paracellular pathway in the nearest future.

In conclusion: 1. The hydrophilic pores in the capillary walls are constituted by focal interruptions in the contact lines, which define the tight junctions between endothelial cells. 2. The plasmalemmal invaginations in endothelial cells are probably elements in a signal-transducing system, which – in conjunction with intracytoplasmic Ca^{2+}-stores – regulate cell responses to various chemical stimuli.

REFERENCES

1. E.H. Starling, The fluids of the body. Constable, London (1909).
2. H.S. Bennett, J.H. Luft and J.C. Hampton, Morphological classifications of vertebrate blood capillaries, *Am. J. Physiol.*, **196**:381-390 (1959).
3. R.R. Bruns and G.E. Palade, Studies on blood capillaries. II. Transport of ferritin molecules across the wall of muscle capillaries, *J. Cell Biol.*, **37**:277-299 (1968).
4. M. Bundgaard, The three-dimensional organization of tight junctions in a capillary endothelium revealed by serial section electron microscopy, *J. Ultrastruct. Res.*, **88**:1-17 (1984).
5. C. Crone and D.G. Levitt, Capillary permeability of small solutes. *In:* "Handbook of Physiology,

Section 2, The Cardiovascular System, Vol. IV, Microcirculation, Pt I," E.M. Renkin and C.C. Michel, eds., Bethesda: *Am. Physiol. Soc.*, pp. 411-466 (1984).

6. C.G.A. Persson and E. Svensjø, Drugs interfering with venular permeability, *In*: "Pharmacology of inflammation, Handbook of Inflammation, Vol. V," I.L. Bonta, M.A. Brai and M.I. Parnham, Eds., pp. 61-82 (1985).

7. S.-P. Olesen, A calcium-dependent reversible permeability increase in microvessels in frog brain, induced by serotonin, *J. Physiol.*, 361:103-113 (1985).

8. M. Bundgaard and J. Frøkjær-Jensen, Functional aspects of the ultrastructure of terminal blood vessels: A quantitative study on consecutive segments of the frog mesenteric microvasculature, *Microvasc. Res.*, 23:1-30 (1982).

9. M.A. Perry, Capillary filtration and permeability coefficients calculated from measurements of inter-endothelial cell junctions in rabbit lung and skeletal muscle, *Microvasc. Res.*, 19:142-157 (1980).

10. S.L. Wissig, Identification of the small pore in muscle capillaries, *Acta Physiol. Scand. Suppl.*, 463:33-44 (1979).

11. J.R. Pappenheimer, Passage of molecules through capillary walls, *Physiol. Rev.*, 33:387-423 (1953).

12. M.J. Karnovsky, The ultrastructural basis of capillary exchanges, *J. Gen. Physiol.*, 52:64-95 (1968).

13. G.E. Palade, M. Simionescu and N. Simionescu, Structural aspects of the permeability of the microvascular endothelium, *Acta Physiol. Scand. Suppl.*, 463:11-32 (1979).

14. B. Rippe and B. Haraldsson, Fluid and protein fluxes across small and large pores in the microvasculature. Application of two-pore equations, *Acta Physiol. Scand.*, 131:411-428 (1987).

15. S.-P. Olesen, An electrophysiological study of microvascular permeability and its modulation by inflammatory mediators, *Acta Physiol. Scand. Suppl.*, in press (1988).

16. S.-P. Olesen and C. Crone, Substances that rapidly augment ionic conductance of endothelium in cerebral venules, *Acta Physiol. Scand.*, 127:233-241 (1986).

17. C. Crone, Modulation of solute permeability in microvascular endothelium, *Fed. Proc.*, 45:77-83 (1986).

18. R. Morgan-Boyd, J.M. Stewart, R.J. Vavrek and A. Hassid, Effects of bradykinin and angiotensin II on intracellular Ca^{2+} dynamics in endothelial cells, *Am. J. Physiol.*, 253:C588-C598 (1987).

19. S.-P. Olesen, Regulation of ion permeability in frog brain venules. Significance of calcium, cyclic nucleotides and protein kinase C, *J. Physiol.*, 387:59-68 (1987).

20. M. Cereijido, I. Meza and A. Martinez-Palomo, Occluding junctions in cultured epithelial monolayers, *Am. J. Physiol.*, 240:C96-C102 (1981).

21. J. Frøkjær-Jensen, Three-dimensional organization of plasmalemmal vesicles in endothelial cells: an analysis by serial sectioning of frog mesenteric capillaries, *J. Ultrastruct. Res.*, 73:9-20 (1980).

22. M. Bundgaard, P. Hagman and C. Crone, The three-dimensional organization of plasmalemmal vesicular profiles in the endothelium of rat heart capillaries, *Microvasc. Res.*, 25:358-368 (1983).

23. M. Bundgaard, Tubular invaginations in cerebral endothelium and their relation to smooth-surfaced cisternae in hagfish (Myxine glutinosa), *Cell Tiss. Res.*, 249:359-365 (1987).

24. Y. Noguchi, Y. Shibata and T. Yamamoto, Endothelial vesicular system in rapid-frozen muscle capillaries revealed by serial sectioning and deep etching, *Anat. Rec.* 217:355-360 (1987).

25. M.S. Forbes, M.L. Rennels and E. Nelson, Caveolar systems and sarcoplasmic reticulum in coronary smooth muscle cells of the mouse, *J. Ultrastruct. Res.*, 67:325-339 (1979).

26. M. Bundgaard, Invaginations of the endothelial cell membrane – a possible clue to their functional significance, *Int. J. Microcirc. Clin. Exp.*, 5:209 (1986).

THEORETICAL MODELING OF FLUID TRANSPORT
THROUGH ENDOTHELIAL JUNCTIONS

Richard Skalak

Bioengineering Institute
Department of Civil Engineering
and Engineering Mechanics
Columbia University
New York, NY 10027, USA

INTRODUCTION

This paper will review some recent theoretical models of the fluid transport through an endothelial cell layer from the standpoint of hydrodynamic theories based on ultrastructural information. These theories attempt to use realistic models of the observed morphology of endothelial cell junctions and realistic estimates of the forces, pressures, and flows that can take place in narrow slits and porous media. The classical system of transendothelial pathways consisting of a small pore system, medium size pores and a few large pores for the passage of macromolecules is well supported by experimental data on filtration measured macroscopically. Excellent summaries of this theory and data are available (eg. Curry, 1984; Michel, 1984; Taylor and Granger, 1984).[1,2,3] However, the possible ultrastructural features of endothelial cells which correspond to the various sizes of pores continue to be refined by electron microscopic and other studies. One of the most striking developments is the demonstration that most vesicles of endothelial cells are attached to cell walls.[4,5] This has led to a concept of a lesser role of vesicular transport and a greater emphasis on the filtration through the endothelial cell junctions.[6,7] In these more recent theories, the classical system of pores is replaced by a system of narrow slits which realistically represent the endothelial cleft and tight junctions, some wider tortuous gaps between protein junctional strands, and transiently open junctions which are associated with the replacement phase of dying endothelial cells.[8]

The geometry of the tight junctions is modeled as two parallel planes, representing the cell walls with a uniform spacing except where the protein strands pull the membranes into closer approximation. A mathematical model based on electrostatic repulsions, van der Waals forces and the membrane bending stiffness allows a detailed computation of the membrane shape at the tight junctions. The minimum gap provides a channel through which water and small solutes, but not macromolecules can pass.

An important feature of the system of slits representing the tight junctions is that the protein strands which maintain the minimum gap are not continuous. This leaves tortuous pathways which wind through the open spaces between protein strands (Fig. 1). These pathways may correspond the medium size pores which allow passage of both water and proteins up to the size of albumin. The largest pores are associated with transiently open junctions that are hypothesized to occur after cell death, during cell replacement.[8] This pathway is most important for macromolecular transport but much less important for fluid filtration.

An interesting and important aspect of filtration through an endothelial cell layer is its interaction with the vessel wall or tissue surrounding the endothelium. Considering the media as a porous matrix allows an estimation of the distribution of pressure drop between the endothelial layer and the rest of vessel wall.[6]

Another aspect of endothelial cell layer filtration is the possible effect of macromolecules in the junctional space between two cell membranes. Such molecules spanning the space may

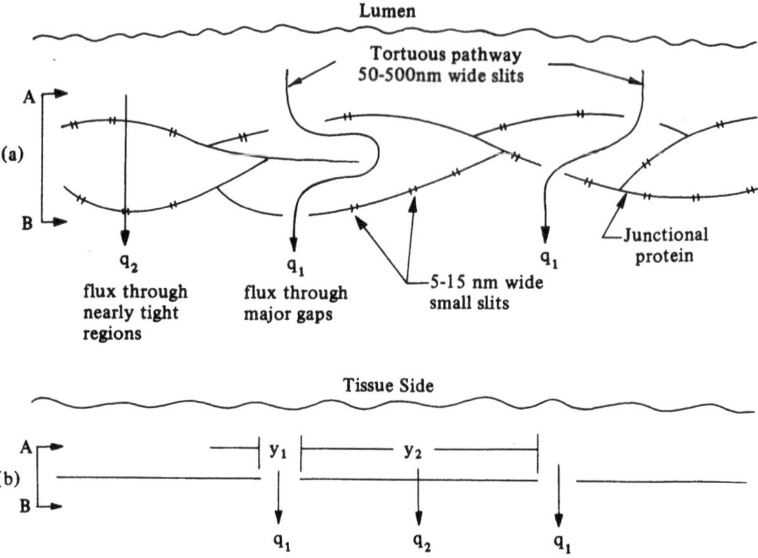

Fig. 1. (a) Diagrammatic sketch of interwoven array of junctional protein strands showing filtration flux q_1, through tortuous wide gap pathway as proposed by [Wissig and Williams, 1987][9] and flux q_2 through tight junction region where the pores are the interstices between junctional proteins. Also shown are the much less frequent 5-15 nm wide small slits formed by occasional missing proteins as suggested by [Bungaard, 1984].[10] (b) Simplifed mathematical model of junctional protein strands, where wide gaps have average length y_1, and interspersed between wide regions of width y_2. (From Weinbaum et al., 1987 by permission).

be responsible for maintaining the very uniform spacing of the membranes observed even in highly convoluted clefts away from the immediate vicinity of tight junction strands.[11] A model of such distributed molecules shows that it would be possible to have a fairly close spacing of adjacent molecules without a large increase of resistance to fluid flow.[12]

MATHEMATICAL MODELS OF INTERCELLULAR CLEFTS

Models of a tight junction between two endothelial cells have been developed based on bending the cell membranes by van der Waals attractive forces associated with the protein strands along the line of minimum membrane spacing.[13,14] In these models, a surface charge density, σ, is assumed on each cell which produces a repulsion of the membranes. Each cell membrane is assumed to behave as an elastic sheet with bending stiffness D, held in equilibrium by the various forces acting. The governing differential equation of the deflection of the membranes is:

$$D \frac{d^4 2\varepsilon}{dx^4} = -F_{vw} + P_e - P_t \tag{1}$$

where D is the bending stiffness of the membrane, 2ε is the membrane spacing, F_{vw} is the van der Waals force, P_e is the electrostatic repulsion and P_t is the difference of the pressure inside the cleft minus the intracellular pressure of the endothelial cell cytoplasm. All terms in (1) are for a unit width along the protein strand, i.e., measured perpendicular to the plane of the cross-section shown in Fig. 2.

The van der Waals force in the normal direction is given by

$$F_{vw} = \frac{6 A_{12}}{\pi^2} \int_{b_1}^{b_2} dx_2 \int_{-\infty}^{\infty} dz_2 \int_{0}^{d} dy_1 \int_{1+d}^{1+2d} \frac{y_2 - y_1}{r^8} dy_2 \tag{2}$$

where subscripts 1,2 refer to the two membranes, A_{12} is the Hamaker constants associated with

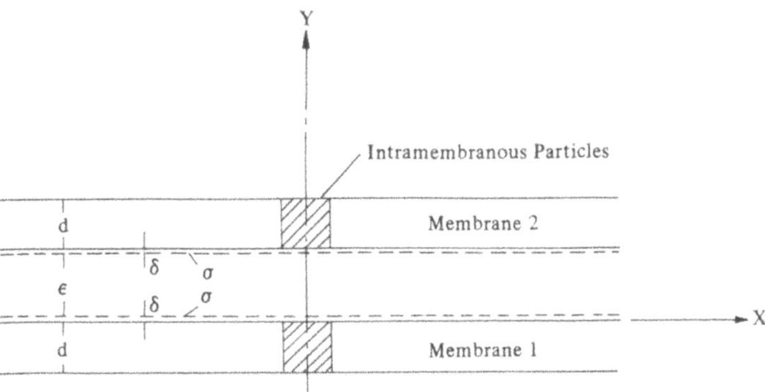

Fig. 2. Cross-section and coordinates used for the analysis of a tight junction of an endothelial cleft. The shaded area represents intramembranous protein particles and the dotted line represents the effective location of surface charges assumed. (From Hsuing and Skalak, 1984, by permission).

these points and r is the distance between them. The Hamaker constant depends on the number density of molecular species present which is taken to be much larger for the protein strands than for the surrounding membrane. This is the factor responsible for the local deformation of the membranes. The repulsive pressure acting on each membrane is

$$P_e(x) = \frac{4\pi\sigma^2}{\beta \sinh^2 K(2\varepsilon - 2\delta)} (1 + \cosh 2K(\varepsilon - \delta))$$ (3)

where σ is the surface charge density, β is the dielectric constant and K^{-1} is the Debye length. The spacing of the membranes is 2ε and δ is the assumed average distance that the charged layer stands off the lipid membrane surface.

The variation of pressure due to fluid flow through the cleft is computed assuming that the velocity distribution may be approximated by a gradually varying Poiseuille flow:

$$u = -\frac{\varepsilon^2}{2\mu} (1 - \frac{y^2}{\varepsilon^2}) \frac{\partial p}{\partial x}$$ (4)

where μ is the viscosity of the fluid and $2\varepsilon(x)$ is the membrane spacing. Eq. (4) can be integrated numerically to find the pressure p if $\varepsilon(x)$ is known. In the computational procedure, the shape of the membranes and the pressure distributions are found by an iterative numerical procedure. The results of one such computation are shown in Fig. 3. The narrowest gap occurs at the intramembranous protein strands and the severe deflection of the membrane is restricted to this vicinity. There is a narrowing of the cleft width downstream of the tight junction due to the decreasing pressure associated with the fluid flow. This narrowing has not been reported in electron-microscopic observations, but this may be because endothelial cells are not usually fixed under pressure. It may also be that the normal spacing of cell membranes in the uniform portion of endothelial cell clefts is enforced by bridging molecules which provide an additional stiffness, but are not visible in the usual transmission elctron microscopic sections.

The fluid flow through a slit of variable width such as shown in Fig. 3 is not sensitive to the precise shape of the gap thickness, but depends on the minimum width of the channel and the longitudinal extent of the constriction primarily. Tzeghai et al. (1985)[6] have suggested a simple cosine distribution for $\varepsilon(x)$:

$$\varepsilon(x) = \frac{1}{2} (\varepsilon_n + \varepsilon_m) + \frac{1}{2} (\varepsilon_n - \varepsilon_m) \cos(\frac{2\pi x}{w})$$ (5)

where $2\varepsilon_n$ nd $2\varepsilon_m$ are the normal and minimum membrane spacings and w is the length over which the constriction, Eq. (4) applies. For the remainder ($\ell - w$) of the channel (total length, ℓ) the

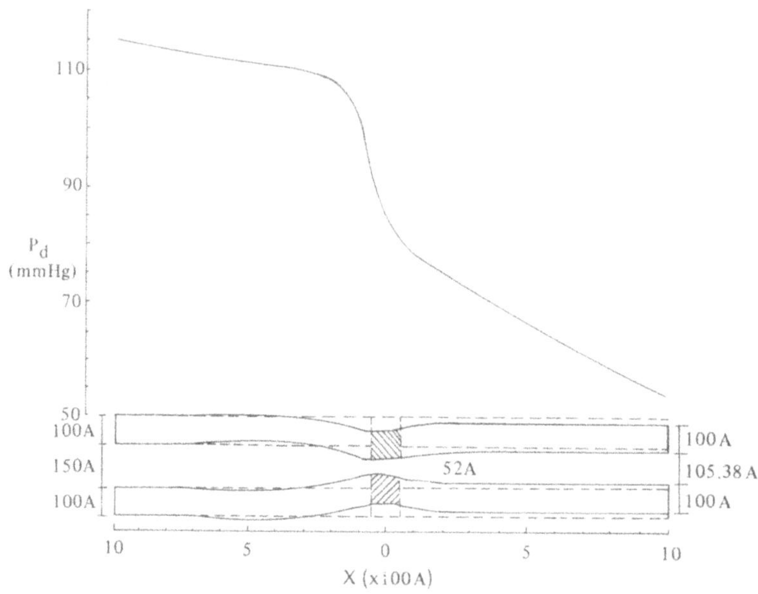

Fig. 3. Pressure distribution and equilibrum configuration of an endothelial tight junction and cleft with the fluid flow through the cleft taken into account. The dotted lines in the lower part of the figure indicate the equilibrium spacing of the membranes in the absence of intramembranous proteins and fluid flow.

width is assumed to be normal uniform width, $2\varepsilon_n$. It can be shown[6] that the constricted channel of the same length, ℓ, and width, $2\varepsilon_o$, is given by

$$\varepsilon_o = \varepsilon_n \left[1 - \frac{w}{\ell} \left(\frac{3 + 2\alpha + 3\alpha^2}{8\alpha^{5/2}} - 1 \right) \right]^{-1/3} \tag{6}$$

where $\alpha = \dfrac{\varepsilon_m}{\varepsilon_n}$ $\tag{7}$

In more comprehensive models, including the media of the vessel wall, the concept of an equivalent uniform slit (6) is useful to simplify the analysis.

INTERACTION OF ENDOTHELIAL CLEFTS AND VESSEL MEDIA

Fluid filtering though the endothelial clefts encounters next the media of the vessel wall which to first approximation may be regarded as a porous medium. The pressure encountered on the abluminal side of the endothelial layer depends on the relative resistance offered by the endothelial clefts and the rest of the vessel wall. In the media, the flow is not a uniform one-dimensional flow, but starts as relatively narrow streams issueing from the endothelial clefts. These streams disperse over a length which is comparable to the width of an endothelial cell, as indicated schematically in Fig. 4. This qualitative picture has been analyzed quantitatively by the boundary value problem illustrated in Fig. 5. In this model the endothelial cell clefts are represented as continuous parallel slits spaced at a distance representing a typical endothelial cell width (Fig. 4). This makes the problem a two dimensional one which is more tractable analytically. The problem is solved assuming the fluid flow in the media is governed by Darcy's law

$$\underline{u} = -\frac{k}{\mu} \nabla p \tag{8}$$

where k is a permeability coefficient of the media and μ is the fluid viscosity; u is the velocity

12

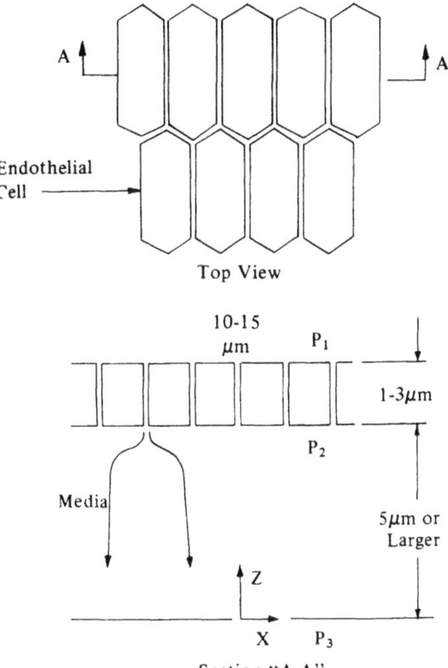

Fig. 4. Schematic enface and cross-sectional view of endothelial cells and media of an artery wall for modeling water filtration. The intercellular clefts are assumed to be an array of two-dimensional parallel channels whose spacing 2ε is roughly the width of the endothelial cells. (From Tzeghai et al. 1985, by permission).

due to the pressure gradient ∇p. It is also assumed that the flow and tissue are incompressible so

$$\nabla \cdot u = 0 \tag{9}$$

It follows that p obeys Laplace's equation:

$$\nabla^2 p = 0 \tag{10}$$

The pressure field is solved in a series form under the boundary conditions illustrated in Fig. 5. In this figure and the solution, all dimensions are non-dimensionalized by the length, L, which is the thickness of the media measured from the abluminal side of the endothelium to the adventia of the vessel wall. The pressure at the adventia surrounding the vessel is assumed to be zero. The pressure and flow from the endothelial clefts and through the porous media are set equal to each other at their junction. This allows a complete solution. The pressure P_2 the total pressure drop from the lumen to adventia is given by

$$P_2 = \beta \phi \, [\, 3\ell \, \xi/\varepsilon^2 + \beta\phi \,] \tag{11}$$

where ξ is half of the cell width and (Weinbaum et al., 1987):[7]

$$\beta = \varepsilon_0^2 \, L/\varepsilon_n k \tag{12}$$

$$\Phi = 1 + \frac{2}{\varepsilon_n^2} \sum_{m=1}^{\infty} \frac{\tanh \lambda_m}{\lambda_\mu} \left(\frac{\sin \lambda_m \varepsilon_n}{\lambda_\mu} \right)^2 \tag{13}$$

where λ_m are the eigenvalues of the roots of $\sin (\lambda_m \xi) = 0$.

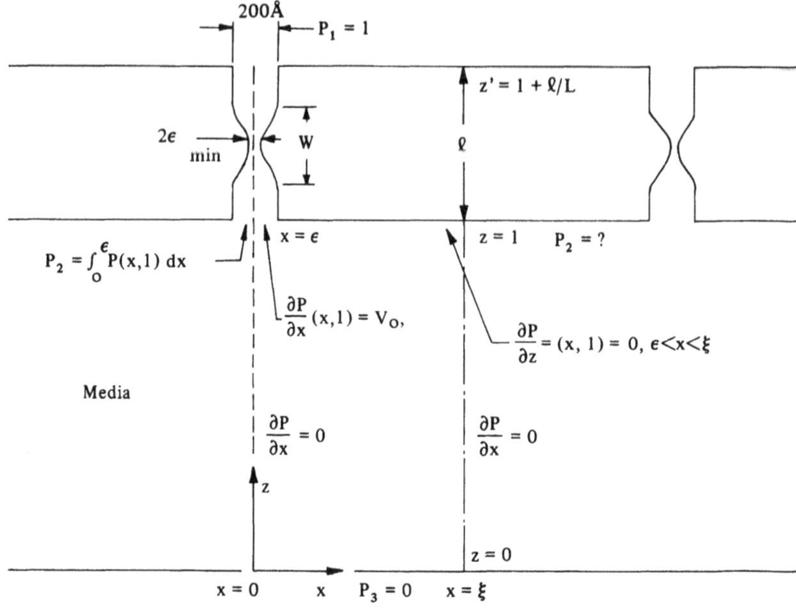

Fig. 5. Sketch of simple mathematical model of vessel wall in cross-section showing boundary value problem for filtration. Interendothelial clefts of depth ℓ with constrictions of depth w are arranged in periodic two-dimensional array obtained by taking a cross-sectional view of the clefts for the simplified model shown in Fig. 4. (From Tzeghai et al. 1985, by permission).

Graphs and some numerical examples based on the above analysis are given by Tzeghai, et al. (1985).[6] The uniform portion of the junction has a width of about $2\varepsilon_v = 20$ nm and the narrowest part of the tight junction is of the order of $2\varepsilon_m = 2.6$ nm. The length of the cleft, ℓ, is 1 to 3 μm. The hydraulic conductivity k is taken to be 1.55×10^{-9} cm³/sec cm H₂O based on data of Vargas et al. (1978).[15] These parameters applied to a thin vessel wall (L = 200 μm) yield a dimensionless pressure $P_2 = 0.50$ at the junction of the endothelium and media. This is in the same range as measured by Vargas et al. (1978)[15] which indicates that the theory gives reasonable results with realistic parameters. Pressure and velocity profiles predicted are given by Tzeghai et al. (1985).[6]

In the above analysis the endothelial junctions are assumed to be uniform at all points around the periphery of each cell. The actual picture is more complex as shown in Fig. 1. There are two principal paths. One is the tortuous pathway which circumvements the protein strands of the tight junctions. This is represented by the length y_1, in Fig. 1b. The width of the pathway is of the order of $2\varepsilon_n = 20$ nm throughout most of its length with a minimum width $2\varepsilon_m = 4$ to 10 nm, so fairly large molecular species can pass this way. The second path is through the nearly tight junctions, represented by length y_2 in Fig. 1b. Fluid and small ions can pass through this path. It is assumed that for purposes of filtration, the flux through these pathways are additive and the complex can be represented by a single uniform cleft of width $2\varepsilon_0$. The percentage of the cell periphery occupied by tight junctions (y_1) may vary from 0.1 in the lung to 0.9 in systemic arteries and nearly 1.0 in brain. When $y_1 < 0.1$, most of the fluid filtration will be through the tight junction strands and the wider tortuous channels contribute 10 to 20% to the total flow.

BRIDGING MOLECULES AND TIGHT JUNCTION STRANDS

Some consideration of the possibilites of molecular dimensions and arrangements in the endothelial clefts are of interest as they may determine the normal cleft spacing and the hydraulic resistance encountered by fluid filtering through the junctions. In the above theory, the flow through clefts was computed as if there were nothing in the clefts besides fluid. In any case, the proteins of the tight junction strands are present and it is possible that large molecules span the normal (20nm) width of a cleft and give it its uniform spacing. Although such molecules are not normally visible in EM, it has been suggested that the cleft contains a fibrous matrix of such molecules which controls the hydraulic resistance observed.[16]

In the model of endothelial permeability in which a molecular matrix in the wider parts of the junction are assumed to be filled by a fibrous network, the junctions are assumed to be uniform around the periphery of each cell. This model does not invoke the tight junctions and tortuous paths which are more open, as illustrated in Fig. 1. In the fiber-matrix theory it is hypothesized that the hydraulic permeability is determined primarily by the open enface area of the junctions. The passage of solutes is assumed to be controlled by the size and distribution of the network of fibrous molecules within the wider parts of the junction.[17] This network is not seen in the usual EM sections, but cytochemical methods have established that endothelial cells have a glycocalyx, at least on the lumenal surface of the cell.[18] The basic reason for the fiber matrix hypothesis is that the equivalent pore radius which describes the selectivity of the capillary wall to various sizes of molecules is smaller than the equivalent pore radius that is necessary to account for the hydraulic conductivity.[19] This fiber matrix provides a steric barrier to molecules over a certain size and a retardation of smaller molecules. If the molecules are small compared to the fiber network openings, then the solute is convected and diffused essentially as in a free fluid. The permeability k (as in Eq. 8) of a fiber matrix is given by (Curry and Michel, 1980)[16]

$$k = \frac{f^2 \, v^3}{20 \, (1 - v)^2} \tag{14}$$

where f is the fiber radius and v is the fractional volume occupied by fluid.

Experimental data on the permeability of frog mesenteric capillaries has been interpreted in terms of a fiber matrix consisting of fibers 0.6nm in radius and occupying a 5% of the junctional volume.[16] These figures show that the fiber matrix theory of endothelial junctions is a realistic possibility. However, it does not take into account that there are alternative pathways (Fig. 1) through the cell junctions, nor does it have a role for the tight junctions formed by protein strands. It implies the narrow regions of the tight junctions offer little resistance to the diffusion of small ions and solutes. While all of these aspects remain as consistent possibilities, the structural details and composition of the hypothesized fiber matrix remain to be demonstrated.

Another possible role of fibers spanning the cleft between two endothelial cells is to establish and maintain the very regular and uniform spacing of the two cell membranes as observed in EM sections, even if the junction itself is convoluted. While electrostatic and van der Waals forces are operative and provide a sufficient system of forces to maintain equilibrium spacing, they would have to be very uniform to maintain the very even spacing observed. It has therefore been suggested that a bridging molecule may be present, attached to both cell membranes, which establishes the membrane spacing by its own characteristic length.[11] This mechanism has been also suggested in the very even spacing of red blood cell membranes in a rouleau.[20] In this case, the spacing is proportional to the length of the dextran molecule causing the aggregation. The charges of each red blood cell surface provide a repulsive force which keeps the bridging molecules taut. In the case of endothelial cells, Silberberg (1987)[11] has suggested that charges distributed on the bridging molecules themselves may keep them extended. Such bridging molecules could be very sparse, perhaps a small fraction of 1% volumetrically and still be effective in maintaining spacing of the membranes because the cell membranes have a certain bending stiffness which will also be small if their volumetric percentage is low. Detailed estimates of the fluid flow past an array of posts between parallel planes have been developed by Lee and Fung (1969)[21] and Hsuing (1984).[12]

REFERENCES

1. F.E. Curry, Mechanics and thermodynamics of transcapillary exchange, in: "Handbook of Physiology," Sec. 2, The Cardiovascular System, Vol. IV, The Microcirculation, pp. 309-374, E.M. Renken and C.C. Michel, eds., Amer, Physiol. Soc., Bethesda (1984).
2. C.C. Michel, Fluid movements through capillary walls, in: "Handbook of Physiology," Sec. 2, The Cardiovascular system, Vol. IV, The Microcirculation, pp. 375-409, E.M. Renkin and C.C. Michel, eds., Amer. Physiol. Soc., Bethesda (1984).

3. A.E. Taylor and D.N. Granger, Exchange of macromolecules across the microcirculation, *in*: "Handbook of Physiology," Sec. 2, The Cardiovascular System, Vol. IV, The Microcirculation, pp. 467-520, E.M. Renkin and C.C. Michel, eds., Amer. Physiol. Soc., Bethesda (1984).

4. M. Bundgaard and Jensen, J. Frokjaer, Functional aspects of the ultrastructure of terminal blood vessels: a quantitative study of consecutive segments of frog mesenteric microvasculature, *Microvasc. Res.*, **23**:1-30 (1982).

5. S. Chien, L. Laufer and D.A. Handley, Vesicle distribution in the arterial endothelium determined with ruthenium red as an extracellular marker, *J. Ultrastruct. Res.*, **79**:198-206 (1982).

6. G. Tzeghai, S. Weinbaum and R. Pfeffer, A steady-state filtration model for transluminal water movement in small and large blood vessels, *J. Biomech. Engra.* **107**:123-130 (1985).

7. R. Tsay, S. Weinbaum and R. Pfeffer, A model for capillary filtration based on junctional protein structure of the interendothelial cleft, submitted *Chemical Engineering Communications* (1988).

8. S. Weinbaum, G. Tzeghai, P. Ganatos, R. Pfeffer and S. Chien, Effect of cell turnover and leaky junctions on arterial macromolecular transport, *Am. J. Physiol.*, **248**:H945-H960 (1985).

9. S.L. Wissing and M.C. Williams, Permeability of muscle capillaries to microperoxidase, *J. Cell Biol.*, **76**:341-359 (1978).

10. M. Bundgaard, The three dimensional organization of tight junctions in a capillary with continuous endothelium revealed by serial section electron microscopy, *J. Ultrastruct. Res.*, **88**:1-17 (1984).

11. A. Silberberg, Passage of macromoleules and solvent through clefts between endothelial cells. Conditions controlling cleft patency, *in*: "Microcirculation, An Update," M. Asano, Y. Mishma and M. Oda, eds., Proceedings of the Fourth World Congress for Microcirculation, Excerpta Medica, Amsterdam (1987).

12. C.C. Hsuing, "Mechanics of Endothelial Cell Junctions," Doctoral dissertation, Columbia University, New York (1984).

13. S. Weinbaum, Theory for the formation of intercellular junctions based on intramembranous particle patterns observed in the freeze fracture technique, *J. Theor. Biol.* **83**:63-92 (1980).

14. C.C. Hsuing and R. Skalak, Hydrodynamic and mechanical aspects of endothelial permeability, *Biorheol.*, **21**:207-221 (1984).

15. B.C. Vargas, F.F. Vargas, J.G. Pribyl and P.L. Blackshear, Hydrolic conductivity of the endothelial and outer layers of the rabbit aorta, *Amer. J. Physiol.*, **236**:H53-H60 (1978).

16. F.-R.E. Curry and C.C. Michel, A fiber matrix theory of capillary permeability, *Microvasc. Res.*, **20**:96-99 (1980).

17. F.-R.E. Curry, Determinants of capillary permeability: a review of mechanisms based on single capillary studies in the frog, *Circ. Res.*, **39**:367-380 (1986).

18. A.S. Charonis, P.C. Tsilibary, R.H. Kramer and S.L. Wissig, 1983, Localization of heparan sulphate proteoglycan in the basement membrane of continuous capillaries, *Microvasc. Res.*, **26**:108-113 (1983).

19. C.C. Michel, M.E. Phillips and R.M. Turner, The effect of native and modified bovine serum albumin on the permeability of frog mesenteric capillaries, *J. Physiol.* **360**:333-346 (1985).

20. S. Chien and K.-M. Jan, Ultrastructural basis of the mechanism of rouleax formation, *Microvasc. Res.*, **5**:155-166 (1973).

21. J.S. Lee and Y.C. Fung, Stokes flow around a circular cylindrical post confined between two parallel plates, *J. Fluid Mech.*, **37**:657-670 (1969).

VARIABILITY IN MICROVASCULAR ESTIMATES OF CAPILLARY SURFACE AREA FOR EXCHANGE

Ingrid H. Sarelius, Tara A. Nealey and Terrence E. Sweeney

Departments of Biophysics and Physiology
University of Rochester
Rochester, NY 14642, USA

INTRODUCTION

A recurring and tantalizing deficiency in many areas of microvascular research is the problem of quantitative reconciliation of measurements made in whole organs (or whole animals) versus those made at the level of individual microvessels. With respect to endothelial cell function, it is recognized that whole organ measurements of capillary filtration coefficient yield values that are 10-20 times lower than single vessel permeability measurements,[1] and that observed transport rates of macromolecules in experimental systems at low volume flows exceed calculations based on the two pore model.[2] It is clear that at least a partial contribution to these discrepancies lies in the assumptions underlying the models or experimental systems. For example, comparison of data collected by whole organ versus single vessel approaches depends on how 'typical' is the single vessel selected for measurement, or on assumptions describing heterogeneity of function in the whole organ approach.

Capillary surface area is a parameter which is normalized out of single vessel experimental data (e.g., Curry et al., 1983)[3] and usually assumed constant in the whole organ approach (e.g., Rippe et al., 1978).[4] The effective capillary surface area for exchange processes is, of course, that surface area which is open to flow. It is well established that in many tissues (striated muscle for example), this effective surface area, defined by the functional capillary density, is significantly less than the anatomical capillary density[5] and can be modified by mechanisms which change capillary blood flow, e.g., changes in tissue oxygen supply or demand.[6] Thus measurements of anatomical and functional capillary density, and hence, by inference, determination of the effective capillary surface area available for exchange, are critical to a proper understanding of the control microvascular permeability.

Methods and controversies in the measurement of both anatomical and functional capillary density are well documented.[7,8,9,10] A common theme in many studies is how to distinguish between open (flowing) versus closed capillaries. In general, capillaries with flow are identified by the presence of a selected flow-based marker; either erythrocytes or ink particles,[5,11,12] or dye or labeled albumin.[10,13] Careful examination of this literature identifies an interesting discrepancy. Usually, measurements of functional capillary density using erythrocytes or ink as the flow marker identify a singificant capillary reserve i.e. there is a finite (tissue-specific) fraction of the total capillary density which remains unperfused by marker after a significant period of time (generally 1-3 minutes), whereas in contrast, plasma-based flow markers fill the capillary bed more completely and more rapidly. As a specific example, a comparison of two studies in gastrocnemius muscle shows that in rat, 100 percent of the anatomical capillary density is filled after 30 sec perfusion with fluorescent dye — a plasma marker,[10] whereas rabbit gastrocnemius, perfused with dialyzed ink, has about 70 percent of all capillaries filled after 90 sec.[14] A similar discrepancy can be identified for rat myocardial capillaries which appear 100 percent filled in 10 sec using plasma marker[13] compared to 60 percent functional capillary density in the steady state identified with red blood cells.[12] Explanations for this discrepancy include differences in species, muscle, experimental design and technique, incomplete particle mixing and the like. However, there is also evidence from other sources to suggest that the apparent difference in plasma versus cells distribution space might be a real phenomenon. For example, capillary hematocrit is lower than expected from predictions based on simple application of established phenomena such as the Fahraeus effect;[15,16] more importantly, hematocrit at the capillary level has a wide and variable distribution[17] which implies that cells and plasma are likely to be distributed in a variable but unequal way.

Based on the preceding rationale, the work reported here was designed to determine whether cellular and non-cellular elements of blood have the same distribution space. Specifically, the study was intended to answer two questions.

1. Do all capillary segments without flowing cells receive plasma flow?
2. At what rate does labeled albumin enter a perfused capillary bed?

METHODS

Observations were made on cremaster muscles of 11 golden hamsters (weight 134 ± 4 g), anesthetized with pentobarbital sodium (70 mg/kg, i.p.), tracheostomized and maintained on supplemental pentobarbital sodium in saline (9 mg/ml at 0.47 ml/hr) infused via a femoral venous catheter. Deep body temperature was maintained between 37 and 38°C.

In each animal the right cremaster muscle was prepared, superfused, viewed and recorded for analysis as described previously.[17,18]

Bovine serum albumin (BSA, Sigma, Fraction V) was labeled with dichlorotriazinyl amino fluorescein (DTAF, Research Organics) for observation of plasma (albumin) distribution space. BSA (100 mg/ml) in borate buffer (pH 9.23) was dialyzed overnight at 4°C against borate buffer containing 0.2 mg/ml DTAF. The BSA-DTAF was then dialyzed against 4 liters of physiological salt solution[18] and filtered through a 0.2 μm millipore filter. Aliquots of 0.5 ml each were frozen for storage and thawed immediately prior to use.

Capillary density was sampled in tissue volumes denfined by the videomonitor; four sites per animal were recorded for a total sampled tissue volume of approximately 0.15 mm^3 per animal. Anatomical (total) capillary density (CD_T) was estimated as the total number of capillary segments observed per sampled volume; functional capillary density (the number of segments with flowing cells, CD_F), was estimated as the number of capillary segments with moving erythrocytes (observed with transillumination at 436 nm to highlight red blood cells); plasma-containing segments (CD_P) were estimated from capillary segments containing BSA-DTAF using epi-illumination with 450-490/515-535 nm filters to excite and observe DTAF fluorescence. Measurements of CD_T, CD_F and CD_P were made in each sampled tissue volume using sequential rapid transfer between trans- and epi-illumination.

In quantitation of CD_F, it is important to determine a criterion for "stopped" flow. This is because, within any sampling period, all capillaries have a finite probability of containing blood flow at a given instant. For these experiments, we defined vessels as "flowing" where observed cell velocities were 20 μm/sec or greater. This cut-off was calculated from cell transit time and path length distributions[18] and excluded from the flowing population those pathways whose cell residence times were greater than 3 times the population median.

Standard statistical techniques were used to compare data sets; significance was assessed at the 95 percent confidence level.[19]

RESULTS AND DISCUSSION

The fractions of CD_T containing either flowing cells or BSA-DTAF are summarized in Table 1. At 30 sec and 3 min after intravenous injection of 35 mg BSA-DTAF, we observed that 70 percent of the total capillary bed contained flow; this is similar to previously reported CD_F in hamster cremaster muscle.[17] At 30 sec, all flowing capillaries contained the labeled albumin; of the total of 579 segments observed to contain moving erythrocytes, 574 contained BSA-DTAF. This confirms that the plasma label was rapidly distributed into those capillaries containing active flow. By 3 min after BSA-DTAF injection all capillaries (99 percent of CD_T) contained the label, whereas CD_F remained unchanged. Furthermore, the majority of capillaries in the CD_F sample at 30 sec remained in the sample at 3 min. In other words, addition of vessels containing BSA-DTAF between 30 sec and 3 min cannot be explained by redistribution of the flowing red blood cells into different capillary segments.

The overall rate of vessel filling with BSA-DTAF was not affected when the tissue was

Table 1. Fraction of Anatomical Capillary Density Containing Flow or Labeled Albumin

	Time after BSA-DTAF	
	30 sec	3 min
Cell Perfused caps (CD_F)	0.70	0.70
Caps Containing Labeled Albumin (CD_P)	0.74	0.99

exposed to 10^{-8} M norepinephrine (Figure 1). Thus, CD_T was completely filled with labeled albumin in the same 3 min time period that we found in control preparations. Parenthetically, we note the similarity between this filling time and the increase in capillary filtration coefficient after about 3 minutes observed in whole organ experiments after stimulation of the sympathetic nervous system, and classically attributed to sympathetic escape.[4] Interpretation of the data summarized in Figure 1 are complicated by our observation of no significant difference in mean cell velocity in the controls (87 ± 11 μm/sec) versus the norepinephrine-exposed group (82 ± 10 μm/sec). This does not imply that we observed no effect of the norepinephrine but rather, based on other work from this laboratory[18,20] and elsewhere,[21] we conclude that the norepinephrine effect is principally on the distribution of flowing versus non-flowing capillaries, achieved by active changes in tone of upstream arterioles, each controlling groups of capillaries. This observation supports our conclusion from the data of Table 1 that distribution of the labeled albumin into the total capillary space is not solely a function of active capillary flow as indicated by erythrocyte behavior.

Possible mechanisms which might contribute to filling this group of capillaries with labeled albumin include asymmetric cell and bulk flow distribution at capillary bifurcations such that vessels receiving flow below a critical velocity receive only plasma.[22] Although such a phenomenon has been observed *in vivo* (Cokelet and Sarelius, unpublished data) it does not ap-

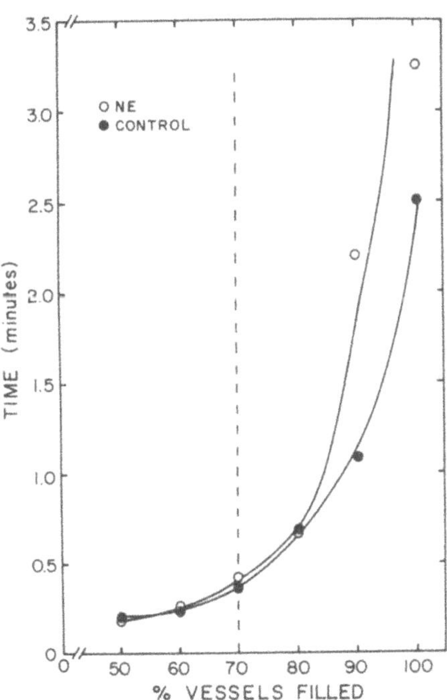

Fig. 1. Rate of filling of CD_T by BSA-DTAF in nor-epinephrine-treated and control muscles. Dotted line indicates functional capillary density.

Table 2. Number of Capillary Segments in Each Category Expressed as Cumulated Total (Column A) or Individual Videofield Means $\pm$ Standard Error (Column B)

	A	B
Total Segments	352	14.7 ± 0.9
Perfused with Cells ("flowing")	274*	11.4 ± 0.7*
Segments Containing Labeled Albumin	339	14.1 ± 0.9
Total With Any Observable Cell Movement	342	14.3 ± 0.9

*$P > 0.05$.

pear likely to be the principal mechanism by which labeled albumin enters this capillary group. We observed that the majority of this subgroup, while not conforming to our definition of "flow", did in fact exhibit one of two general classes of cell movement. 1. A finite, very short episode of cell movement in a vessel with otherwise stationary cells. 2. Extremely slow, continuous cell movement with cell velocities of 5 μm/sec or less. Vessels in these two categories account very closely for the number of capillaries receiving BSA-DTAF in excess of CD_F (Table 2).

The episodic flow pattern might be accounted for by such phenomena as transient shifts in blood cells (leukocytes, erythrocytes) which have plugged vessels previously, but we have no obvious explanation for the "creeping flow" observed in the second vessel category. In many of these vessels the rate of entry of BSA-DTAF was of the order of 0.5 μm/sec or less, which is substantially slower than the corresponding cell velocity observed in this vessel group. Thus it seems likely that the expected ratio of cell to bulk velocity of 1.3[23,24] cannot hold in these vessels and some other explanation must be sought.

In summary, we interpret these data as indicating that the perfused capillary volume defined by flowing erythrocytes is separable from a functional distribution space (defined by BSA-DTAF) which contains a population of vessels with minimal flow, but which cannot have zero intravascular pressure and which therefore must contribute to the effective surface area for transvascular exchange. While this area is relatively small in cremaster, it is reasonable to assume that a similar phenomenon is likely in other tissues with a significantly larger capillary reserve, such as the majority of skeletal muscle.

ACKNOWLEDGMENTS

We thank Sharon M. Morrissey for her assistance. Supported by NIH grants HL 29929 and HL 18208.

REFERENCES

1. C. Crone and O. Christensen, Transcapillary transport of small solutes and water, *Int. Rev. Physiol.* **18**:149-213 (1979).
2. E.M. Renkin, Capillary transport of macromolecules: pors and other endothelial pathways, *J. Appl. Physiol.* **58**:315-325 (1985).
3. F.E. Curry, V.H. Huxley and I.H. Sarelius, Techniques in the microcirculation: measurement of permeability, pressure and flow, in: "Techniques in the Life Sciences," vol. P3/1, R.S. Linden, eds., pp. 1-34, Elsevier, New York (1983).
4. B. Rippe, A. Kamiya and B. Folkow, Simultaneous measurements of capillary diffusion and filtration exchange during shifts in filtration-absorbtion and at graded alterations in the capillary permeability surface area product (PS), *Acta Physiol. Scand.* **104**:318-336 (1978).
5. A. Krogh, The number and distribution of capillaries in muscles with calculations of the oxygen pressure head necessary for supplying the tissue, *J. Physiol.* **52**:409-415 (1919).
6. B. Klitzman, D.N. Damon, R.J. Gorczynski and B.R. Duling, Augmented tissue oxygen supply during striated muscle contraction in the hamster: relative contributions of capillary recruitment, functional dilation and reduced tissue PO_2, *Cir. Res.* **51**:711-721 (1982).
7. S.D. Gray and E.M. Renkin, Microvascular supply in relation to fiber metabolic type in mixed skele-

tal muscles of rabbits, *Microvasc. Res.* **16**:406-425 (1978).

8. I.H. Sarelius, L.C. Maxwell, S.D. Gray and B.R. Duling, Capillarity and fiber types in the cremaster muscle of rat and hamster, *Am. J. Physiol.* **245**:H368-H374 (1983).

9 P.F. McDonagh, R.W. Gore and S.D. Gray, Perfused capillary surface area in postural and loco-motor skeletal muscle, *Microvasc. Res.* **24**:142-157 (1982).

10. S.R. Kayar and N. Banchero, Sequential perfusion of skeletal muscle capillaries, *Microvasc. Res.* **30**:298-305 (1985).

11. E.M. Renkin, Flow and distribution of India ink in microvessels of the frog, *Microvasc. Res.* **29**:32-44 (1985).

12. L. Henquell and C.R. Honig, Intercapillary distances and capillary reserve in right and left ventricles: significance for control of tissue PO_2, *Microvasc. Res.* **12**:35-41 (1976).

13. F. Vetterlein, H. dalRi and G. Schmidt, Capillary density in rat myocardium during timed plasma staining, *Am. J. Physiol.* **242**:H133-H141 (1982).

14. E.M. Renkin, S.D. Gray and L.R. Dodd, Filling of microcirculation in skeletal muscles during timed India ink perfusion, *Am. J. Physiol.* **241**:H174-H186 (1981).

15. G.R. Cokelet, Speculation on a cause of low vessel hematocrits in the microcirculation, *Microcircula-tion* **2**:1-18 (1982).

16. B.R. Duling, I.H. Sarelius and W.F. Jackson, A comparison of microvascular estimates of capillary blood flow with direct measurements of total striated muscle blood flow, *Int. J. Microcirc. Clin. Exp.* **1**:409-424 (1982).

17. I.H. Sarelius, D.N. Damon and B.R. Duling, Microvascular adaptations during maturation of striated muscle, *Am. J. Physiol.* **241**:H317-H324 (1981).

18. I.H. Sarelius, Cell flow path influences transit time through striated muscle capillaries, *Am. J. Physiol.* **250**:H899-H907 (1986).

19. G.W. Snedecor and W.G. Cochran, "Statistical Methods," 6th ed., Iowa State University Press, Ames. IA (1967).

20. T.E. Sweeney and I.H. Sarelius, Does location within a microvascular network influence arteriolar function? *Proc. Int. Union Physiol, Sci.* **16**:526 (Abstract) (1986).

21. N. Lund, D.H. Damon, D.N. Damon and B.R. Duling, Capillary grouping in hamster tibialis anterior muscles: flow patterns and physiological significance, *Int. J. Microcirc. Clin. Exp.* **5**:359-372 (1987).

22. R.T. Yen and Y.E. Fung, Effect of velocity distribution on red cell distribution in capillary blood vessels, *Am. J. Physiol.* **235**:H251-H257 (1978).

23. P. Gaehtgens, K.U. Benner, S. Schickendantz and K.H. Albrecht, Method for simultaneous deter-mination of red cell and plasma flow velocity in vitro and in vivo, *Pflugers Arch.* **361**:191-195 (1976).

24. M.C. Starr and W.G. Frasher, In vivo cellular and plasma velocities in microvessels of the cat mes-entery, *Microvasc. Res.* **10**:102-106 (1975).

ATRIAL NATRIURETIC PEPTIDE (ANP)-INDUCED INCREASE IN CAPILLARY ALBUMIN AND WATER FLUX

Virginia H. Huxley and D. Joseph Meyer, Jr.

Department of Physiology
University of Missouri-Columbia
Medical School
Columbia, MO 65212, USA

INTRODUCTION

Circulating levels of atrial natriuretic peptide (ANP) rise in response to acute hypervolemia and during chronic conditions such as congestive heart failure or arterial hypertension.[1,2,3] Intravenous infusion of the peptide depresses mean arterial blood pressure and elevates hematocrit in both normal and hypertensive subjects.[4,5] Although ANP is a potent vasorelaxant and reduces peripheral vascular resistance, recent studies suggest that ANP-induced hypotension results primarily from a drop in cardiac output.[6,7,8] ANP infusion reduces plasma volume in normotensive rats; which may account, at least in part, for the change in cardiac output.[9,10] Investigations thus far have failed to identify a direct inotropic effect of the peptide on cardiac muscle[6].

Infusion of ANP reduces blood pressure and raises hematocrit to the same degree in nephrectomized rats as in normal rats.[10] Thus, enhanced fluid filtration across non-renal circulatory beds may account for ANP-induced vascular fluid losses.[11] The present study addresses the hypothesis that ANP directly induces an alteration in exchange microvessel permeability properties to water and macromolecules. Single perfused microvessel techniques were used to quantitatively assess the action of the peptide. To measure the transcapillary movement of water, the modified Landis technique was used.[12] Paired determinations of hydraulic conductivity (Lp) were made on single perfused microvessels of frog mesentery under control conditions and in the presence of ANP. Protein flux in individual vessels was measured as a function of hydrostatic pressure by microscope fluorometry.[11] The advantages of these methods are that changes in water or solute flux are measured independent of changes in vascular surface area under conditions of known capillary pressure.

This manuscript is a report of studies in progress. Our results, to date, demonstrate that the petide, ANP, can reversibly increase the hydraulic conductance of exchange microvessels at doses as low as 10 pM.[13] The protein permeability of the microvascular bed can likewise be elevated in the presence of 100 nM ANP. In both cases, though, whether water or macromolecule flux, a subclass of vessels remain unresponsive to the peptide. Thus far we have found no common feature to distinguish "responsive" from "unresponsive" vessels.

METHODS

Animals. All experiments were performed on mesenteric microvessels of the frog (male *rana pipiens*, 6.5-7.5 centimeters body length, supplied by J.M. Hazen, VT). The frogs were housed in fresh water tanks at 15—18°C. One to 5 days prior to use, the animals were transferred to a holding tank at 24-26°C.

Experimental preparation. The brain of the frog was destroyed by pithing; the spinal cord was left intact. The skin on the right side of the abdomen was dissected away and the abdominal cavity opened. A loop of intestine was then floated out over a polished quartz pillar and lightly secured so that the mesentery lay over the top of the pillar. Transillumination of the pillar under the microscope (Leitz, Diavert) allowed examination of the mesenteric microvasculature. For the duration of all experiments, the mesentery was superfused with air equilibrated frog Ringer's, pH 7.4 ± 0.1 and $15 \pm 1°C$.

Vessel Selection and Classification. Only one vessel was used per frog. The type of vessel studied (ie. arterial, true, or venular capillary) was recorded according to the classification scheme of Chambers and Zweifach (1944).[14] Vessels chosen were free of leukocyte sticking or rolling on the walls. Long (>900 μm), unbranched vessels were chosen for hydraulic conductivity measurements. "Y" shaped vessels were chosen for protein permeability studies in order to allow dual cannulation.

Determination of hydraulic conductivity, Lp. Hydraulic conductivity measurements were made using the modified Landis microocclusion technique. The method is described in detail in a number of publications.[12,15,16,17] Perfusion micropipettes, drawn from 1.5 mm OD glass (WP Instruments), were beveled on an air-driven grinding stone with 0.3-3.0 μm grit abrasive film (Thomas Scientific) to an inside tip diameter of 5-25 μm. Just prior to use, the pipette was filled with frog Ringer's albumin solution containing a small number of human erythrocytes as flow markers. The micropipette was connected to a water manometer for control of perfusion pressure (ΔP). The image of the cannulated, perfused capillary was recorded by close-circuit television (DAGE-MTI 650 camera, Panasonic AG-6300 video recorder) along with the image of a videotimer (FOR-A).

The vessel was occluded downstream from the cannulation site with a second micropipette. The marker cell velocity ($d\ell/dt$) following each occlusion was determined by replaying the video tape frame-by-frame. Cell position was measured from the image of a stage micrometer as a function of time following occlusion. Assuming the vessel dimensions approximated those of a right cylinder, initial transcapillary water flow per unit area of capillary ($Jv/S)_i$, was calculated from the initial cell velocity, $(d\ell/dt)_i$, the capillary radius r, and the distance from the marker cell to the site of occlusion ℓ.

$$(Jv/S)_i = (d\ell/dt)_i \ (r/2\ell) \tag{1}$$

Lp is the slope of the relationship between $(Jv/S)_i$ and hydrostatic pressure, ΔP.

$$(Jv/S)_i = Lp(\Delta P - \sigma\Delta\pi) \tag{2}$$

The reflection coefficient, σ, is a measure of the mean selectivity of the vessel wall to macromolecular transit, $\Delta\pi$ is the osmotic pressure gradient.

For each Lp measurement, 3-4 occlusions were made at each of a minimum of three pressures.

Measurement of Permeability, P. Details of the methods and calibrations for measuring solute flux (Js) in single capillaries are found in several current papers.[11,18] In brief, light intensity was monitored (Leitz MPV compact) from a small rectangular window defining a perfused capillary segment downstream from a "Y" branch. The two arms of the "Y" were cannulated and perfused: one pipette contained Ringer's-albumin solution, the second contained fluorescently labeled Ringer's-albumin solution. Each pipette was connected to a water manometer such that flow could be controlled. The tissue was epi-illuminated (75 W Xenon) allowing excitation of the fluorophore (tetramethyl rhodamine isothiocyanate, TRITC) at its maximum absorbance wavelength (554 nm) and detection of emission at its maximum emission wavelength (573 nm). Dual cannulation enabled a rapid change between control and labeled solutions. Dye concentration and window size were set so that fluorescence intensity (I_f) was a linear function of the number of fluorescent molecules in the window.

Initially, the vessel was perfused with control solution while monitoring the fluorescence intensity. The perfusate was then switched to the second pipette. As labeled perfusate entered the vessel, a step increase in fluorescence (ΔI_f) occured. Subsequent diffusion of labeled solute across the vessel wall and into the tissue resulted in a further, initially linear, increase in fluorescence, $(dI_f/dt)_i$. The flux per unit surface area and concentration was calculated as:

$$Js/S\Delta C = (dI_f/dt)_i \ 1/\Delta I_f \ (r/2) \tag{3}$$

The Hertzian equation describing the net flux resulting from both diffusive and convective forces is given as:

$$Js = PS\Delta C\ Pe/(e^{Pe} - 1) + Jv(1 - \sigma)C_1 \tag{4}$$

The Peclet number, Pe, is an expression of the imposed (convective) solute velocity relative to the diffusive solute velocity. Thus:

$$Pe = Lp\ S\ (1 - \sigma)\ \Delta P/(PS) \tag{5}$$

The reflection coefficient, σ, in these expressions refers to the mean selectivity of the pathway across which solute and water are coupled. Likewise Jv is the water flux across this coupled pathway. In the hydraulic conductivity studies outlined above (Eqns. 1&2), Jv is the water flux across all fluid pathways. Under conditions of low volume flux, Equation 4 is an expression of the Fick diffusion where:

$$Js = PS\ \Delta C; \quad Pe = 0 \tag{6}$$

Equation 4 given in terms of Lp, P and σ, when $C_1 = \Delta C$ is:

$$Js/S\Delta C = P\ Pe/(e^{Pe} - 1) + Lp(1 - \sigma)\ \Delta P \tag{7}$$

Thus, the flux of solute, Js/SΔC, measured at each of two capillary hydrostatic pressures, ΔP, provides sufficient information to solve for P and Lp($1 - \sigma$). To this end, four measurements of solute flux were made at a minimum of three hydrostatic pressures.

Solutions. Frog-Ringer's solutions, prepared daily, contained (in mM):NaCl 111, KCl 2.4, $MgSO_4$ 1.0, $CaCl_2$ 1.1, glucose 5.0, $NaHCO_3$ 0.03. The Ringer's solution was buffered to pH 7.4 at 15°C with 5 mM N-2-hydroxy-ethyl-piperazine-N'-2-ethanesulfonic (HEPES) acid/Na-HEPES salt. The pH was adjusted by changing the ratio of HEPES acid to Na-HEPES salt.

All perfusate solutions contained 10 mg/ml bovine serum albumin, BSA, (Sigma A7638, Lot #25F-9405) in frog Ringer's. To remove low molecular weight contaminants, protein solutions were dialyzed against 4 liters of frog Ringer's in 2 liter amounts for 48 hours (12,000 MW cut-off dialysis tubing, Spectropor). Final protein concentration was checked by absorption spectroscopy at 280 nm.[19]

Perfusate solutions containing atrial natriuretic peptide (ANP) were prepared by dilution of a stock suspension of 10 μM Human Atrial Natriuretic Peptide, ANP, (Bachem, 28 amino acids, MW 3083, Lot #140A).

A small number of human red blood cells were suspended in perfusate solutions for use as flow markers during Lp measurements. Prior to addition, the cells were washed three times by centrifugation in frog-Ringer's to remove the buffy-coat and plasma layers.

Protein Labeling. 60 mg of protein was dissolved into 10 ml 0.05 M Borate buffer ($Na_2B_4O_7$-10H_2O, pH 9.24, 20°C) containing 0.4 M NaCl. The high salt/protein solution was put into washed dialysis tubing (12,000 MW cutoff, Spectropor). Dye solution was prepared by dissolving 10 mg of TRITC in 50 ml 0.05 M Borate buffer. The dialysis bag was suspended in the dye overnight at 6°C. The protein was then dialyzed against 2 liters of glucose-free frog-Ringer's solution at 6°C. The dialysate was changed after 24 hour to 2 liters fresh frog-Ringer's solution. While a slight pink tinge was observed following the first wash, analysis of the second dialystate in a spectrofluorometer (Farrand) failed to show free dye.

Experimental Design. In all vessels studied, initial measurements of Lp or Js/SΔC were made with frog-Ringer's perfusate containing 10 mg/ml BSA. In this manner each vessel served as its own control. The control Lp measurement in each of 32 vessels was followed by recannulations and determinations of Lp at one or more ANP concentrations (10 pM – 10 μM). Jv/S measurements were initiated 1-2 minutes following each cannulation. In 14 of the 32 vessels, a final Lp measurement was obtained with return to control perfusate. In 7 vessels, control measurements of Js/SΔC were followed by recannulation and measurement of protein flux in the presence of 100 nM perfusate ANP. Js/SΔC measurements were initiated 2-5 minutes after cannulation.

RESULTS

Transcapillary water flux. Figure 1 shows the changes in Lp in a single 24 μm vessel with

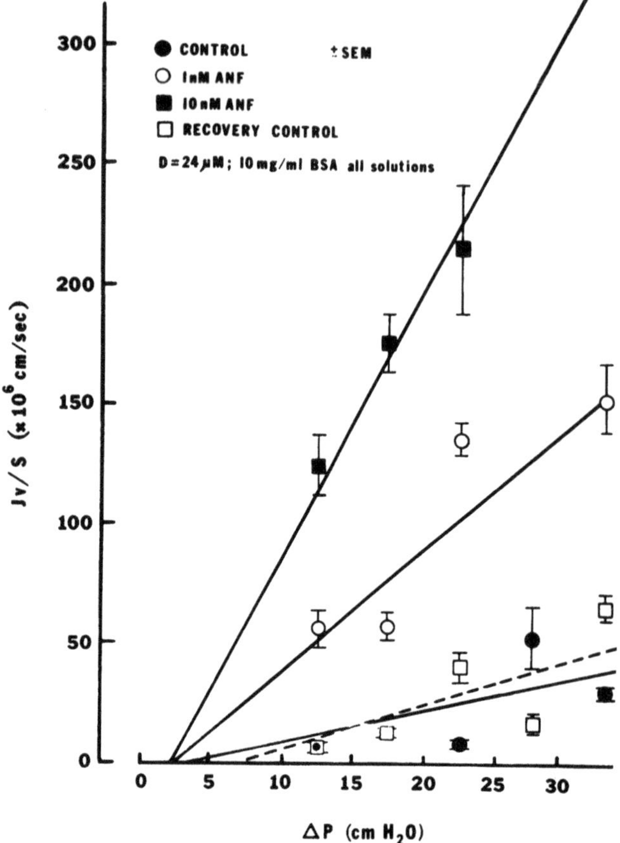

Fig. 1. Capillary water flux (Jv/S) in a single vessel is plotted as a function of capillary hydrostatic pressure (ΔP) at two doses of ANP. Control measures (closed circles) of Jv/S were made with peptide-free perfusion. Repeated measures were made with 1nM ANP (open circles) followed by perfusion containing 10 nM ANP (closed squares) and finally under control conditions (opens squares). All solutions contained 10 mg/ml dialyzed bovine serum albumin.

exposure to ANP. A control Lp (closed circles) of 13.6×10^{-7} cm sec^{-1} cmH$_2$O^{-1} was measured during perfusion with frog-Ringer's containing 10 mg/ml dialyzed BSA. Lp increased to 52.9×10^{-7} cm sec^{-1} cmH$_2$O^{-1} (open circles) with addition of 1 nM ANP. The Lp rose further to 115.2×10^{-7} cm sec^{-1} cmH$_2$O^{-1} (closed squares) when the peptide concentration was elevated to 10 nM ANP. Finally, removal of ANP from the perfusate returned Lp to 19.5×10^{-7} cm sec^{-1} cmH$_2$O^{-1} (open squares), statistically indistinguishable from the initial Lp ($P \leqslant 0.10$).

The ratios of test Lp to control Lp for 50 paired trials (in 32 vessels) are plotted against the log of the peptide concentration in Figure 2. These data demonstrate that Lp is a graded function of ANP concentration. Further, ANP was able to increase Lp at concentrations as low as 10 pM.

In 14 of the 32 vessels, a final (recovery) Lp measurement was made in the absence of ANP. In each case, the recovery Lp was indistinguishable from the control Lp ($P \leqslant 0.10$) indicating a reversible response to the peptide.

Comparison of control and test Lp's by Student's t-test showed an Lp ratio less than or equal to 2.0 was indistinguishable from a ratio of 1.0 ($P \leqslant 0.10$). By this criterion, 19 of 50 trials (representing 15 of the 32 vessels) failed to show a significant response to ANP as illustrated in Figure 3. Lp ratios greater than 2.0 are plotted in the upper curve (circles); those less than 2.0 are plotted in the lower curve (triangles).

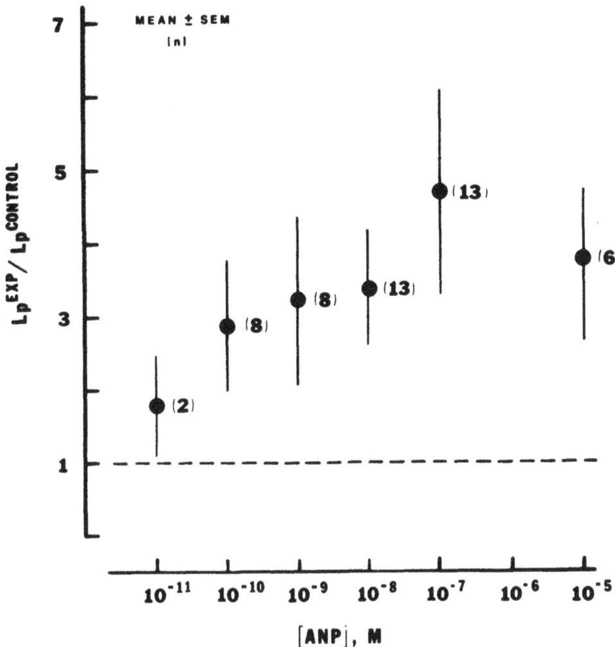

Fig. 2. The ratio of capillary water filtration coefficient with ANP (Lp^{exp}) to control filtration coefficient in the absence of peptide (Lp^{control}) is plotted as a function of peptide concentration. The ratios are given as the mean ± SEM.

Analysis of the data obtained thus far has failed to reveal a correlation between Lp response to ANP and a) initial Lp value, b) vessel diameter, or c) vessel classification.

Transcapillary albumin flux. In Figure 4, albumin flux per unit surface area and concentration is plotted as a function of the capillary hydrostatic pressure. These data are the composit data from three vessels perfused first with no peptide (triangles) and then with 100 nM ANP (circles). No effect of the peptide was discerned in these vessels.

Figure 5, by contrast, shows the response of 4 additional vessels. A marked increase in protein flux occurred upon exposure to ANP. In the absence of ANP, a mean Js/SΔC of 5.4×10^{-6} cm/sec was measured at 11.5 cmH$_2$O perfusion pressure. This flux increased to 16.2×10^{-6} cm/sec during ANP perfusion. Lp$(1-\sigma)$ approximated by simple linear regression, yeilds slopes of 1.7×10^{-7} cm sec^{-1} cmH$_2$O^{-1} and 5.2×10^{-7} cm sec^{-1} cmH$_2$O^{-1} for the control and ANP perfusion data, respectively.

CONCLUSION

Infusion of ANP is known to markedly enhance renal glomerular filtration.[20] An additional action of the peptide has been proposed: that of modulation of non-renal fluid filtration. The hypothesis arose from the observation of an equivalent ANP-induced elevation in systemic hematocrit in both normal and nephrectomized rats.[9,10] The hydraulic conductance data in the present study support this hypothesis: ANP markedly enhanced fluid transport across select microvessels of frog mesentery. The albumin flux data independently demonstrate that the peptide, at a dose that can maximally elevate trancapillary flux, can increase exchange microvessel permeability to albumin.

In the transcapillary water studies, individual microvessels varied considerably in their sensitivity to peptide. Sensitivity, though, did not follow an identifiable pattern. Response to the peptide did not correlate with initial value of Lp, vessel diameter or vessel classification. In the solute flux studies, on the other hand, the behavior of the vessels studied thus far fell into two consistent patterns (Fig. 4 versus Fig. 5). Coupling of solute and water flux was greater in

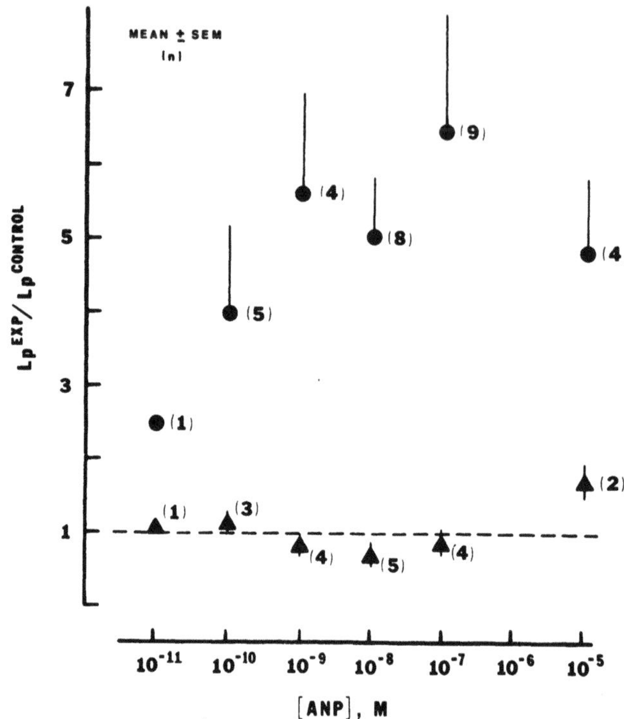

Fig. 3. Microvessels showing a significant (P>0.1, circles) or an insignificant (P<0.1, triangles) change in Lp as a function of peptide concentration. The ratio of microvessel water conductivity in the presence of peptide (Lp^{exp}) relative to the control, peptide-free filtration coefficient ($Lp^{control}$) is plotted on the y-axis.

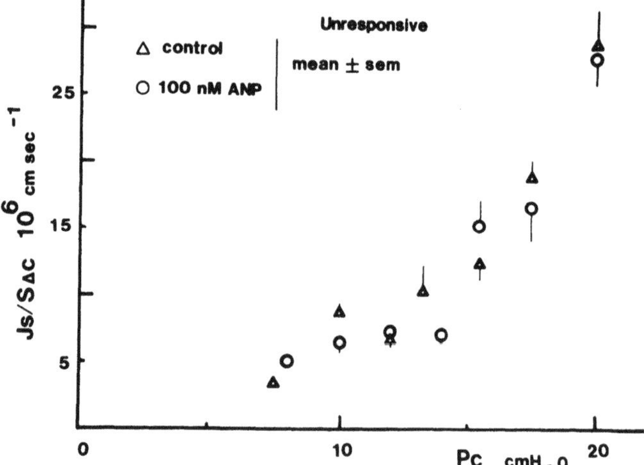

Fig. 4. Transcapillary solute flux as a function of capillary pressure. Data are composit responses from three vessels perfused first with peptide-free solution (triangles) and then with 100 nM ANP (circles).

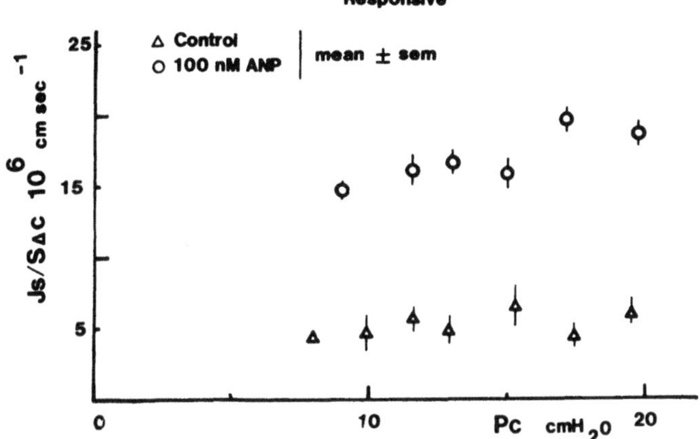

Fig. 5. Capillary albumin flux as a function of capillary pressure. Data are from four vessels perfused first with peptide-free solution (triangles) and then with solution containing 100 nM ANP (circles).

the ANP-insensitive vessels. Under control conditions and low perfusion pressures, similar solute fluxes were measured in all vessels. At higher perfusion pressures (>15 cmH$_2$O) significantly higher fluxes were detected in the "unresponsive" than in the "responsive" vessels. These preliminary data suggest that the solute flux studies may be used to distinguish ANP-sensitive from ANP-insensitive vessels.

Two-fold and greater elevations in Lp can occur with exposure to ANP at concentrations as low as 10 pM. In addition, the decrease in capillary resistance to water flow is a graded function of the peptide concentration. The maximum change appears to occur at 100 nM ANP (Fig. 3). Thus ANP is able to induce non-renal capillary hyperfiltration, in part at least, by a direct action on capillary endothelia. Removal of peptide from the capillary perfusate was accompanied by a decrease in water filtration coefficient to control levels. Thus exposure of the vessels to peptide concentrations as high as 10 μM did not irreversibly alter the vascular barrier with respect to water movement. These studies of total capillary hydraulic conductivity, though, only provide information on the movement of water. Conclusions on transcapillary barrier integrity with respect to macromolecules cannot be drawn from these studies. Indeed, elevation of microvascular water conductivity need not be accompanied by an alteration in microvascular protein permeability.

Assessment of the peptide action on the permeability and selectivity of the exchange microvessel wall was initiated with the direct measurement of fluorescently labeled albumin flux in individual microvessels. Macromolecules normally move across the capillary wall by simple diffusion (Eqn. 6) and/or by solvent drag. Under conditions of solvent drag, the movement of protein is "coupled" to the movement of water. Coupling of solute to water flux is demonstrated by measuring flux as a function of capillary pressure (Eqn. 7). Little to no coupling is observed if capillary permeability to the molecule is much greater than capillary water conductivity (e.g. PS $>>$ Jv$(1-\sigma)$ and Pe < 1). Conversely if the vessel permeability is of the same order, or less than Jv$(1-\sigma)$, (e.g. Pe > 1) then solute flux will rise with rising pressure. Convective movement of solute predominates when Jv$(1-\sigma)$ is 3-fold greater than PS.

The capillaries in Fig. 4 show a significant solvent drag component in the presence or absence of peptide. In contrast, the vessels in Fig. 5 show only a small convective component. For reasons as yet unknown, the behavior of the vessels in Fig. 4 remained unchanged with the peptide perfusion. The vessels in Fig. 5 demonstrate two behaviors upon perfusion with ANP. First, the flux of TRITC-albumin was elevated from control over the range of pressure tested. Second, the solvent drag component of the transcapillary flux was increased.

Elevation of albumin flux with ANP perfusion could arise by more than one mechanism. The flux of albumin could be elevated by increasing the number of macromolecule conducting pathways, thereby elevating capillary permeability to albumin and water without changing the selectivity of the capillary wall (e.g. σ remains unchanged). A second mechanism for an elevated flux at a given hydrostatic pressure is an increase in the size of the macromolecule conducting pathways. This would serve to elevate capillary permeability, as well as water conductivity and

29

to decrease selectivity. A third mechanism involves the alteration in the chemical or morphologic structure of the macromolecule conducting pathways whereby the permeability to albumin is elevated without altering water flow. One example would be the rearrangement of a fiber matrix thereby decreasing selectivity, elevating permeability and leaving water conductivity unchanged.[21,16] Additional experimental data are required to make definitive statements on the mechanisms whereby vascular permeability is elevated when ANP is present. The following statements can be made about the data thus far.

Under conditions of low volume flux ($Jv \cong 0$), the true diffusive permeability to the vessel wall determines solute flux (Eqn. 6). These conditions are approximated at low perfusion pressures. In the simplest model of a homoporous microvessel [21] solution of Eqn. 6 yields a 3-fold increase in P to albumin with 100 nM ANP (Fig. 5). The vessels in Fig. 4 show no ANP-induced change in albumin flux at any pressure tested. Thus, the peptide elevates albumin permeability in a select subset of microvessels.

As perfusion pressure is increased, the slope, of solute flux on capillary pressure, approaches a limiting value of $Lp(1 - \sigma)$ (Eqn. 7). An homoporous analysis of the data allows an approximation of $Lp (1 - \sigma)$ in the presence and absence of ANP. A 3-fold increase in $Lp(1 - \sigma)$ was detected, implying that ANP elevated the convective coupling across the protein permeable pathways in these vessels.

The magnitudes of elevation in albumin permeability and in $Lp(1 - \sigma)$ are similar: three-fold. To a first approximation this behavior is consistent with an increase in the number of pathways conducting water and solute. To make an unequivocal statement to distinguish if the elevation in permeability results from decreased selectivity and/or the formation of additional "leaks" further experiments must be performed. Solute reflection coefficient or total vessel Lp, as well as solute flux, need to be measured in the same exchange microvessel. The measurement of microvessel solute flux with solutes of different sizes are required to define the degree to which the exchange microvessels are "homoporous" or "heteroporous". Without these data we are, as yet, limited in the ability to define the mechanisms whereby ANP alters microvessel permeability.

Atrial natriuretic peptide reduced plasma volume, presumably by shifting fluid into the extravascular space. Starling's relationship (Eqn. 2) indicates enhanced fluid filtration may result from one or more of the following conditions: an increase in the hydrostatic pressure gradient across the capillary wall, an elevation in vessel wall hydraulic conductance or a decrease in trancapillary osmotic gradient ($\sigma \Delta \pi$). Our studies demonstrate that ANP enhances both total water conductivity (Lp) and microvessel permeability (P) in select microvessels. The rise in protein permeability may or may not be associated with a change in mean capillary selectivity (σ). Nevertheless, $\sigma \Delta \pi$ decreases as protein leaves the vascular space. ANP also increases the coupling of solute and water flow across albumin permeable pathways i.e. elevates $Lp(1 - \sigma)$. Whether this observation results from an increase in the hydraulic conductance of albumin permeable pathways or from a decrease in σ remains to be determined.

ACKNOWLEDGMENTS

The research in this laboratory is supported by NIH Research Grant HL 34872. V.H.H. is an Established Investigator of the American Heart Association. The authors thank Bill O'Connell for typing the manuscript.

REFERENCES

1. R.E. Lang, H. Tholken, D. Ganten, F.C. Luft, H. Ruskoaho and T. Unger, Atrial natriuretic factor — a circulating hormone stimulated by volume loading, *Nature* 314:264-266 (1985).
2. R.E. Lang, R. Dietz, A. Merkel, T. Unger, H. Ruskoaho and D. Ganten Plasma atrial natriuretic peptide values in cardiac disease, *J. Hypertension* 4 (suppl. 2):S119-S123 (1986).
3. M. Epstein, R.D. Loutzenhiser, E. Freidland, R.M. Aceto, M.J.F. Camargo and S.A. Atlas, Increases in circulating atrial natriuretic factor during immersion-induced central hypervolemia in normal humans, *J. Hypertension* 4 (suppl. 2):S93-S99 (1986).
4. T. Maack, D.N. Marion, M.J.F. Camargo, H.D. Kleinert, J.H. Laragh, E.D. Vaughan and S.A. Atlas, Effect of auriculin (atrial natriuretic factor) on blood pressure, renal function, and the renin-aldosterone system in dogs, *Am. J. Med.* 77:1069-1075 (1984).
5. J. Biollaz, J. Nussberger, B. Waeber and H.R. Brunner, Clinical pharmacology of atrial natriuretic (3-28) eicosa-hexapeptide, *J. Hypertension* 4 (suppl. 2):101-108 (1986).
6. U. Ackerman, Cardiovascular effects of atrial natriuretic extract in the whole animal, *Federation*

Proc. **45**:2111-2114 (1986).

7. R.W. Lappe, J.F.M. Smits, J.A. Todt, J.J.M. Debets and R.L. Wendt, Failure of atriopeptin II to cause arterial vasodilation in the conscious rat, *Circ. Res.* **56**:606-612 (1985)

8. B.L. Pegram, M.B. Kandon, N.C. Trippodo, F.E. Cole and A.A. MacPhee, Atrial extract: hemodynamics in Wistar-Kyoto and spontaneously hypertensive rats, *Am. J. Physiol.* **249**:H265-H271 (1985).

9. A.F. Almeida, M. Suzuki and T. Maack, Atrial natriuretic factor increases hematocrit and decreases plasma volume in nephrectomized rats, *Life Sci.* **39**:1193-1199 (1986).

10. J.P. Fluckiger, B. Waeber, G. Matsueda, B. Delaloye, J. Nussberger and H.R. Brunner, Effect of atriopeptin III on hematocrit and volemia of nephrectomized rats, *Am. J. Physiol.* **251**:H880-H883 (1986).

11. V.H. Huxley, V.L. Tucker, K.M. Verburg and R.H. Freeman, Increased capillary hydraulic conductivity induced by atrial natriuretic peptide, *Circ. Res.* **60**:304-307 (1987).

12. C.C. Michel, J.C. Mason, F.E. Curry and J.E. Tooke, A development of the Landis technique for measuring the filtration coefficient of individually perfused capillaries of frog mesentery, *Q.J. Exp. Physiol.* **59**:283-309 (1974).

13. D.J. Meyer and V.H. Huxley, Atrial natriuretic peptide increases capillary water conductivity in a graded manner (abstract), *Fed. Proc.* **46**(4):1536 (1987).

14. R. Chambers and B.W. Zweifach, Intercellular cement and capillary permeability, *Amer. J. Anat.* **75**:173-205 (1944).

15. F.E. Curry, V.H. Huxley and R.H. Adamson, Permeability of single capillaries to intermediate sized colored solutes, *Am. J. Physiol.* **245**:H495-H505 (1983).

16. C.C. Michel, Fluid movements through capillary walls, *In*: "Handbook of Physiology, Cardiovascular System." Bethesda, MD: Am. Physiol. Soc. Sect. 2, Vol IV, Chapt. 9, pp. 375-409 (1984).

17. V.H. Huxley, F.E. Curry and R.H. Adamson, Quantitative fluorescence microscopy on single capillaries: α-lactalbumin transport, *Am. J. Physiol.* **252**:H188-H197 (1987).

18. F.E. Curry, V.H. Huxley and I.H. Sarelius, Techniques in the Microcirculation: Measurement of permeability, pressure and flow, *In*: "Techniques in the Life Sciences." R.J. Linden, Ed., Vol. P3/1, Elsevier, New York, pp. 1-34 (1983).

19. H.K. Schachman and S.J. Edelstein, Ultracentrifuge studies with absorption optics. IV. Molecular weight determination at the microgram level, *Biochem.* **5**:2681-2691 (1966).

20. R.H. Freeman, J.O. Davis and R.C. Vari, Renal response to atrial natriuretic factor in conscious dogs with caval constriction, *Am. J. Physiol.* **248**:R495-R500 (1985).

21. F.E. Curry, Mechanics and thermodynamics of transcapillary exchange, *In*: "Handbook of Physiology. Cardiovascular system. Microcirculation." Bethesda, MD; Am. Physiol. Soc., Sect. 2, Vol IV, Chpt. 8, pp. 309-374 (1984).

22. R.M. Arendt, A.L. Gerbes, D. Ritter, E. Stangl, P. Bach and J. Zahringer, Atrial natriuretic factor in plasma of patients with arterial hypertension, heart failure or cirrhosis of the liver, *J. Hypertension* **4** (suppl. 2):S131-S135 (1986).

ROLE OF ENDOTHELIUM IN ATHEROGENESIS

COMPUTERIZED 3-D RECONSTRUCTION OF SMALL BLOOD VESSELS FROM HIGH VOLTAGE ELECTRON-MICROGRAPHS OF THICK SERIAL CROSS SECTIONS

L. Horn*, W.S. Krajewski**, P.K. Paul**, M.J. Song† and M.J. Sydor**

*Department of Physiology, UMDNJ-New Jersey Medical School
Newark, NJ 07103, USA
**Grad. Div. of Biomed. Engineering, NJIT, Newark, NJ 07102, USA
†Wadsworth Center for Laboratories and Research
New York State Department of Health
Empire State Plaza, Albany, NY 12201, USA

INTRODUCTION

Every cell and organ system in the body depends on the circulation of blood for appropriate nutrients, humoral message exchange, and removal of waste. The heart and the large blood vessels are indispensable as pump and plumbing. Blood flow according to tissue needs, however, and body weight economy in terms of total blood volume, requires complex control mechanisms and an intricate distribution system peripherally, particularly in the microcirculation which consists of vessels less than 100 μ. The smallest arteries and arterioles are generally considered the key vessels mediating the distribution of flow by changing their diameters and thus flow resistance. The structural aspects of these vessels thus become crucial for the understanding of the mechanisms that allow the system to operate in optimal harmony — the harmony that we call good health.

Despite its ancient anatomical roots[1,2,3,4] and more recent intravital microscopy,[5,6,7,8,9] the detailed knowledge of the cytostructural and histoarchitectural aspects of the network of microvessels have remained largely descriptive and qualitative. However, the techniques have allowed us to further our knowledge about "the vessels architectural design and their strict adaptation to the function performed in the organs involved".[8] Substantial advances have been made in the knowledge of microcirculation within the last thirty years. A combination of innovative methods and technology has made it possible to describe microvascular behavior in more precise quantitative terms. These methodologies are microtechniques, electronmicroscopy (EM) and modern data handling procedures. Some of these microtechniques and computer-assisted analysis of video images have enabled us to use intravital microscopy to subject individual segments of the microcirculation vessel system to more accurate analysis and to use such information to reconstruct the operational characteristics of an entire microvascular bed.[10]

The use of the electron microscopy for study of the microvasculature by early workers[11,12,13] and in particular by Rhodin,[14,15] produced new information on both the structural arrangement and on the ultrastructural details of most vascular elements in the microcirculation. The fact remains, however, that after all this effort our knowledge of the structural detail is still quite incomplete. The importance of real and accurate quantitative information on the cellular elements that constitute this network can hardly be overestimated.

The influence of paravascular elements, in particular nerves and mast cells, have long been recognized to control or affect blood flow in the microcirculation, and over the past few decades so have some of the formed elements of the blood. WBC and platelets have received attention as producing potent mediators that modify microcirculatory behavior.[16,17]

Recently, prominent and important research focus has been on a constituent of the vessel itself, the endothelium. For a long time these cells have been considered a smooth lining of the vessels, and related basically to permeability properties of the very smallest exchange vessels. However, during the last few years the focus of attention has changed from the endothelium merely being an exchange counter for substance and information exchange, between the parenchymal elements, the vascular smooth muscle and the blood, to being an important participant in blood flow control. Today the endothelium is recognized as a large, multifarious regulatory organ and factory of potent vasoactive and vasotrópic mediators. The most notable, endothelial derived relaxing factor (EDRF), was discovered less than a decade ago[18] and the endothelium is today recognized as a key organ in eicosanoid metabolism.[19] An interaction between the endothelium and the vascular smooth muscle was not entirely unexpected after the first EM observations of pseudopods or processes of endothelium penetrating the internal lamina forming cell to cell contact with the vascular smooth muscle.[15]

For decades the flow properties of the vessels, their permeability, and the contractile properties of the vascular smooth muscle, related to ionic and electrical membrane properties of vascular smooth muscle, and the biochemical aspects of its force development have been vigorously pursued. Only recently has attention been bestowed on other aspects of the microvessels. Althought the last few years scientific literature contains numerous examples of diversity in terms of size, shape, surface to volume ratios, nuclear to cytoplasonic volume ratios for different cell constituents, particularly the vascular smooth muscle, a systematic assessment of these important parameters is lacking. Both teaching and most interpretations of physiological experimentation are based on generalizations and transposition of data between species, vessel sizes, age and specific pathologies which often are erroneous, misleading, or at best include large margins of error.[20]

One of the main reasons for the paucity in systematic detailed and comprehensive description of these paramenters is the tedious and costly collection of such data. The major difficulty is not that we don't know how to get the detailed data, but the sheer work involved in such endeavors.

Attempts to find practical and relieable methods to assess morphological vascular and particularly microvascular changes in detail during normal angiogenesis, pathogenesis, or in manifest chronic disease have been and still are quite difficult, cumbersome and time consuming.

Our purpose is, therefore, to provide a method that will devise an accurate, versatile and time economical assessment of detailed dimensional description of the cellular compartments and architectural features of microvascular vessels. Such a method should be amenable to both numerical calculations of the parameters of the cell wall compartments, and provide for image reconstruction of the vessel in solid or transparent mode that can be viewed from any chosen angle, and allow for computerized dissection.

The state-of-the-art technological capabilities together with reliable tissue fixation techniques, high resolution electronmicrography, image digitization, and fast computer handling of data provide a whole range of choices.[21,22,23] However, the greater the sophistication the more time consuming and costly the methods become; and may thus, as mentioned, have discouraged investigators from attempting a detailed quantitative description of the morphological aspects of microcirculation. We have tried to choose the simplest salient features of the available technological capabilities to fulfill the purpose stated above.

MATERIALS AND METHODS

Mesenteric vascular tissue was obtained from acute surgical exteriorization of the intestine of pentobarbital anesthetized 18-20 kg mongrel dogs of unknow age. The dogs had been operated on, and instrumented 30 days earlier, and permanently catheterized to monitor the conscious dogs' aortic and vena cava pressures. One group of dogs had the left renal artery permanently narrowed by a 3 mm wide silver loop-clip that would permit roughly 15%-20% of normal renal blood flow. The blood pressure of this group clearly established renovascular hypertension (1 clip-2 kidney Goldblatt) after 2-3 weeks. The control dogs had been operated on and instrumented identically, except that the clip was removed within minutes of installation (normotensive controls). On the day of specimen collection the superior mesenteric artery (SMA) and vein (SMV) were dissected free and a 10 cm wide segment of small intestine, 5 cm proximal to the ileocolic junction, was isolated. After this procedure the SMA was cannulated and perfusion was started with oxygenated, modified Ringer's solutions at 37°C and a hydrostatic pressure of 100 cm of water. All branches of SMA outside the segment that showed blanching were tied off. After ten minutes perfusion of the segment, the SMV was cut, and the solution was switched to 3% glutaraldehyde in cacodylate buffer, adjusted to pH 7.2. After ten minutes *in situ* fixation perfusion, the small intestine was excised from the segment, the remainder of the segment removed and transferred to a large Petri dish filled with primary fixing solution. It remained in this solution for two hours. Two rectangular sections of mesentery, 3 mm × 8 mm, longitudinally parallel to the main large blood vessel from the pedicle and about 2 cm from the peripheral cut of the segment, were sampled.

The mesenteric samples were then washed in diluted cacodylate buffer, post fixed for one hour with 1% osmium tetroxide, washed again and slowly dehydrated with increasing concentrations of ethyl alcohol and gradually infiltrated with increasing Spurr medium concentrations, followed by final polymerization at 60 degrees Celsius.

We used small arterioles, about 50 μm in diameter, from the mesenteric microcirculatory beds of these dogs. Collection of specimens was standardized, i.e. sampling location, perfusion fixation, embedding, staining and sectioning by methods proven to preserve in vivo dimensions and ultrastructure of the specimens.[24] To examine the ultrastructure, we used high voltage electronmicroscopy (HVEM).

For thick section HVEM a straight vessel was selected after microscopic examination of the vascular bed through the Spurr medium block and 0.5 μm thick sections were cut from a mesa formed by hand under a stereomicroscope to give: a) perpendicular cross sections as small as possible to avoid unnecessary compression; b) with leading and trailing edges of the block face perfectly parallel.[21]

Placement of up to 50 such sections on slot grids with Formvar support films was accomplished. Five or more 1.0 MeV electronmicrographs at 2500× were taken to cover the individual cross sections.

Glossy prints of the electronmicrographs, linearly enlarged (3×) were made into photomontages of the sections, with a final magnification of 7500, and all contours of the smooth muscle layer (VSM), the endothelium (E), nuclei (N), and the internal lamina (IL) were traced in color on a clear plastic overlay with orientation coordinates.

The plastic overlay was then transferred to a GTCO digitizing pad and the various polygons digitized, labelled, and stored in a computer filing system. See Figures 1 and 2.

Solid and transparent image reconstructions and computerized dissection of cell compartments were performed using software from Multidimensional Computing, Inc.[25] Compartment volumes of VSM, IL, E and N, and nuclear/cytoplasmic ratios were calculated. It should be noted that the images shown are unedited and were photographed from the computer monitor. They can be viewed at any angle, rotated around X, Y, and Z axes.

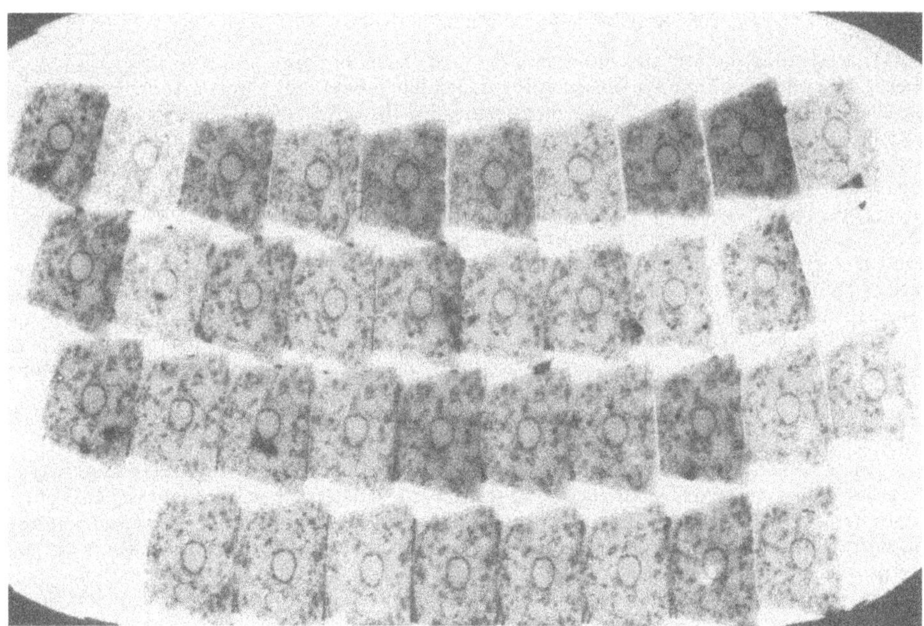

Fig. 1. This HVEM low mag mode (63×) shows a montage of slot grid 7A with sections 123 to 160 of the experimental vessel. Total magnification is 94.5×.

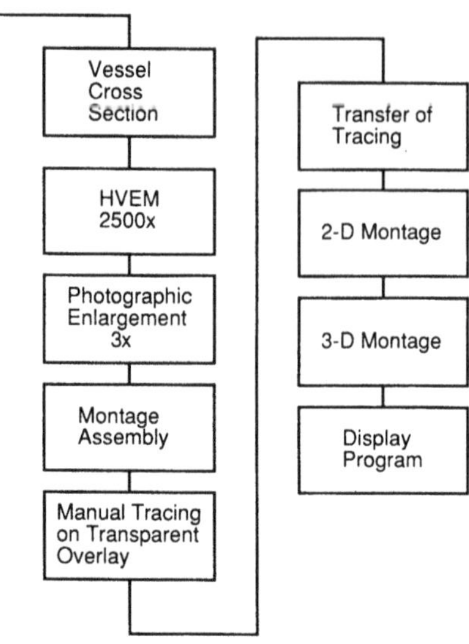

Fig. 2. This is a flow diagram illustrating the steps from sectioning to the display program in our three dimensional reconstruction procedure.

We have also reconstructed an endarteriole, about 15 μm in diameter, from the hypertensive dog. The VSM coat of this vessel is not continuous and so we have only reconstructed the endothelium. Due to the small diameter of the vessel we used direct enlargement of the electronmicrograph without making montages.

RESULTS

Display of all the contours in transparent mode gives an image of the vessel that is too unwieldy, and all the contours in solid mode (hidden line mode) only shows a short uninteresting tube. We, therefore, go to the solid mode and show the VSM layer in the experimental vessel with the outer membranes removed or peeled off; see Figure 3. This figure show the inner surface of the VSM layer in green with the nuclei in red. For this reconstruction 10 sections were lost due to Formvar buckling and have been replaced with 5 replicas of the last section before the hiatus, and 5 replicas of the first full section after the hiatus.

Figure 4 shows the luminal surface of the endothelium of the experimental vessel in yellow and the nuclei in red. Judging from nuclear orientation in Figure 3, the VSM appear circumferentially or helically oriented with a pitch of from 5° to about 30-35°, whereas the endothelial cells appear to be oriented parallel to the longitudinal axis of the vessel in Figure 4.

The next two figures show analogous dissection of the control vessel. Green is the inner surface of the VSM layer, and the nuclei are in red; see Figure 5. Figure 6 shows the luminal endothelial surface in yellow with the nuclei in red.

We note that the pitch of the VSM is less than in the experimental vessel and also that the endothelial nuclei appear shorter than in the experimental vessel.

The reconstruction of the endarteriole SV is depicted in the next two illustrations. Figure 7 shows the beginning of reconstruction in transparent mode. We notice that the "fit" of the contours is better than in the previous images of the montages. Figure 8 shows the complete reconstruction in solid mode of 165 sections. We notice the oval appearance of the nuclei and the lack of any distinct axial orientation.

It should be emphasized that the precision of the orientation of the individual wire frame contours as they appear in the images on the monitor and illustrated here does not affect the calculated parameters. These images serve basically as visual aid to monitor reconstruction. Accurate and esthetically pleasing images can be obtained with more elaborate and sophisticated

Table 1

DESCRIPTION	VSM		IL		ENDO		ENDO
	E	C	E	C	E	C	SV
Avg. outer diameter (μ)	43.90	53.06	40.12	50.08	39.38	49.42	16.70
Avg. inner diameter (μ)	40.12	50.08	39.38	49.42	37.40	48.52	15.56
Avg. layer thickness (μ)	1.89	1.49	0.37	0.32	0.99	0.45	0.57
Avg. volume % of the total wall volume	60.08	66.64	11.24	14.19	28.68	19.16	
Avg. number of cells per 100 μ length	45.54	43.07			31.68	21.53	17.34
Avg. nucleus volume (μ^3)	89.98	65.99			70.38	32.91	35.54
Avg. cell volume (μ^3)	547.87	561.39			375.95	322.85	201.34
Ratio of nuclear volume to cell volume	0.1642	0.1175			0.1871	0.1019	0.2144
Ratio of nuclear volume to cytoplasm	0.1965	0.1332			0.2303	0.1135	0.2729

E = 2-KGH, C = Control, SV = Small Vessel 2-KGH

techniques and equipment[21] as shown in Figre 9, which beautifully illustrates a solid mode reconstruction of a single astrocyte from cat brain.

DISCUSSION AND CONCULSION

We have calculated and tabulated the various parameters for the specimens shown and there are some distinct differences between the hypertensive and normotensive samples. However, before discussing and comparing the data we must caution that they represent only two samples and that the differences may be fortuitous rather than characteristic changes that occur as a result of chronic hypertension, however plausible they may appear, see Table 1.

If we first look at the outer diameter, we see that the one of the experimental specimen is about 20% less than that of the control, whereas the wall thickness is about 30% greater, due to about the same number of VSM cells of similar cell volumes and apparently both hypertrophy and hyperplasia of the endothelium. It is also apparent that the nuclear to cytoplasmic volume ratios are much larger in the hypertensive vessel cells than those of the control. In determining the pitch of the cell, it is assumed that the nuclei are oriented along the long axis of the VSM cells.[26] The greater pitch of the VSM in Figure 3 may possibly indicate slight vasoconstriction. This speculation may perhaps also be supported statistically by a more irregular (wrinkling or corrugation) and larger total contour (greater length) of the IL in sections of the experimental sections, despite the lesser diameter than in the controls, data not shown.

When all three wall compartments in the experimental vessel are normalized to those of the control diameters, the total difference in wall thickness almost disappears (less than 3%), and the perplexing fact appears that only endothelial changes remain, and that the IL as percent of wall volume is even reduced. Again, due to the limitation of the data, further speculation is quite fruitless. However, the purpose of the table is to show that the program can handle the number crunching and make comparison simple and accurate.

Also, attempts to use HVEM 1000$\times$ only, and photographic enlargement to 7500$\times$, have yielded data that are almost identical to those of the montages ($P < 0.05$). Attempts are being made to increase cross section thickness to 1.0 μ and use only one micrograph of each section. This reduces the work of reconstruction to less than 20% of the rather efficacious method described, and would permit us to start detailed quantitative descriptions of whole microvascular beds in terms of cellular parameters.

In conclusion we have shown that HVEM and computerized reconstruction of thick serial cross sections of small blood vessels provide a powerful and reliable method for studying and assessing hypertrophy, hyperplasia and changes that may clarify the pathogenesis of chronic hypertension or other angiopathy, as well as studying architectural angiogenesis.

40

SUMMARY AND CONCLUSION

Morphological analysis of compartments in terms of volumes and the orientation of the cells and their nuclei within very small mesenteric arteries and arterioles is being carried out. Samples were from simultaneously sham operated and instrumented control and one-clip two kidney Goldblatt sustained (30 days) hypertensive dogs. Collection of specimens was standardized, i.e. sampling location, perfusion fixation, embedding, staining, and sectioning by methods proven to preserve in vivo dimensions. Serial thick cross sections (0.5 μ) were subjected to high voltage electromicrography (1.0 MeV) at 2500× and then linearly enlarged 3× photographically. The glossy micrographs (7500×) were made into montages and the contours of the smooth muscle layer (vascular smooth muscle), the endothelium (E), nuclei (N), and the internal lamina (IL) were digitized on a large GTCO digi-pad with input to a microcomputer (PC-Limited, Turbo) equipped with a 20 MB hard disk and coprocessor. Solid and transparent image reconstructions and computerized dissection of cell compartments were performed. Compartment volumes of vascular smooth muscle, IL, E and N, and individual cell and nuclear volumes, as well as nuclear/cytoplasmic ratios were calculated. Image reconstructions are presented. The emphasis is on methods and these are discussed in terms of useability for determining accurate microvessel morphology in health and disease, with particular emphasis on assessment of hypertrophy and hyperplasia in experimental hypertension, and architectural angiogenesis in general.

ACKNOWLEDGMENTS

Thanks are due to the director of the HVEM National Biotechnology Resource, Dr. D.F. Parsons and his staff, Dr. F.P.J. Diecke of UMDNJ for continued support, and Mr. G. Powell for typing this manuscript. This research was aided in part by NIH Grants 2 S07 RR05393, 7R01 HL31880, PHS Grant RR01219, DHHS, generous gifts from CP Chemicals, Inc. and Multidimensional Computing, Inc.

REFERENCES

1. M. Malphigi, De Pulmonibus. Trans. by J. Young 1929, *Proc. Roy. Soc. Med.* **23**:1-4 (1661).
2. M. Hall, A critical and experimental essay on the circulation of the blood. R.B. Seeley and W. Burnside, *London*. p. 22 (1831).
3. F. Arnold. Handbuch der Anatomie des Menschen, Zweite Bd. Abt., Emmerling, Freiburg in Br. (1847).
4. W. Spalteholz, Die Vertheilung der Blutgefasse in der Haut, *Arch. f. Anat. u. Entwicklungsgesch.* (Anat. Abst.) 1-54, Leibzig (1893).
5. A. Krogh, The Anatomy and Physiology of Capillaries, *Yale Univ. Press* New Haven (1929).
6. B.W. Zweifach, The structure and reaction of the small blood vessels in amphibia, *Am. J. Anat.* **60**:473-514 (1937).
7. R. Chambers and B.W. Zweifach, The topography and function of the mesenteric capillary microcirculation, *Am. J. Anat.* **75**:173-205 (1944).
8. M.H. Knisely. The histopathology of peripheral vascular beds. In F.R. Moulton (ed.) Blood, Heart, and Circulation, pp. 303-307. Publ. No. 13, A.A.A.S. *The Science Press*, Lancaster, PA.
9. P.I. Brånemark and E. Eriksson, Method for studying qualitative and quantitative changes of blood flow in skeletal muscle, *Acta Physiol, Scand.* **84**:284-288 (1971).
10. B.W. Zweifach, Introduction, Perspectives in microcirculation. In Kaley, G. and B.M. Altura (eds.) Microcirculation. Vol. 1; *Univ. Park Press.* Baltimore (1977).
11. H.S. Bennett, J.H. Luft and J.C. Hampton, Morphological classifications of vertebrate blood capillaries, *Am. J. Physiol.* **196**:381-390 (1959).
12. D.W. Fawcett, The fine structure of capillaries and small arteries. In S.R.M. Reynolds and B.W. Zweifach (eds.), THE MICROCIRCULATION. Univ. Illinois Press, *Urbana, IL.* pp. 1-13 (1959).
13. G.E. Palade, Blood capillaries of the heart and other organs, *Circulation* **24**:368-384 (1961).
14. J.A.G. Rhodin, Ultrastructure of mammalian venous capillaries, venules, and small collecting veins, *J. Ultrastruc. Res.* **25**:452-500 (1968).
15. J.A.G. Rhodin, The ultrastructure of mammalian arterioles and precapillary sphincters, *J. Ultrastruc. Res.* **18**:181-223 (1967).
16. J. Björk, Microvascular reactions in acute inflammation. An intravital microscopy study in the hamster, Acta Univ. Upsaliensis, Thesis, ISSN 0345-0058, ISBN 91-554-1551-2, Upsala, Sweden (1984).

17. *J.T. O'Flaherty, Biology of Disease. Lipid mediators of inflammation and allergy, Lab. Invest.* 47:314-329 (1982).

18. R.F. Furchgott, The role of endothelium in the responses of vascular smooth muscle to drugs, *A. Rev. Pharmac. Tox.* 24:175-197 (1984).

19. N. Chung Welch, D. Shepro, B. Dunham and H.B. Hectman, Prostacylclin and prostaglandin E_2 secretion by bovine pulmonary microvessel endothelium cells are altered by changes in culture conditions, *J. Cell Physiol.* In press (1988).

20. M.E. Todd, C.G. Laye and D.N. Osborne, The dimensional characteristics of smooth muscle in rat blood vessels. A Computer-Assisted Analysis, *Circ. Res.* 53:319-331 (1983).

21. M. Marco, A. Leith and D.F. Parsons, Three-dimensional reconstruction of cells from serial sections and whole-cell mounts using multilevel contouring of stereo micrographs, *J. Electron Microsc. Tech,* In press (1988).

22. E.R. Macagno, C. Levinthal and I. Sobel, Three-dimensional computer reconstruction of neurons and neuronal assemblies, *Ann. Rev. Biphys. Bioeng.* 5:323-351 (1979).

23. M.S. Braverman and I.M. Braverman, Three dimensional reconstructions of objects from serial sections using a microcomputer graphics system, *J. Investig. Dermatology* 86:290-294 (1986).

24. J.A.G. Rhodin, Perfusion and superfusion fixation effects on rat mesentery microvascular beds. Intravital and electron Microscope Analyses, *J. Submicrosc. Cytol.* 18:453-470 (1986).

25. E.K. Fram, 3-D Reconstruction, Seeing Beyond, *PC Magazine,* August 20, pp. 170-174 (1985).

26. P.B. Canham, R.M. Henderson and M.W. Peters, Coalignment of the muscle cell and nucleus, cell geometry and Vv in the tunica media of monkey cerebral arteries, by electron microscopy, *J. Microsc.* 127:311-319 (1982).

CORRELATION OF LASER-DOPPLER-VELOCITY MEASUREMENTS AND ENDOTHELIAL CELL SHAPE IN A STENOSED DOG AORTA

D.W. Liepsch, M. Levesque*, R.M. Nerem* and S.T. Moravec**

Hal B. Wallis Research Facility
Eisenhower Medical Ctr. 39000 Bob Hope Drive
Rancho Mirage, CA 92270, USA
*Department of Mechanical Engineering
University of Houston, TX 77058 USA
**Labor für Fluidmechanik, Fachhochschuile
München FB05, West Germany

INTRODUCTION

Apart from chemical factors, hemodynamics play a major role in atherosclerosis and aging. It has been suggested that vascular geometry may affect the atherogenic process by its influence on the hemodynamic environment which the intima is exposed to.[1,2] Rodkiewicz[3] demonstrated very clearly the shear stress on the wall at flow separation and stagnation points. Several flow studies were done in artery models to find out the influence of hemodynamic forces on the vessel wall and on the blood cells; only a few shall be mentioned here.[4,5,6,7,8] The vessel wall is very resistant against pressure perpendicular to the wall. Pressure on the vessel wall is usually between 10,000 to 20,000 N/m^2. These forces are compensated by the elastin or collagen fibers in the wall. However, forces which are tangential-shear stresses attack the endothelial cells and their resistance is much less. At shear stresses from 20 to 40 N/m^2 the endothelial cells are sheared away. This can lead to an injury of the inside vessel wall. Usually, the shear stresses on the endothelial cells are about 1-2 N/m^2. Thus, the effect of such forces upon endothelial cells is therefore of great interest.

Davis et al.[9] studied the endothelial turnover by exposing contact-inhibited confluent cell monolayers in a cone-plate viscosimeter. In the presented study, the influence of shear stresses on the endothelial cell geometry and orientation are demonstrated.

EXPERIMENTAL STUDIES

Model Preparation: The vascular casting technique was used to construct an elastic silicone rubber model. A cast of a dog aortic stenosis was used where the severity of the stenosis was 71% based on the area. The stenosis in the dog aorta was prepared by wrapping a cotton band around the aorta. The band was tightened until the presence of a thrill or a bruit was felt distal to the band. Twelve weeks later the animal was sacrificed and the aorta was prepared using the vascular casting procedure.[10] From these vascular casts, the cross-sectional area was calculated. Micrographs of endothelial cells were obtained from the ventral aspect of the cast. Endothelial cells were analyzed with a video plan image analyzer. Models for the velocity measurements were prepared in the following way: A plaster of Paris form was made from the cast. This plaster of Paris form was divided into two parts. Wax was then placed in the plaster of Paris form to obtain a wax cast. A 1 mm thick copper layer was galvanized around the wax cast. After that, a second plaster of Paris form was prepared from the galvanized model. A second wax form was prepared in the first plaster of Paris form. This wax model was put into the second plaster of Paris form with distance rings. Silicone rubber was injected under vacuum into the

"

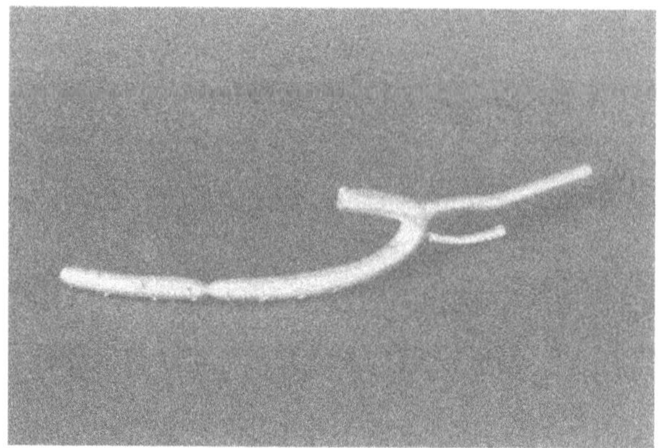

Fig. 1. Cast of the dog aorta

gap between the wax cast and the second plaster of Paris form. Figure 1 shows the cast of the dog aorta. Figure 2 shows an enlarged area which has a 71% constriction of the aorta. The whole silicone rubber model with the aortic arch and the constriction is shown in Figure 3. It has a diameter of 10 mm and a wall thickness of 1 mm. This resulted in elasticity of E = 1.1 × 10^6 dynes/cm^2 and provided for distensibility and wall motion that were a reasonable approximation of those of the dog aorta. The fluid used in the laser Doppler anemometer (LDA) studies was a glycerol-water solution with a dynamic viscosity of η = 8.5 cP. This viscosity is higher than that of blood; however, it was necessary to use it in order to achieve the same refractive index for the fluid as the wall of the silicone rubber model had. The refractive index of the silicone rubber model is n = 1.413. The entire model was embedded in the same fluid so that the path of the laser beam would not be deflected. A non-Newtonian fluid that was a mixture of AP 30 (0.05%) and AP 45 (0.04%) with MgCl$_2$ (0.01%) and 4% isopropanol was mixed together in a ratio of 3:1. Magnesium chloride and isopropanol stabilized the mixture of the polyacrylamide solution. The complex viscosity was determined with a Haake rotating viscosimeter of the Couette type. Blood shows thixotropic viscoelastic behavior, thus, we have used a polyacrylamide mixture to simulate human blood. Human blood cannot be used in models with those diameters because the laser light will be absorbed by the red cells. It is only possible to measure the velocity by using human blood in tubes up to a diameter of 0.5 mm. This non-Newtonian polyacrylamide mixture shows over a wide shear rate range nearly the same viscosity as human blood with a hematocrit of 45%. The viscous component for this fluid corresponds to that for blood, whereas the elastic component is a little higher. The representative viscosity was calculated[7] using the measured viscosity curvature.

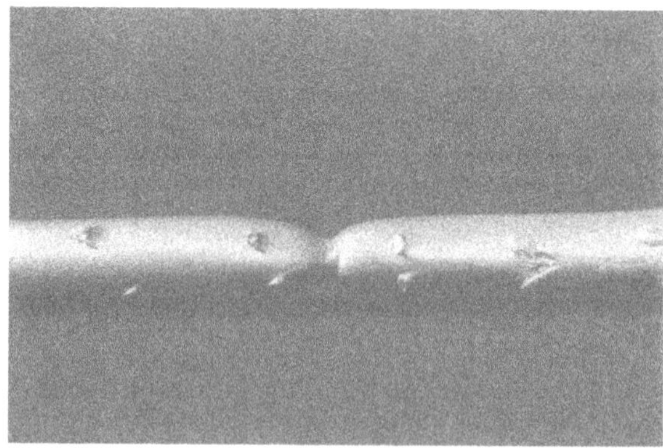

Fig. 2. Constriction of the aorta

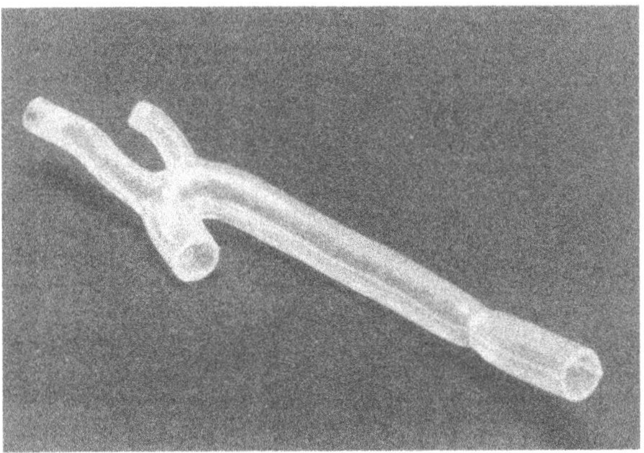

Fig. 3. Silicone rubber model

LASER DOPPLER VELOCITY MEASUREMENTS

Velocity measurements were carried out using a laser-Doppler-anemometer perpendicular to the center line. The laser-Doppler-anemometer has been described in detail several times[8,11]. A one-component laser-Doppler-anemometer with a 5 mW He-Ne laser was used to measure the local flow velocities in the axial direction. These measurements were carried out using the forward scattering method. The direction of the flow velocity was determined by producing a frequency shift between two beams by means of acoustic-optic modulation using two Bragg cells. The laser anemometer was mounted on an X-Y table. By shifting the anemometer perpendicular to the center line of the model, a complete velocity profile covering the entire diameter or lumen of the model vessel was obtained. These velocity profiles were plotted on line to provide a continuous representation of the variation of velocity with position across the lumen of the model vessel. The average velocity and the RMS velocity fluctuations, over several periods at one measurement point and at a constant phase angle, were obtained and recorded on a magnetic tape. Flow studies were carried out with a Newtonian and non-Newtonian blood-like fluid with a Reynolds number Re = 450 proximal to the stenosis. The mean pressure was 100 mm Hg, the mean pressure gradient was 1480 Pa/m, and the superimposed sinusoidal oscillation had an amplitude of ± 20 mm Hg with a pressure amplitude drop of 1950 Pa/m for the pulsatile flow studies. The frequency used for these studies was 1.23 Hz; the Womersley parameter was $\alpha = 6.5$. Starting with the center-point, 3 points in each direction towards the vessel wall were selected as measuring points.

The velocity gradients near the wall were determined from the velocity measurements for steady flow and the shear stress calculated.

RESULTS AND DISCUSSION

Figure 4 shows the viscosity over shear rate for an aqueous polyacrylamide mixture (0.05% Separan AP 30 and 0.04% Separan AP 45 in a rate of 3:1 and added 0.01% magnesium chloride and 4% isopropanol) compared to human blood with a hematocrit of 45%. No difference could be seen over a wide shear rate range between this mixture and human blood. This mixture also shows a thixotropic flow behavior similar to blood.

Figure 5 shows the velocity profiles for steady flow of the glycerol water solution and the non-Newtonian polyacrylamide mixture in the model with a stenosis. The dotted line shows the Newtonian fluid and the solid line shows the non-Newtonian velocity distribution. The presence of a stenosis in an artery alters the flow locally and distally. The velocity in the stenosed area increases and the pressure decreases. Distal to the stenosis, flow separation from the wall and the recirculation zone is found at a Reynolds number Re = 450. Although there are some differences between the Newtonian and non-Newtonian velocity profiles, these fluids create flow separation distal to the stenosis. The separation zones and the location of the reattachment points depend on the shape of the stenosis and the proximal Reynolds number.

Proximal to the stenosis, the flat profile of the non-Newtonian fluid can be seen. Distal

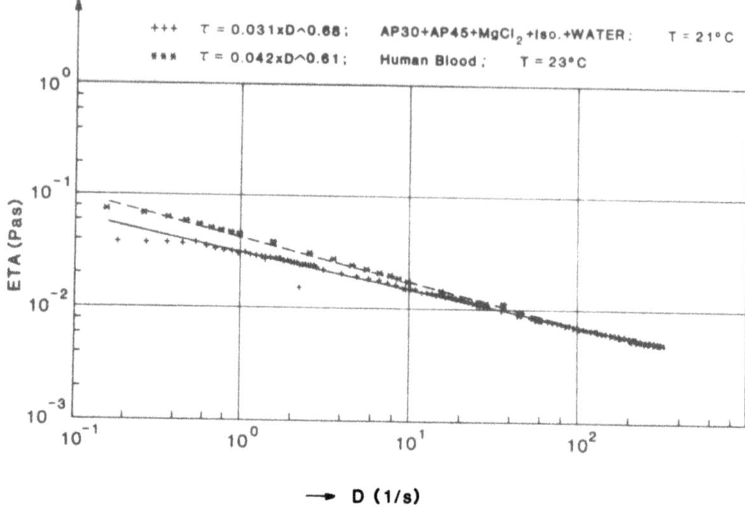

Fig. 4. Viscosity versus shear rate for a polyacrylamide mixture (AP 30 0.05%
and AP 45 0.04% + 4% isopropanol + 0.01% MgCl$_2$ and human blood at 21°C
and 23°C, respectively.

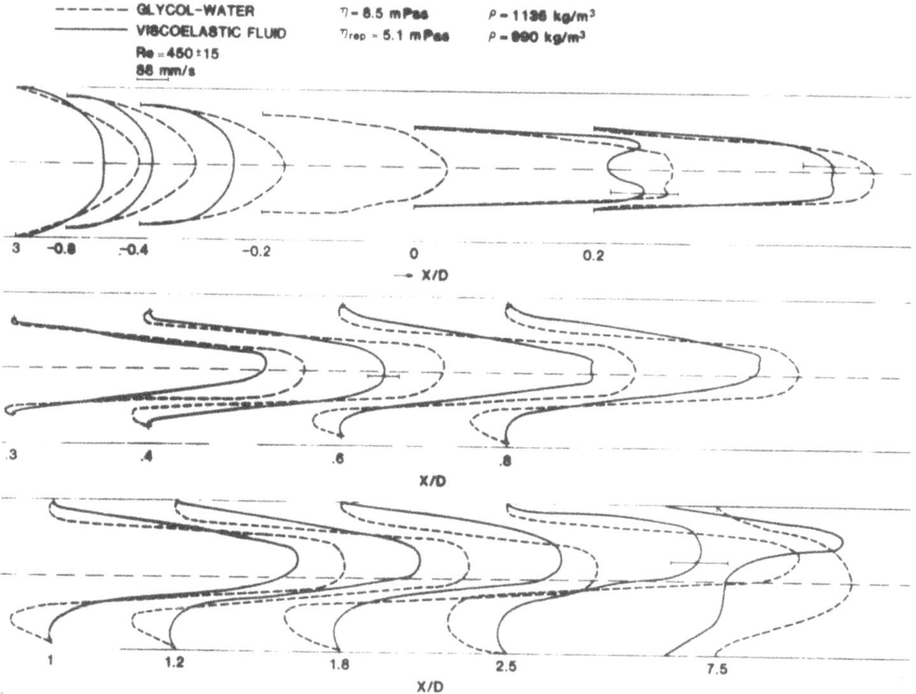

Fig. 5. Velocity profiles for steady flow of a Newtonian and non-Newtonian fluid through the model
with a stenosis X/D = distance proximal and distal to the stenosed area as a ratio of diameter of
an unstenosed vessel.

to the stenosis some smaller differences can be observed between the Newtonian and non-Newtonian fluid, but on the whole, flow behavior is similar.

Micrographs of endothelial cell patterns show that the cells are smaller and more elongated in the throat. In the region immediately distal to the stenosis, the endothelial cells are larger and have a rounder appearance.[11]

The results for the pulsatile flow of a Newtonian fluid were already reported.[11] Figure 6 shows the results for a non-Newtonian fluid at pulsatile flow as a function of the phase angle. The different velocity profiles throughout the model stenosis are shown for selected positions both proximal and distal to the stenosis. The Womersely parameter was 6.5 and the frequency was 1.23 Hz.

Levesque and Nerem calculated the shape index which is the surface of the cell divided by the gradient of the perimeter of the cell. They showed that the value of the shape index decreases rapidly in the convergent part of the stenosis. At the very point of the constriction, an extreme increase of this value can be seen. Distal to the constriction in the divergent part, the values decrease rapidly. Further downstream the values reach the same level they had upstream. We have calculated the shear stresses close to the wall from the steady flow of the Newtonian and non-Newtonian velocity profiles and used the inverse shape index to compare our measurements with the elongation and the shape index of the endothelial cells. Figure 7 shows the inverse shape index verses the position through the model stenosis X/D which means the distance proximal and distal to the stenosed area ratio to the diameter of the unstenosed vessel and the shear stress τ_w/τ_0. For the calculation of wall shear stress, the measured velocity profiles of the Newtonian and non-Newtonian fluid of Figure 5 were used. Figure 8 shows the correlation of the inverse shape index of endothelial cells over the calculated mean wall shear stress obtained from the steady profiles of the Newtonian (Figure 8a) and non-Newtonian (Figure 8b) velocity measurements for steady flow. The endothelial cells distal to the stenosis, are larger and rounder in the area where flow separation was found. At low shear stresses less than 1 Pa, the cells are rounded. The change of the shear stress of only 1 Pa is high enough to elongate the cells. Further results and discussions are given by Levesque et al.[11]

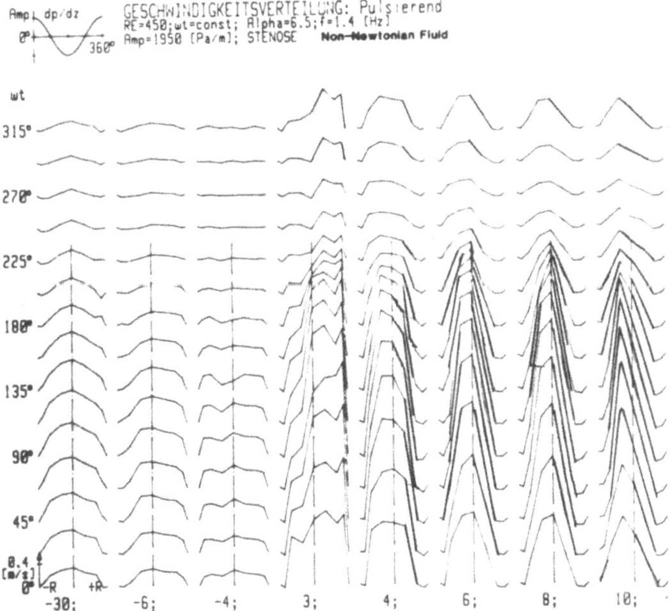

Fig. 6. Velocity profiles for pulsatile flow of the non-Newtonian fluid through the model stenosis at several positions proximal and distal to the stenosis. Upper left corner shows the pressure drop of the sinusoidal pressure. The Womersley parameter was $\alpha = 6.5$ and the frequency $f = 1.23$ Hz.

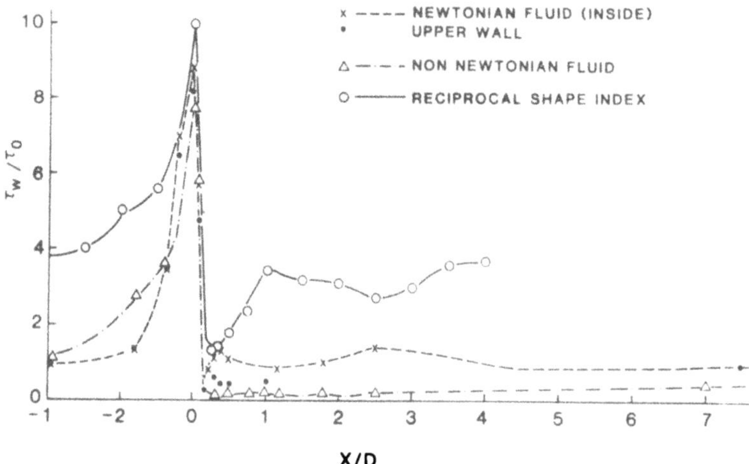

Fig. 7. Inverse shape index of endothelial cells and calculated wall shear stress versus position in a model stenosis. The wall shear stress is calculated from the Newtonian and non-Newtonian velocity profiles of Figure 5. X/D = distance proximal and distal to the stenosed area rationed to the diameter of the unstenosed vessel.

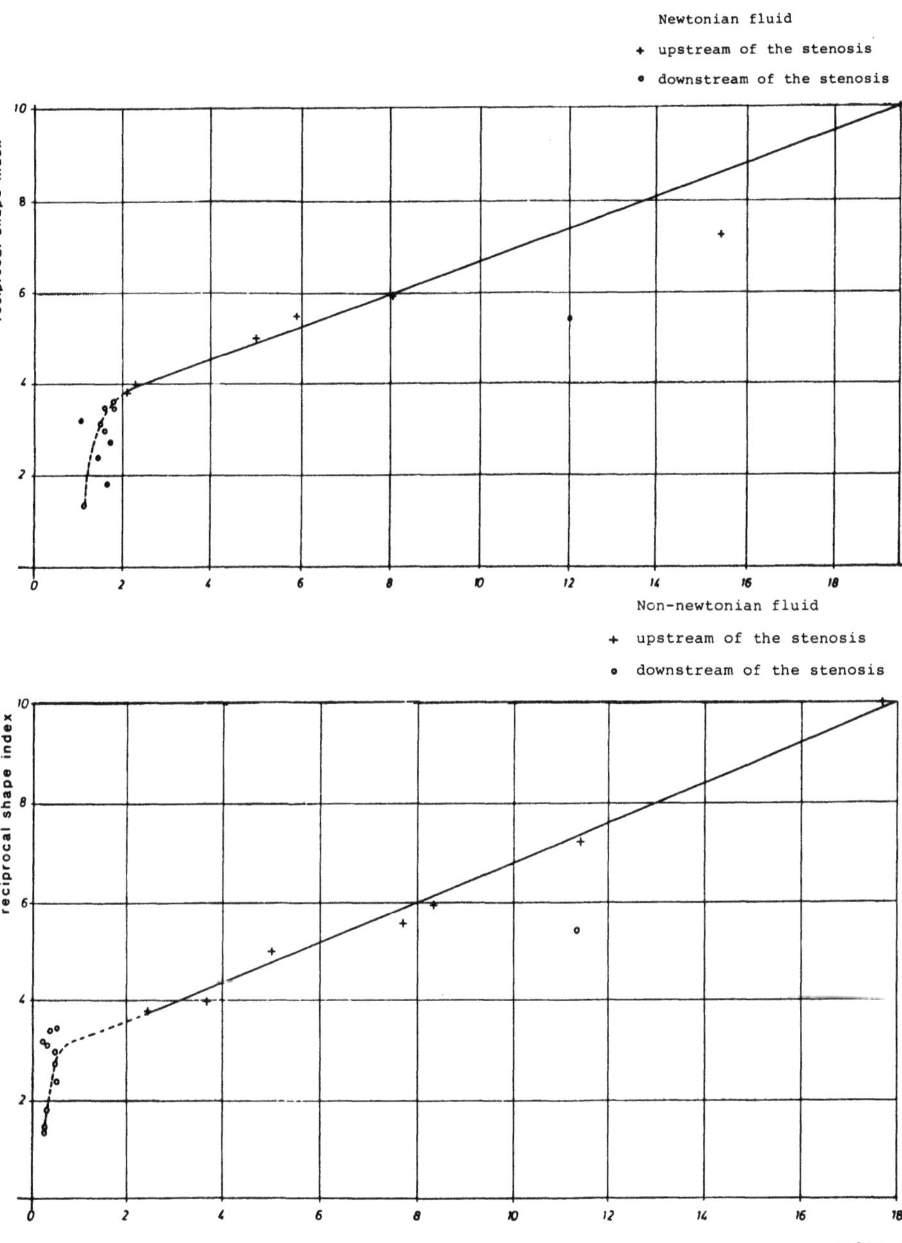

Fig. 8a,b Correlation of the inverse shape index of endothelial cells with the calculated mean wall shear stress obtained from the steady velocity profiles of the Newtonian (a) and non-Newtonian (b) fluid.

49

SUMMARY

Laser-Doppler-velocity measurements were carried out in an elastic 1:1 true-to-scale silicone rubber model of a dog aorta with stenosis. The model was constructed from a cast of a severely stenosed dog aorta (71% of its area). The stenosis in the dog aorta was prepared by wrapping a cotton band around the aorta. This band was tightened until the presence of a thrill or a bruit was felt distal to the band. Twelve weeks later the animal was sacrificed and a cast was prepared from the aorta. From this vascular cast, the cross-sectional area was calculated. Endothelial cell geometry and orientation was studied using computerized analysis to determine the cell area and shape index. An elastic silicone rubber model was prepared from the cast to measure the velocity profiles and to estimate the local wall shear stress. Velocity measurements were done at steady and pulsatile flow using a Newtonian aqueous-glycerol solution and a non-Newtonian blood-like fluid. From those velocity measurements the velocity gradients near the wall were determined and the shear stress calculated. The flow distal to the stenosis separates from the wall at physiological conditions. The endothelial cells are smaller and more elongated in the throat; distal to the stenosis they are larger and rounder. The shape index distribution along the stenosed aorta is correlated with the level of wall shear stress. It is shown that even low changes in the wall shear stress have an influence on the orientation of the endothelial cells.

REFERENCES

1. R.M. Nerem and M.J. Levesque, The case for fluid dynamics as a localizing factor for atherogenesis, *In*: Fluid Dynamics as a Localizing Factor for Atherosclerosis. G. Schettler, R.M. Nerem, H. Schmid-Schonbein, H. Morl, C. Diehm eds., Berlin: Springer-Verlag (1983).
2. M.H. Friedman, O.J. Deters, F.F. Mark, C.B. Bargeron and G.M. Hutchins, Arterial geometry affects hemodynamics - a potential risk factor for atherosclerosis, *Atherosclerosis* **46**:225 (1983).
3. C.M. Rodkiewicz, Arteries and arterial blood flow. Biological and physiologic aspects. CISM Courses and Lectures No. 270 Wien: Springer (1981).
4. D.N. Ku and D.P. Giddens, Pulsatile flow in a model carotid bifuration, *Atherosclerosis* **3**:37 (1983).
5. D.W. Liepsch and St. Moravec, Pulsatile flow in distensible models of human arteries, *Biorheology* **21**:571 (1984).
6. P. Stein, A physical and physiological basis for the interpretation of cardiac ausculation. New York, Futura Publishing Co. (1981).
7. D.W. Liepsch, Flow in tubes and arteries - a comparison, *Biorheology* **23**:395 (1986).
8. D.W. Liepsch, Stromungsuntersuchungen an Modellen menschlicher Blutgefaess-systeme. VDI - Fortschrittberichte Reihe 7: Stromungstechnik, Dusseldorf, VDI - Verlag. Nr. 113 (1986).
9. P.F. Davis, A. Remuzzi, E.J. Gordon, C.F. Dewey and M.A. Gimbroune, Turbulent fluid shear stess induces vascular endothelial cell turnover in vitro, *Proc. Natl. Acad. Sci.* **83**:2114 (1986).
10. M.J. Levesque, J.F. Cornhill and R.M. Nerem, Vascular casting: a new method for the study of the arterial endothelium, *Atherosclerosis* **34**:457 (1979).
11. M.J. Levesque, D.W. Liepsch, St. Moravec and N.M. Nerem, Correlation of endothelial cell shape and wall shear stress in a stenosed dog aorta, *Atherosclerosis* **6**:220 (1986).

ROLE OF HEMODYNAMIC FACTORS IN ATHEROGENESIS

Takeshi Karino, Toshihisa Asakura and Shoji Mabuchi

McGill University Medical Clinic
Montreal General Hospital
Montreal, Quebec, Canada H3G 1A4

INTRODUCTION

Clinical and postmortem studies indicate that atherosclerotic lesions on the vessel wall develop not randomly, and not everywhere in the circulation, but at particular localized sites in the arterial tree such as bifurcations, T-junctions, and curved segments of arteries where the blood flow is disturbed and formation of eddies is likely to occur. Thus, to elucidate the possible connection between blood flow and the localized genesis and development of atherosclerosis, a considerable amount of work has been carried out in recent years.[1,2] Theoretically, through the development of computational techniques, it has now become possible to simulate the blood flow through various channels, but the analysis is still limited to only those vessels having over-simplified geometries. Experimentally, due to the difficulties in visualizing the detailed flow patterns *in vivo*, most of the flow studies have been conducted *in vitro* using various models of arteries[3-5] and arterial molds.[6-8] However, even with the high quality casting and molding techniques available today, it is still not easy to precisely duplicate the complex geometry of the vessel lumen encountered in various regions of the circulation.

To solve the problem, we recently developed a new method to prepare isolated transparent natural blood vessels from animals and humans postmortem.[9] This has, for the first time, enabled us to simultaneously study the exact locations and sizes of atherosclerotic plaques and wall thickenings, and the detailed characteristics of the flow prevailing at such sites by directly observing and photographing the behavior of suspended tracer particles and hardened blood cells flowing through the transparent natural arteries and veins. Using the above method, we have previously studied the detailed flow patterns through venous valves in dog saphenous veins[10] and at the carotid artery bifurcation in man[11] because of the high incidence of thrombogenesis and atherogenesis at these respective sites. The study has since been extended to the major arteries of the cardio- and cerebrovascular systems.

In this paper, we summarize our latest findings on the detailed flow patterns and the exact sites of atherosclerosis observed in major arteries of the human coronary and intracranial cerebral circulations.

MATERIALS AND METHODS

Preparation of Transparent Arterial Segments

Isolated transparent segments of human coronary arterial trees and intracranial cerebral arterial networks containing the whole or parts of the circle of Willis were prepared as follows by a modification of the method described by Karino and Motomiya.[9]

Coronary arterial trees. The human hearts were obtained at autopsy from subjects in whom the major cause of death was not coronary artery disease. The aorta was cut at about 5-7 cm downstream of the aortic valve and cannulated with a 10 cm long plastic cylinder having a diameter approximately the same as the inner diameter of the aorta to provide an inlet to the coronary arteries. The aortic valve was sealed by inserting a tightly fitting plastic disk into the aorta proximal and adjacent to the valve cusps and tying the surrounding aortic tissues over it. The end of the plastic cylinder was connected to a head tank via flexible plastic tubing. The aorta and the coronary arteries were perfused with isotonic saline to wash out the blood. The left and right coronary arteries and their major branches having diameters greater than 1.5 mm were exposed and separated from the heart to the point of cannulation by dissecting the heart muscles and removing the surrounding tissues. After cannulating all the major branches with blunt syringe needles, and ligating or coagulating all the microvessels, the aorta and the coronary arteries were firmly fixed onto a 3-dimensional stainless steel frame to maintain the original geometrical configuration of the heart and the arteries. The arterial tree, still attached to the heart, was then fixed by perfusing it with a mixture of 2% glutaraldehyde and 4% formaldehyde in isotonic saline at the physiological mean perfusion pressure of $\sim$ 100 mm Hg, and at the same time, immersing it in the same fixing solution. The arterial tree, together with the aorta, was then isolated from the heart, dehydrated with ethanol and suspended in oil of wintergreen containing 5% ethanol to render the vessel transparent. Special care was taken to maintain the geometrical configurations (orientations, curvatures, lengths and diameters) as closely as possible to the *in vivo* diastolic conditions by perfusing the arteries at the physiological transmural pressure and supporting the arterial tree in a 3-dimensional frame throughout the entire process of preparation. Finally, the whole arterial tree, mounted on a supporting frame, was installed in a transparent glass chamber filled with oil of wintergreen containing 5% ethanol.

Circle of Willis. The human brain was obtained at autopsy from subjects in whom the major cause of death was not a cerebrovascular episode. After cannulating the branches of the arterial network of the circle of Willis, the whole network was firmly fixed onto a 3-dimensional supporting frame, perfused with isotonic saline to wash out the blood cells and fixed under the mean physiological pressure. The whole network was then isolated from the brain, dehydrated and rendered transparent. Finally, it was installed in a transparent glass chamber filled with oil of wintergreen containing 5% ethanol.

The transparent blood vessels prepared by the above method lose their elasticity during the process of fixing and rendering them transparent. However, this new method gives the following advantage; since the vessel walls are so well soaked in the suspending phase liquid (oil of wintergreen), they become transparent without any optical distortion even in the presence of atherosclerotic thickening of the vessel wall. Thus, one can make observations and measurements of the flow in both normal and diseased vessels, and from any direction without the errors arising from optical distortions (due to the difference in the refractive index between the vessel wall and the suspending liquid) which are inevitable when glass models and plastic casts are used.

Experimental Procedure and Analysis

The transparent blood vessel, mounted on a supporting frame and suspended in oil of wintergreen (containing 5% ethanol) in a transparent glass chamber, was firmly installed on the vertically mounted stage of a microscope and was illuminated with either low intensity light from a tungsten filament lamp, or high intensity light from a 200 W d.c. mercury arc lamp with a filter to eliminate ultraviolet illumination. Steady and pulsatile flow was obtained using a head tank system in combination with an oscillatory flow pump. Suspensions of 15 to 150 μm diameter polystyrene microspheres (density: 1.06 g/cm³, the size depending on the vessel diameter) in oil of wintergreen containing 5% ethanol (density: 1.16 g/cm³, viscosity: 0.026 g/cm sec) were subjected to steady or pulsatile flow through the vessel. The behavior of individual suspended tracer microspheres flowing in a steady or pulsatile fashion through various regions of the transparent artery was observed through a zoom lens ($1 \times$ to $5 \times$) attached to a cine camera, and photographed on 16 mm cine films using a Hycam 16 mm camera at speeds from 500 to 3000 frames/sec. The developed films were subsequently projected onto a drafting table and the movements of individual tracer particles were analyzed frame by frame with the aid of a stop-motion 16 mm movie projector to obtain the detailed flow patterns and distributions of fluid velocity and shear rate (or shear stress).

RESULTS

In each of five human coronary arterial trees and more than twenty arterial networks of the human circle of Willis prepared and studied, atherosclerotic plaques and wall thickenings were found to be localized almost exclusively on the outer wall (hip) of one or both daughter vessels at major bifurcations and T-junctions, and along the inner wall of curved segments where wall shear stresses are expected to be low. Figures 1 and 2 illustrate some examples of such

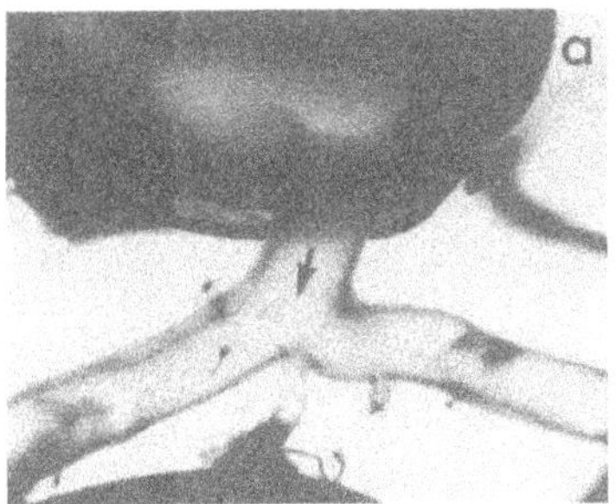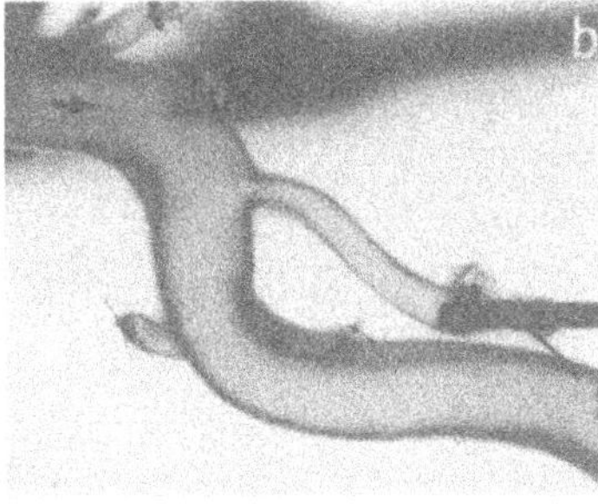

Fig. 1. Photographs of isolated transparent human coronary arteries taken from a 61 year old man, showing the exact location of atherosclerotic wall thickenings at (a) the branching site of the left main coronary artery, and (b) a curved segment in the right coronary artery.

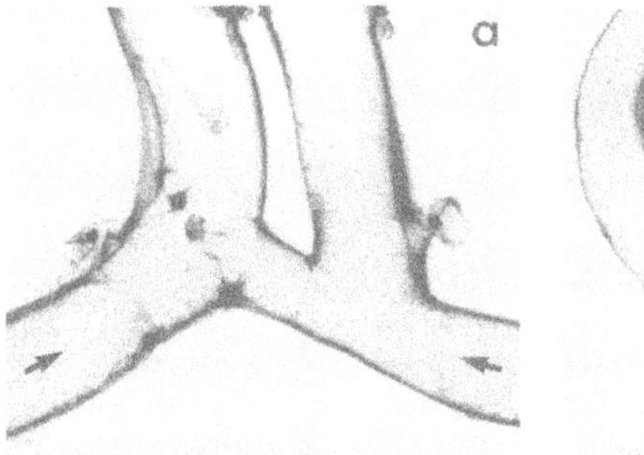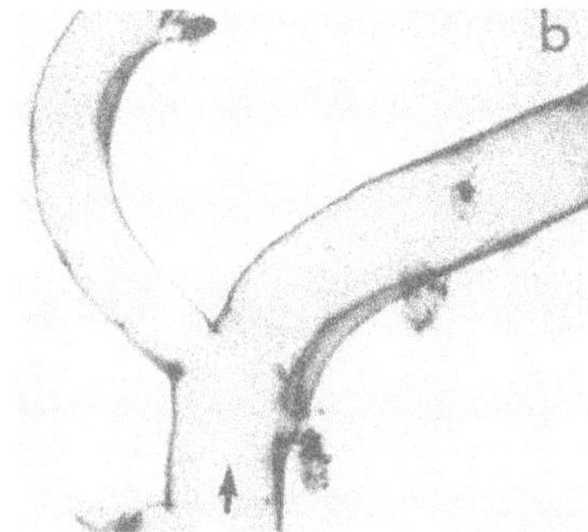

Fig. 2. Photographs of isolated transparent human cerebral arteries taken from an 83 year old man, showing the exact location of atherosclerotic wall thickenings at (a) the junction of the anterior communicating artery and the left and right anterior cerebral arteries, and (b) the first bifurcation of the middle cerebral artery.

case observed in the human coronary arteries and intracranial cerebral arteries respectively. Furthermore, when flow patterns were studied in detail in such vessels, it was discovered that both in steady and pulsatile flow, these sites were the very places where flow was either slow (low shear region) or disturbed and formation of secondary and recirculation flows were dominant. In no instance were atherosclerotic plaques and wall thickenings found in high shear regions such as downstream of flow dividers (inner walls) of bifurcations and T-junctions where the formation of initial atherosclerotic lesions has been reported in experimental animals fed high cholesterol diets.[12-14]

In the left main coronary artery (LMC), formation of a recirculation zone was observed in three vessels right at the entrance of the artery. In all three cases, eddies were formed along the lower wall due to a sudden change in flow direction at the sharp-angled lower leading edge of the main coronary artery which stemmed off the aortic sinus. Also in three cases the strong deflection of the main flow from the LMC at the flow divider of the left anterior descending branch (LAD) and the left circumflex branch (LCx) resulted in the formation of recirculation zones in one or both daughter vessels around the outer wall (hip) of the bifurcation at the very sites where atherosclerotic plaques and wall thickenings were localized. In the LAD, atherosclerotic lesions were found along the inner (lower) wall of the gently curved segment of the proximal portion of the LAD which overlay the myocardium where the fluid velocity and wall shear stress were relatively low compared to that at the outer wall. In the right coronary artery, as shown in Figure 3, most of the atherosclerotic lesions were confined to the curved segments along the inner wall where flow was either disturbed with formation of a recirculation zone or very slow. It was also noted that in both left and right coronary arteries, the frequency and degree of severity of atherosclerotic lesions tended to decrease with increasing distance

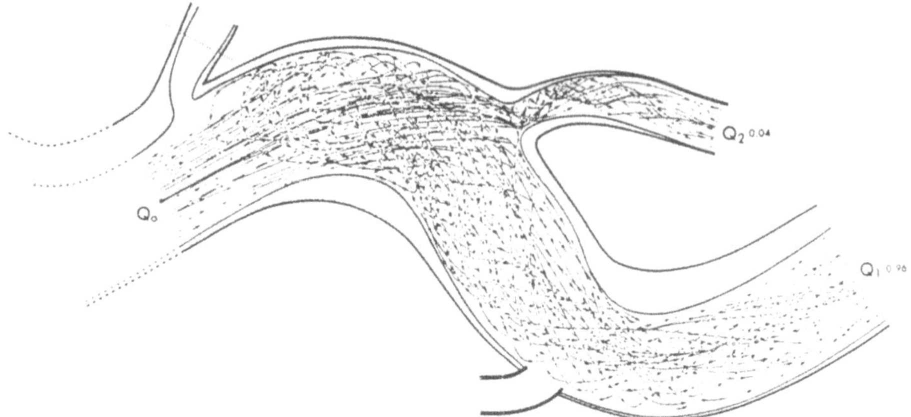

Fig. 3. Tracings of particle paths showing the formation of recirculation zones and secondary flows at a curved segment of the human right coronary artery (shown in Fig. 1) in steady flow at Re_o = 994, Q_o = 335 ml/min and U_o = 686 mm/sec. The solid lines are the paths of particles in or close to the common median plane, and the dashed lines are the paths which are far away from the common median plane (projection of the particle paths on the common median plane).

from the origin of each artery from the aortic sinus.

In intracranial cerebral arteries, the results revealed several important facts which suggested the direct involvement of local flow patterns in the localization of atherosclerosis.

It was found that in each of the five middle cerebral artery bifurcations studied, atherosclerotic thickening of the vessel wall was localized around the hips of the bifurcation. When the flow patterns were studied in detail in these vessels, it was discovered that a standing recirculation zone, very similar to that previously observed in the carotid artery bifurcation,[11] was formed along the outer wall of one or both daughter vessels (depending on the Reynolds number in the parent vessel and the flow ratios in the two daughter vessels) at the exact locations where the atherosclerotic thickening of the vessel wall occurred. Furthermore, under the normal physiological range of flow rates and flow ratios tested, there was an apparent positive correlation between the longitudinal length of the regions of disturbed flow and that of the atherosclerotic wall thickening. Figures 4 and 5 show the detailed flow patterns observed in steady flow in one of the bifurcations having an almost perfectly symmetric structure and spatial arrangement of the daughter vessels. As evident from Figure 4, even when the flow in the parent vessel was distributed equally to the two daughter vessels, the region of disturbed flow (formed along the outer walls of the bifurcation) was much longer in the right side branch where the region of atherosclerotic wall thickening was also longer than that in the left side branch where the wall thickening was confined to only a very narrow area. Furthermore, as illustrated in Figure 5, the size of the backflow region remained almost unchanged even when the flow rate in the left daughter vessel was reduced to 21% of the inflow rate in order to facilitate the formation of a large recirculation zone in that branch. The region of disturbed flow was still confined to a narrow area adjacent to the site of wall thickening, suggesting a strong correlation between the size of the regions of disturbed flow and that of the atherosclerotic lesions found at such sites. In pulsatile flow, the complex spiral secondary flows and the recirculation zones oscillated in phase with the pulsatile flow velocity, and the locations of the stagnation and separation points situated on the outer walls of the bifurcation moved back and forth along the vessel wall. However, the general flow patterns remained the same as those observed in steady flow. This was true for all five vessels studied. A similar observation was made at an arterial bend located further downstream from the middle cerebral artery bifurcation shown in Figure 2b. Here, a recirculation zone was formed along the inner wall of the bend slightly downstream from the apex at the very site of atherosclerotic wall thickening.

CONCLUSION

We have described our latest findings on the exact sites of atherosclerosis and detailed flow patterns existing in such regions in human coronary and intracranial cerebral arteries in

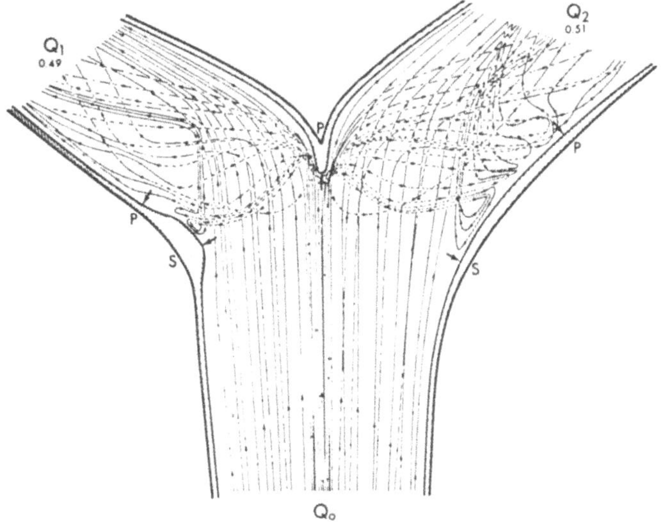

Fig. 4. Detailed flow patterns at the middle cerebral artery bifurcation taken from a 73 year old woman, showing the formation of secondary flows and recirculation zones along the outer walls of the bifurcation in steady flow at $Re_o = 452$, $Q_o = 147$ ml/min and $U_o = 325$ mm/sec. The arrows at S and P denote the respective locations of the separation and stagnation points.

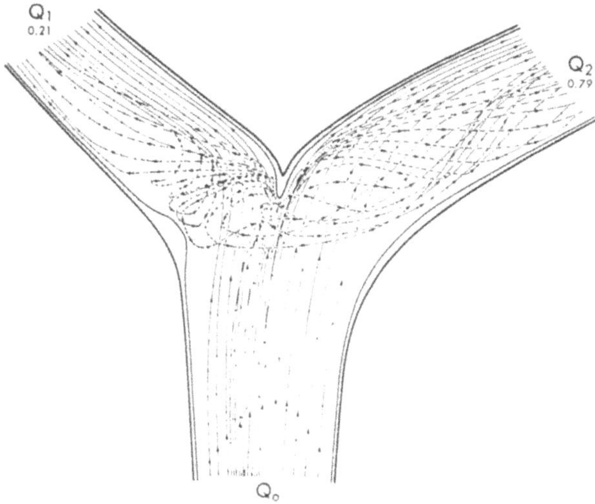

Fig. 5. Tracing of particle paths as in Fig. 4, showing changes in flow patterns when the flow rate in the left daughter vessel was reduced to 21% of the inflow rate in the parent vessel while maintaining the same Re_o and Q_o as in Figure 4.

relation to the localization of atherosclerosis in the human circulation. The results demonstrated convincingly that the flow separation and formation of secondary flows and standing recirculation zones, previously observed in various models of branching vessels,[15-17] do occur also in natural blood vessels in both steady and pulsatile flow. Furthermore, it was confirmed repeatedly that preferred sites for the formation of atherosclerotic plaques and wall thickenings were localized not at flow dividers (high shear region) as observed previously by several investigators in experimental animals by feeding them diets containing high levels of cholesterol,[12-14] but almost exclusively on the outer wall (hip) of one or both daughter vessels at major bifurcations and T-junctions and along the inner wall of curved segments where flow was either slow (low shear region) or disturbed with formation of secondary and recirculation flows. These results indicate that there is a strong correlation between the sites of flow disturbance and the preferred sites for the genesis and development of atherosclerosis in man. What is not clear at present is what factor or factors of disturbed flows are really responsible for atherogenesis. It is possible that in regions of disturbed flow where the translational velocity and wall shear stress are very low, platelets and lipids may have a greater opportunity to interact for longer periods with the vessel wall than elsewhere. This, in turn, may lead to and enhance the deposition of platelets, release of certain chemical agents such as the platelet-derived growth factor for smooth muscle cells, and the uptake of atherogenic lipoproteins by the endothelial cells located in such regions. It is also possible that since vascular endothelial cells are sensitive to flow and exhibit certain morphological changes corresponding to the direction and magnitude of the local shear stress, [18,19] being round shaped in regions of low shear and elongated in regions of high shear,[20,21] endothelial cells in different regions may have different metabolic functions. It is speculated that localization of atherosclerosis may have its origin in either or both of the above two mechanisms.

ACKNOWLEDGMENTS

This work was supported by Grant MT-7084 from the Medical Research Council of Canada, Grant HL-29502 from the National Heart, Lung and Blood Institute, N.I.H., U.S.A., and the Quebec Heart Foundation.

REFERENCES

1. H.L. Goldsmith and T. Karino, Mechanically induced thromboemboli, *in*: "Quantitative Cardiovascular Studies — Clinical and Research Applications of Engineering Principles," N.H.C. Hwang, D.R. Gross and D.J. Patel, eds., University Park Press, Baltimore, (1978).
2. G. Schettler, R. Nerem, H. Schmid-Schönbein, H. Mörl and C. Diehm, eds., "Fluid Dynamics as a Localizing Factor for Atherosclerosis," Springer-Verlag, Heidelberg (1983).
3. B.K. Bharadvaj, R.F. Mabon and D.P. Giddens, Steady flow in a model of the human carotid bifurcation, Part I — flow visualization, *J. Biomechanics* **15**:349 (1982).
4. T. Fukushima and T. Azuma, The horseshoe vortex: A secondary flow generated in arteries with stenosis, bifurcation and branchings, *Biorheology* **19**:143 (1982).
5. R. Rayman, R.G. Kratky and M.R. Roach, Steady flow visualization in a rigid canine aortic cast, *J. Biomechanics* **18**:863 (1985).
6. S. Moravec and D. Liepsch, Flow visualization in a model of a three-dimensional human artery with Newtonian and non-Newtonian fluids, Part I, *Biorheology* **20**:745 (1983).
7. O.J. Deters, F.F. Mark, C.B. Bargeron, M.H. Friedman and G.M. Hutchins, Comparison of steady and pulsatile flow near the ventral and dorsal walls of casts of human aortic bifurcations, *ASME J. Biomechanical Engineering* **106**:79 (1984).
8. F.J. Walburn, H.N. Sabbah and P.D. Stein, Flow visualization in a mold of an atherosclerotic human abdominal aorta, *ASME J. Biomechanical Engineering* **103**:168 (1981).
9. T. Karino and M. Motomiya, Flow visualization in isolated transparent natural blood vessels, *Biorheology* **20**:119 (1983).
10. T. Karino and M. Motomiya, Flow through a venous valve and its implication in thrombus formation, *Thrombosis Research* **36**:245 (1984).
11. M. Motomiya and T. Karino, Flow patterns in the human carotid artery bifurcation, *Stroke* **15**:50 (1984).
12. M.R. Roach, The effects of bifurcations and stenoses on arterial disease, *in*: "Cardiovascular Flow Dynamics and Measurements," N.H.C. Hwang and N.A. Normann, eds., University Park Press, Baltimore, pp. 489-539 (1977).
13. M.R. Roach, J.F. Cornhill and J. Fletcher, A quantitative study of the development of sudanophilic lesions in the aorta of rabbits fed a low-cholesterol diet for up to six months, *Atherosclerosis* **29**:259 (1978).
14. M.R. Roach, and J. Fletcher, Alterations in distribution of sudanophilic lesions in rabbits after cessation of a cholesterol-rich diet, *Atherosclerosis* **32**:1 (1979).
15. M.R. Roach, S. Scott and G.G. Ferguson, The homodynamic importance of the geometry of bifur-

cations in the Circle of Willis (glass model studies), *Stroke* **3**:255 (1972).

16. T. Karino, H.H.M. Kwong and H.L. Goldsmith, Particle flow behavior in models of branching vessels: I, vortices in 90° T-junctions, *Biorheology* **16**:231 (1979).

17. T. Karino and H.L. Goldsmith, Particle flow behavior in models of branching vessels: II, effects of branching angle and diameter ratio on flow patterns, *Biorheology* **22**:87 (1985).

18. J.T. Flaherty, J.E. Pierce, V.J. Ferrans, D.J. Patel, W.K. Tucker and D.L. Fry, Endothelial nuclear patterns in the canine arterial tree with particular reference to hemodynamic events, *Circ. Res.* **30**:23 (1972).

19. C.F. Dewey, S.R. Bussolari, M.A. Gimbrone and P.F. Davies, The dynamic response of vascular endothelial cells to fluid shear stress, *J. Biomech. Eng.* **103**:177 (1981).

20. M.A. Reidy and D.E. Bowyer, Scanning electron microscopy of arteries, *Atherosclerosis* **26**:181 (1977).

21. M.J. Levesque, D. Liepsch, S. Moravec and R.M. Nerem, Correlation of endothelial cell shape and wall shear stress in a stenosed dog aorta, *Atherosclerosis* **6**:220 (1986).

THE ROLE OF ARTERIAL ENDOTHELIAL CELL MITOSIS IN MACROMOLECULAR PERMEABILITY

Shu Chien*,**, Shing-Jong Lin*,**, Sheldon Weinbaum†, Mary M.L. Lee**
and Kung-Ming Jan*,**

*Institute of Biomedical Sciences
 Academia Sinica
 Taipei, Taiwan 11529, ROC
**Department of Physiology and Cellular Biophysics
 College of Physicians and Surgeons
 Columbia University
 New York, NY 10032, USA
†Department of Mechanical Engineering
 City College of the City University of New York
 New York, NY 10031, USA

INTRODUCTION

Atherosclerosis is characterized by focal areas of lipid accumulation and intimal smooth muscle cell proliferation. Atherosclerotic lesions tend to develop in preferential areas in the aortic tree,[1] where transendothelial macromolecular permeability is high as indicated by an enhanced uptake of the protein-binding azo dye Evans Blue in vivo.[2-4] These so-called blue areas have been shown to be associated with an increased rate of endothelial cell turnover[3,5] and an enhanced permeability to low density lipoproteins (LDL).[6] The subendothelial accumulation of unesterified cholesterol has been hypothesized to be an initial event in atherogenesis.[7] The mechanism by which macromolecules such as LDL or albumin enter the arterial wall, however, is still not completely understood.

Endothelial cell injury has been suggested to be responsible for the enhanced endothelial permeability in atherogenesis,[8] but extensive morphologic studies have failed to reveal overt endothelial denudation in normal, hyperlipidemic or endotoxin-treated animals.[9-11] Electron microscopic studies also showed that isolated dying endothelial cells are gradually sloughed off from below by the migration of neighboring healthy endothelial cells without a detectable denudation. The absence of overt endothelial denudation in vivo suggests that some functional change of endothelial cells, rather than their denuding injury, might account for the locally enhanced permeability.

A local increase in macromolecular permeability has been found in areas where endothelial cells have an accelerated turnover as indicated by a higher fraction of endothelial cells with ³H-thymidine uptake.[3] However, experiments that were conducted as a prelude to the present investigation have shown that the cells with ³H-thymidine incorporation are often not the cells with increasing permeability. This lack of correlation suggests that the permeability change might occur in a narrow time window of the cell cycle, rather than the whole cycle of ³H-thymidine labeling.

Although it has been suggested that endothelial cell mitosis following mechanical trauma to veins may account for the increased permeability of growing microvessels,[12] there is still no direct evidence linking the endothelial cell mitosis to permeability. As a result of our recent theoretical studies,[13] the hypothesis has been formulated that an increase in permeability around endothelial cells undergoing mitosis is responsible for the local enhanced transport of macromolecules into the artery wall. Exploration of the quantitative feasibility of this hypothesis using the theoretical model has demonstrated that a small population of endothelial cells corresponding to physiologically observable cell turnover rates could lead to a near doubling of the steady state macromolecular permeability in the larger arteries. The model predicted that these open junctions need only to occupy less than one part in 10^5 of the endothelial surface for the observed enhancement in permeability to occur.

Recently we have developed a more refined model[14,15] which could also predict the time-dependent spread of the tracer in the subendothelial space and the role of the elastic lamina in determining the rapid lateral diffusion in the intima. The results presented in this communication were obtained from experimental studies[16] designed to specifically test the hypothesis that the endothelial cells undergoing mitosis are the ones with enhanced permeability, and these results have been subjected to theoretical analysis using our new time-dependent model.[14,15] The close correlation between endothelial cell mitosis and enhanced permeability found in this study provides direct experimental evidence in support of the hypothesis, and the results may have significant implications in atherogenesis.

MATERIALS AND METHODS

Preparation of Evans Blue-Albumin Conjugate

The Evans Blue-Albumin (EBA) conjugates were prepared by adding 140 mg Evans Blue (EB) to 10 ml of a solution of 100 mg/ml bovine serum albumin (BSA) in 0.85% NaCl. The EBA solution was purified by passing through a Sephadex G-25M column using 0.85% NaCl as an elutant with a final volume of 20 ml.

Animal Experiments

Twelve male Wistar rats weighing approximately 500 gm were used. The experiments were performed under pentobarbital anesthesia (30 mg/kg i.p.). The right femoral artery and the left femoral vein were cannulated with 22G needle catheters. EBA (1.5 ml) was injected into the left femoral vein. Approximately 4 min later, 1,000 international units of heparin was injected intravenously, the chest was opened quickly and the heart was exposed. At 5 min after EBA injection, the rat was sacrificed with an overdose of pentobarbital injected intravenously; at the same time, a 22G needle catheter was placed in the left ventricle via a cardiac puncture and connected to a pressure reservoir set at a physiological pressure of 100 mmHg. The catheter placed in the right femoral artery was used as an egress route for perfusion. A buffered saline solution was perfused first via the left ventricular needle catheter at 100 mmHg pressure until the emergence of clear fluid from the egress site (approximately 10 sec). The perfusate was then switched to a fixative solution. For fluorescence microscopy, a 10% formaldehyde solution was perfused for 10 min. This was followed by an 1-min perfusion with $AgNO_3$ by a method modified from that of Zand et al.[17] in order to stain endothelial cell borders in the rat aorta. Briefly, the 10 min of perfusion fixation with 10% formaldehyde was followed by a 3-min perfusion with 5% glucose solution, an 1-min perfusion with 0.088% $AgNO_3$, another 3-min perfusion with 5% glucose solution, and an 1-min perfusion with bromides (an equal mixture of 1% NH_4Br and 3% CoBr). Finally, the perfusate was switched back to 10% formaldehyde for another 10 min.

Fluorescence Microscopy

After perfusion fixation, the aorta was excised between the aortic root and the diaphragm. The cane-shaped specimen was immersed in 10% formaldehyde overnight. The thoracic aorta was then excised, cut open longitudinally and pinned onto a dental plate with the endothelial surface facing up. The specimens were stained with Harris' hematoxylin. The adventitial tissue was carefully removed and the specimen was mounted wet onto a glass slide, coverslipped, and then viewed under a Nikon fluorescence microscope. Evans Blue fluorescence was studied with an excitation filter at 450-490 nm, a dichroic mirror at 510 nm and a barrier filter at 520 nm, or alternatively, with an excitation filter at 510-516 nm, a dichroic mirror at 580 nm and a barrier filter at 590 nm. The fluorescence intensity in the vessel wall was scanned with the aid of a video-digitizer (EyeCom II) attached to a minicomputer (PDP 11/23), a method which has been developed in our laboratory and applied to studies on the mapping of Evans Blue dye distribution in the arterial wall.

RESULTS

Aortic segments stained with hematoxylin were examined with the fluorescence microscope. The total endothelial surface of each aortic segment was systematically scanned. The number of endothelial cells scanned was determined by dividing the endothelial surface area of each aortic segment by the average surface area of a single endothelial cell, which had been determined to be 520 μm^2. Table I shows the association of EBA permeability with mitotic and non-mitotic endothelial cells in the aorta of twelve rats. The average number of endothelial cells scanned in each rat was 2.94 $\times$ 10^5. Of these large number of endothelial cells scanned, only an average of 41 dividing cells were found per rat. Although mitosis was rarely found in these aortic endothelial cells, nearly all (98.9%) of the mitotic cells were leaky to EBA. In contrast, only 0.03% of the non-mitotic cells were leaky. All phases of endothelial cell mitosis were found to be associated with EBA leaky spots. As shown in Table II, the largest percentage of dividing cells (33.9%) was found in the telophase (and immediately after cleavage).

Figure 1 shows the photomicrograph of a specimen of aortic endothelium with cell boundaries outlined by $AgNO_3$ and cell nuclei identified by hematoxylin. No mitotic figure or EBA leaky spot was found in this area. Association of EBA leaky spots with endothelial cell mitosis is shown for the anaphase (Figs. 2 and 3); similar results were obtained in metaphase, telophase, and immediately after cleavage. The EBA leaky spot was usually larger than the size of one endothelial cell, with a dividing cell located approximately at the center of the spot. Stomata and stigmata were usually found at the equator or along the cell boundary during all phases of endothelial cell mitosis.

The fluorescence intensity of the EBA leaky spots was determined with the aid of the EyeCom II video-digitizer. Figure 4 shows the results of scanning of the fluorescence micrograph of Fig. 2 along the long axis of the dividing cell. The fluorescence intensity shows two peaks at both ends of the cell. The video-digitizer was also used to outline the iso-intensity lines of fluorescence surrounding the dividing endothelial cells at five different intensity levels. As shown in Figs. 5 and 6, which correspond to the pictures in Figs. 2 and 3, respectively, the dividing endothelial cells are located in the center of the iso-intensity profiles. The center of these fluorescence profiles is found to be around the equator of the dividing cell. It seems that EBA leaked initially from the boundaries of the dividing cell, most likely from the site of cleavage, and then spread laterally in the subendothelial space.

Table 1. The association of Evans Blue-albumin (EBA) permeability with mitotic and non-mitotic endothelial cells in aortae of twelve rats (From him et al.[16])

Rat No.	No. cells scanned	Mitotic cells			Non-mitotic cells		
		No. cells found	No. cells with EBA spot	% cells with EBA spot	No. cells found	No. cells with EBA spot	% cells with EBA spot
1	1.85×10^5	36	36	100%	1.85×10^5	28	0.0151%
2	1.97×10^5	50	50	100%	1.97×10^5	27	0.0137%
3	3.76×10^5	4	4	100%	3.76×10^5	48	0.0128%
4	2.20×10^5	26	26	100%	2.20×10^5	26	0.0118%
5	4.39×10^5	42	40	95%	4.39×10^5	51	0.0116%
6	2.31×10^5	26	26	100%	2.31×10^5	32	0.0139%
7	2.54×10^5	29	29	100%	2.54×10^5	187	0.0736%
8	3.34×10^5	89	89	100%	3.34×10^5	252	0.0754%
9	2.12×10^5	26	26	100%	2.12×10^5	146	0.0689%
10	3.37×10^5	54	54	100%	3.37×10^5	71	0.0211%
11	3.82×10^5	63	59	94%	3.82×10^5	92	0.0241%
12	3.61×10^5	43	42	98%	3.61×10^5	180	0.0499%
Mean	2.94×10^5	40.7	40.1	98.9%	2.94×10^5	95.0	0.0327%
S.D.	0.87×10^5	21.9	21.5	2.2%	0.87×10^5	77.2	0.0263%

Table 2. The phases of endothelial cell mitosis associated with Evans Blue-albumin (EBA) permeability

Rat No.	No. dividing cells with EBA spot	Prophase	Metaphase	Anaphase	Telophase
1	36	8	8	4	16
2	50	11	15	6	18
3	4	1	2	0	1
4	26	10	3	6	7
5	40	12	2	11	15
6	26	7	6	6	7
7	29	13	8	1	7
8	89	26	21	11	31
9	26	6	4	3	13
10	54	22	4	9	19
11	59	16	14	8	21
12	42	17	10	7	8
Total	481	149	97	72	163
% total	100%	31.0%	20.0%	15.0%	33.9%

From Lin et al.[16]

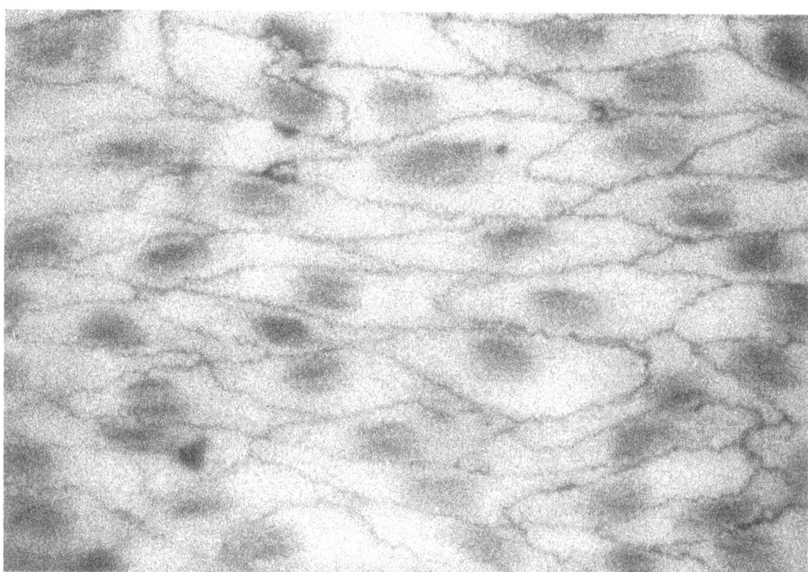

Fig. 1. Light micrograph of en face preparation of rat thoracic aorta showing normal aortic endothelium with cell boundaries outlined by silver nitrate and cell nuclei identified by Harris' hematoxylin. No mitosis or EBA leaky spot was found.

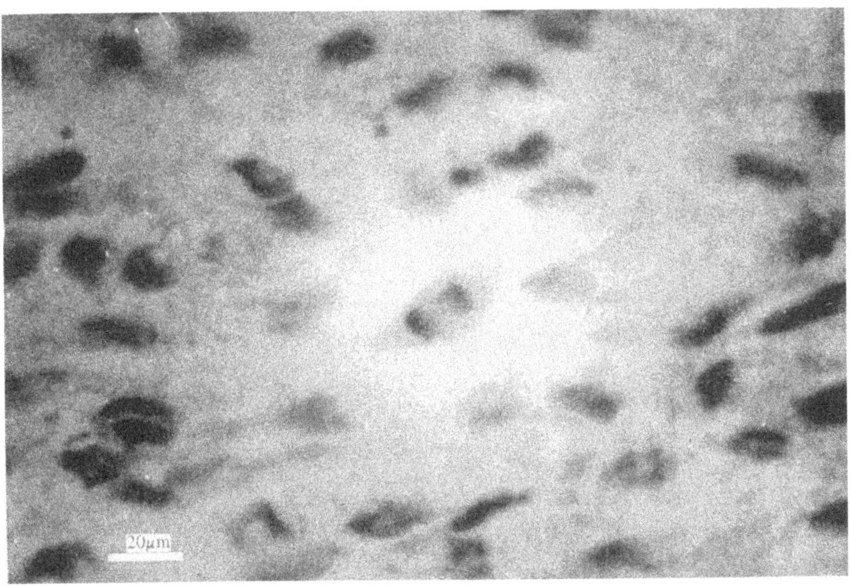

Fig. 2. A dividing endothelial cell in anaphase within an EBA leaky spot. En face preparation stained with hematoxylin.

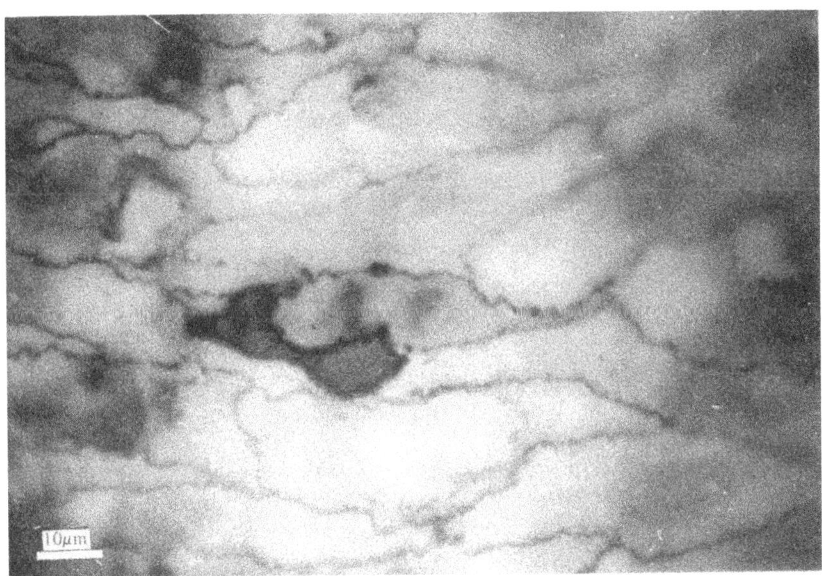

Fig. 3. A dividing endothelial cell in anaphase associated with an EBA leaky spot. Note the stigmata (arrowhead) on one side of the cell at the equator and a probable dead cell (arrow) attached to the side of the dividing cell. En face preparation. Silver nitrate and hematoxylin staining.

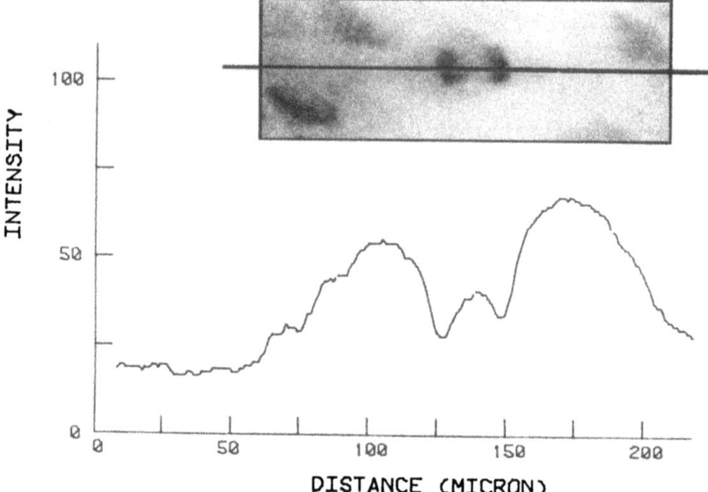

Fig. 4. Scanning of the fluorescence intensity of the EBA leaky spot in Fig. 2 along the long axis of the dividing endothelial cell with the EyeCom II video-digitizer. Note the two peaks of intensity at both ends of the cell. The intensity was suppressed by the cell itself and even more by the nuclear staining. The black line represents the scanning line.

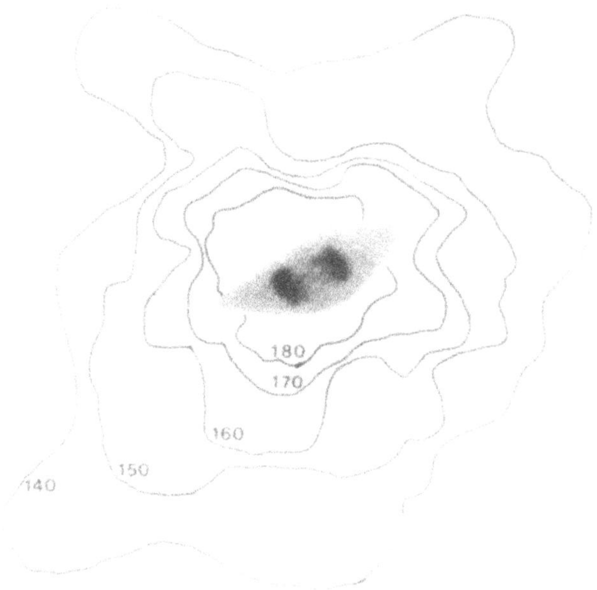

Fig. 5. Iso-intensity profile of fluorescence surrounding the dividing endothelial cell in Fig. 2, obtained by scanning with the video-digitizer at 5 different intensity levels. The values represent relative fluorescence intensities of Evans Blue. The center of the iso-intensity rings is located near the equator of the dividing cell.

64

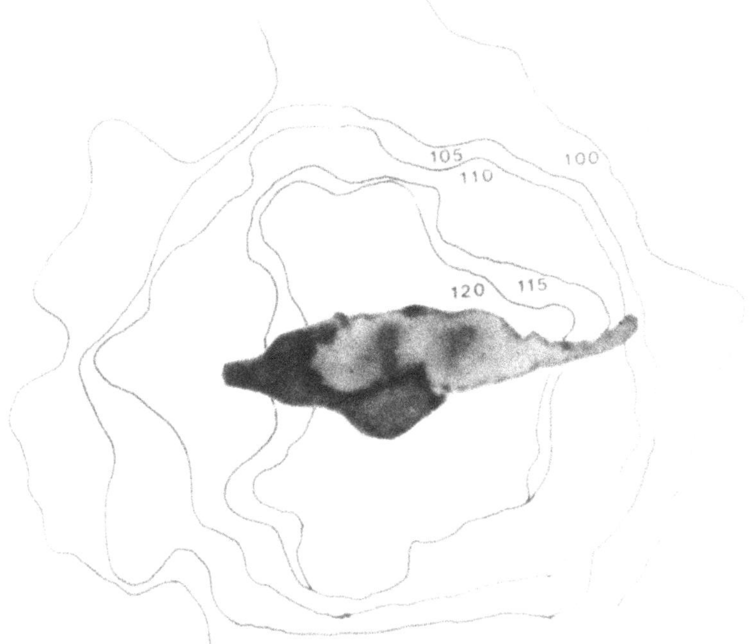

Fig. 6. Five different iso-intensity lines of fluorescence surrounding the dividing endothelial cell in Fig. 3, obtained by scanning with the video-digitizer. The center of the iso-intensity rings is located near the equator of the dividing cell.

Several experiments were performed in which horseradish peroxidase (HRP) was administered as the tracer macromolecule instead of EBA, and the aorta was perfusion-fixed with 2% glutaraldehyde and processed for electron microscopic examination. Figures 7A and 7B show the transmission electron micrographs taken from two thin sections of the same endothelial cell. The nuclear pattern of this cell indicates that it is undergoing mitosis. In Fig. 7B, the junction to the right of the dividing endothelial cell shows abnormal widening and is filled with the electron-dense HRP reaction product. Fig. 7C shows an enlargement of this leaky junction.

THEORETICAL ANALYSIS

Figure 8 shows a schematic drawing of our recently developed time-dependent theoretical model[14,15] which is briefly summarized below. In the model the artery wall is divided into periodic units. In the center of each unit there is a shaded cell (labeled "mitotic") with a transiently open junction at its border. This cell is assumed to be leaky during one or more phases, e.g. the M phase, of the cell cycle during cell turnover. Each cell with a transiently open junction is surrounded by a circle of radius $r = \xi$ composed of healthy cells with normal junctions which allow the passage of water and smaller solutes through dispersed small slits with 4 nm gap heights.[18]

The time-dependent model shown in Fig. 8 contains two important refinements that were not present in the steady-state prototype model we first proposed.[13] First, it is assumed that junctions open and close gradually with time and that the fraction of the cell cycle length (value of ϕ) during cell turnover which permits the passage of a given molecule varies inversely with molecular diameter. This is accounted for in the refined model by introducing a diffusion coefficient D_j which controls the passage of the tracer molecule through the open cleft as shown in the insert of Fig. 8. Second, instead of treating the subendothelial tissue as being isotropic, two coefficients D_r and D_z are introduced to describe the diffusion in the subendothelial tissue in the directions parallel and perpendicular to the endothelial surface, respectively. Ultrastruc-

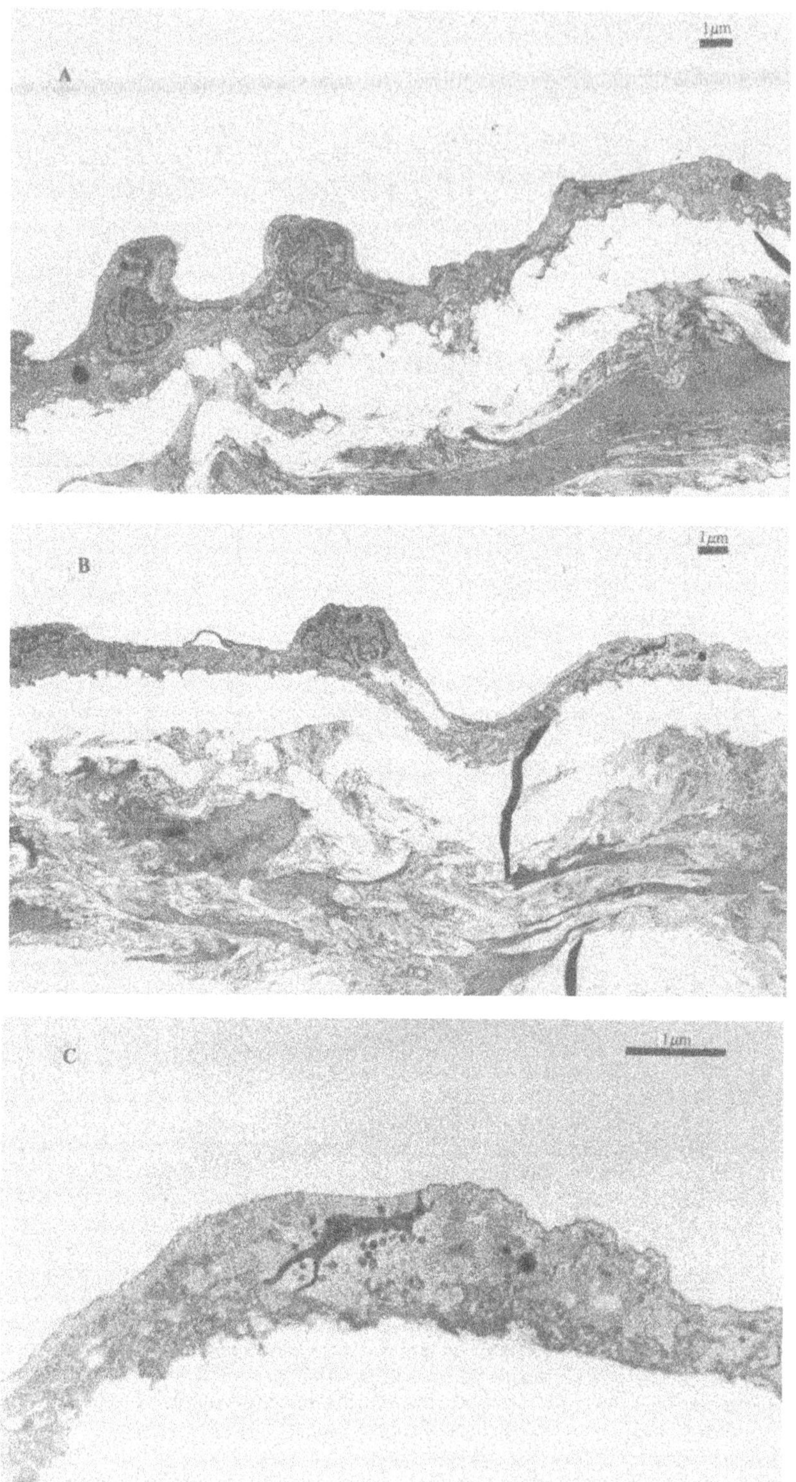

Fig. 7. Electron micrographs of rat aortic endothelium showing a dividing cell. A and B were taken on thin sections of the same cell. In B, on the right side of the dividing cell is a junction (containing horseradish peroxide) which has been widened to a bizarre shape. C shows an enlargement of this junction.

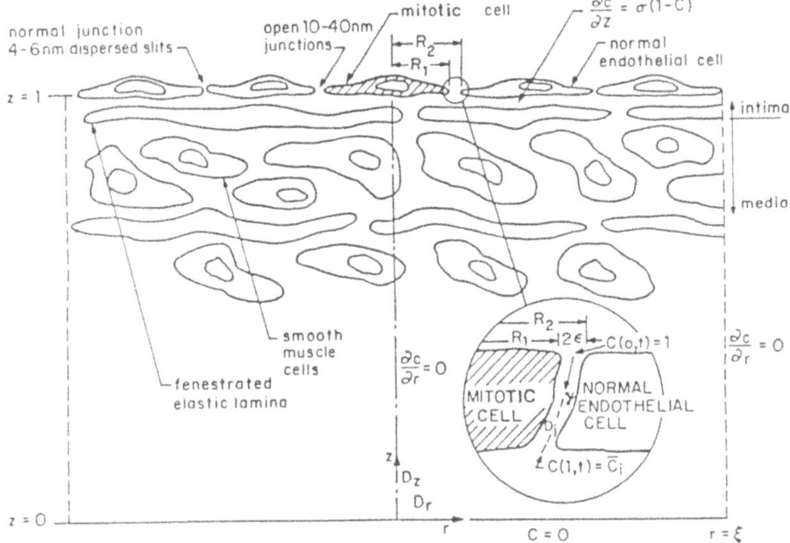

Fig. 8. Schematic illustration of the mathematical model to describe the time-dependent diffusion of inert tracer macromolecules in a vessel wall having periodically distributed mitotic endothelial cells.

tural[19] and uptake studies[20,21] have indicated that the internal elastic lamina (IEL) could present an important barrier to subendothelial diffusion, and hence the spread in the perpendicular direction is much slower than that in the parallel direction. The theoretical predictions in Weinbaum et al.[14] indicate that the value of D_r/D_z for mammalial aorta is between 10 and 100. The two diffusion coefficient ratios D_j/D_z and D_r/D_z determine the time-dependent evolution of the subendothelial concentration at the leakage site, the rapidity of the lateral spread of the tracer macromolecule in the subendothelial space, and thus the difference in behavior of tracer macromolecules with different molecular sizes (e.g., HRP, albumin and LDL).

The model predictions indicate that a tracer with a molecular diameter of about 5 nm (e.g. HRP) can pass through a transient open junction even when it is only slightly widened, since its dimensions are just borderline for the passage through a normal junction.[22] There is, therefore, a relatively small drop in concentration across the cleft and a large concentration driving potential for the subendothelial spread of this tracer from the open junction leakage site. A slightly larger tracer, e.g. the 6 nm albumin, is essentially impermeable through a normal junction; thus a transiently open junction must first widen to a significant extent in order for an initial leakage to occur. Therefore, in comparison to HRP, albumin would have a lower concentration at the cleft exit and a lower chemical activity potential for the lateral spread in the subendothelial space. Another consideration is that the D_r of albumin is smaller due to its larger effective molecular diameter. Each of these two effects is much more pronounced for LDL (22 nm). These considerations provide the explanations for (a) the more localized distribution of albumin in the present study than HRP (Stemerman et al.[23]) and (b) the greatly increased concentration of LDL in the HRP reaction foci observed by Stemerman et al.[23] The theoretical predictions for the time-dependent increase in cleft exit concentration ($\bar{C}$) for these three molecules (HRP, albumin and LDL) are shown in Fig. 9. The results indicate that, for $Dx/Dz = 100$ (i.e. $Dx = Dr$), after the initial rapid increase C_{HRP} is about three times $\bar{C}_{alb}$, and $\bar{C}_{alb}$ is about seven times $\bar{C}_{LDL}$.

In our theoretical models[13-15] the ratio of the number of cells with transiently open junctions to the number of cells with normal mature junctional strands is ϕ. According to our hypothesis, it is the change in ϕ that determines the regional variations in endothelial permeability. Prior to the present study, there had been no direct measure of this parameter. Indirect indices such as ³H-thymidine or IgG labeling had been used as a substitute for this important missing information. Since ϕ reflects the leakage which occurs in a particular phase in the turnover cycle, it may not bear a definitive relationship to these indirect indices. The present results in

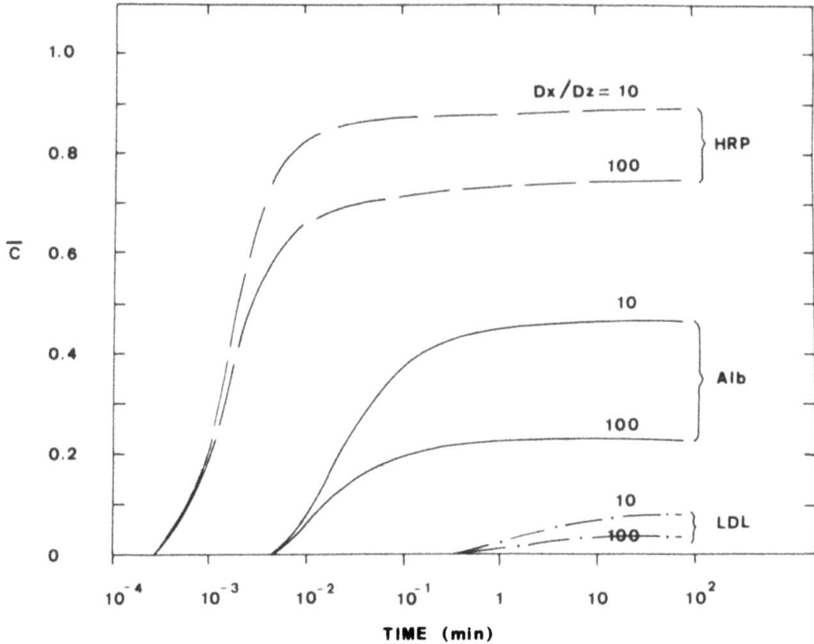

Fig. 9. Results of theoretical computation showing increases in cleft exit concentration ($\overline{C}$) of macromolecules of different sizes (HRP, albumin and LDL) as a function of time.

Table I show that the background value for ϕ, including both mitotic and non-mitotic cells, is 4.6×10^{-4}. Using our new time-dependent model, the effects of ϕ on the steady state macromolecular flux ψ_s/ψ_i or uptake ratio u_s/u_i can be derived as shown in Fig. 10, where the subscript i denotes an intact endothelium with no transient open junctions ($\phi = 0$). For the background ϕ value obtained in the present experiments of 4.6×10^{-4}, the flux and uptake ratios are essentially unity. When ϕ is increased by one order of magnitude to 4.6×10^{-3}, for a D_r/D_z ratio between 10 and 100, the predicted increase in permeability is approximately 50%, as observed experimentally for albumin.[2,6]

The value ϕ of 4.6×10^{-4} obtained in the present study is about an order of magnitude lower than the background value for the thymidine index (approximately 3×10^{-3}) obtained in quiescent endothelium in most arterial vessels.[24] Tritiated thymidine is a measure of DNA synthesis and is thus a quantitative index for the fraction of cells that have entered S phase during the period of study (24 hr). A value of 3×10^{-3} day^{-1} implies that on the average an endothelial cell would enter S phase in 333 days, and hence we can obtain an estimate of the average life-time of an endothelial cell. If the statistical frequency of cells with leakage sites is 4.6×10^{-4}, then this leaky junction turnover index also provides the fractional time in the total cell cycle that an average cell will have transiently open junctions large enough to permit the passage of albumin. Therefore, the average duration of the leakage for albumin is $(4.6 \times 10^{-4}) \times 333$ days or 3.7 hr. As reasoned above, this leakage time should vary inversely with molecular size since the gap height of the leaky junction varies dynamically with time as the junction is first disrupted and then reformed during the cell turnover process. This dynamic relation between the physical state of the junction and the permeability to macromolecules of different sizes is summarized in Fig. 11. The curve for albumin is drawn based on the present study, and that for LDL is based on unpublished experiments by Lin et al.

While the fraction of leaky endothelial cells is 4.6×10^{-4}, the fraction of mitotic cells is only 1.4×10^{-4}. Therefore, the average duration of mitosis is only about one-third of that of leakiness, i.e. 67 min. The fractional distribution of various stages of mitosis reflects the fractional duration of these stages in mitosis. Therefore, the durations of prophase, metaphase, anaphase and telophase of mitosis of arterial endothelial cells are estimated to be 21, 14, 10 and 22 min, respectively.

68

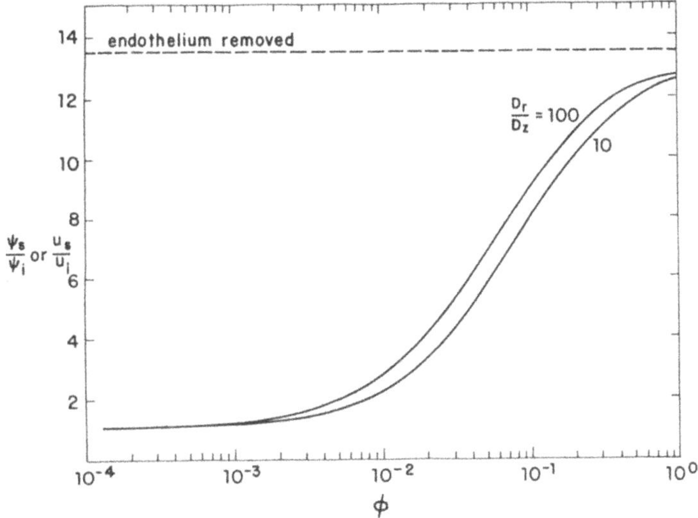

Fig. 10. Average steady-state flux perpendicular to the endothelium (ψ_s/ψ_i), or total uptake (u_s/u_i), as a function of lesky cell fraction (ϕ). The value of D_j/D_z of 87.5 is used for albumin transport in major arteries. The curves obtained for D_r/D_z = 10 and 100 are shown. The computation is based on data for the rabbit aorta.[15]

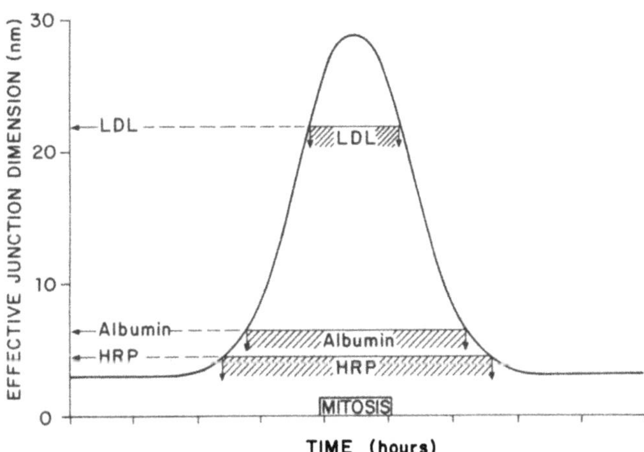

Fig. 11. Hypothetical plot of effective junction dimension in the portion of endothelial cell cycle near the period of mitosis. The junction is shown to start widening approximately two hours before the beginning of mitosis, reach a peak size of close to 30 nm in the middle of mitosis, and gradually recovers to the resting dimension by two hours after the end of mitosis. The time window in which various macromolecular tracers (LDL, albumin and HRP) can pass through the leaky junction varies inversely with the molecular size. The curve is drawn in such a way that albumin is permeable through the junction in a time period approximately three times as long as the duration of mitosis, based on the finding of the present study. The time window for LDL permeability is approximately 50% longer than the duration of mitosis, based on the unpublished findings of Lin et al.

DISCUSSION

The integrity of vascular endothelium serves to limit the entry of macromolecules into the subendothelial artery wall. This endothelial function is especially important for the prevention of excessive entry of native LDL, a major element in atherogenesis. Endothelial permeability to macromolecules is not uniform along the aortic tree. In vivo studies with the protein-binding dye Evans Blue and with LDL have shown that there are local variations in arterial wall permeability in normal animals.[2-4,6] Regions of the arterial tree with normally occurring enhanced permeability have been shown to be associated with a high rate of endothelial turnover, as measured by ^{3}H-thymidine incorporation.[3]

Prior to the starting of the present experiments, we performed preliminary studies to correlate ^{3}H-thymidine labeling with EBA leakage in the rat aorta. In agreement with the findings of previous investigators,[3,5] we did observe an increase in the density of ^{3}H-thymidine labeling spots in aortic regions with enhanced endothelial permeability. However, examination of individual endothelial cells showed that less than 20% of endothelial cells with ^{3}H-thymidine incorporation were associated with EBA leaky spots (Lin et al., unpublished data). The interpretation of the ^{3}H-thymidine data must take into account the time period of labeling (24 hr in this study); therefore all endothelial cells entering the S phase during this period would be labeled, including not only those still in the S phase, but also those already entering the subsequent phases following the initial labeling. These findings prompted us to correlate EBA leakage with a more selective time window in the cell cycle when the junctions are most likely to be disrupted. Therefore, the present study was performed by concentrating on the mitotic phase of the cell cycle, when the chromosomes are segregated, the cell shape is changed and the junctions around the cell are disrupted and remodeled. Following the division of the cell into two daughter cells, normal junctions are formed again.

The most striking result of the present study is that nearly all (99%) of endothelial cells in the mitotic phase were associated with EBA leaky spots. The observation that the mitotic figures and the cleavage site were usually located in the center of EBA leaky spots suggests that most of the leakage of albumin occurred through junctions between two daughter cells or around a single cell prior to cleavage. Therefore, the present study provides experimental evidence in support of the hypothesis that macromolecular leakage occurs in a specific time window of the cell cycle. An electron microscopic picture of a junction around a dividing endothelial cell reveals unusual junctional widening and the leakage of HRP (Fig. 7B), further supporting the contention that the endothelial cell junction becomes leaky to macromolecules during mitosis.

In contrast to the very high percentage of leakiness in mitotic cells, only 0.03% of the non-mitotic endothelial cells showed an increased permeability to EBA. It is to be noted that although EBA leaky spots are very rare in non-mitotic endothelial cells on a percentage basis, in absolute terms about two-thirds of the EBA leaky spots were associated with them. These results suggest that, while nearly all endothelial cells become leaky during the mitotic phase, the leakiness also occurs in periods preceding and following mitosis. Such leakiness may occur in cells in the period preceding mitosis if the junction has already become widened as a result of rearrangement in the F-actin filaments on the cell border, as seen in tissue culture studies of a proliferating endothelial monolayer,[25,26] as well as in cells which have completed their division but still do not have fully reformed junctions. Another possibility is that the junctions around dying endothelial cells may become leaky to macromolecules. Our transmission electron microscopic study (Fig. 12), however, showed that there was no leakage of HRP across the junction surrounding a dying endothelial cell, which had lost its membrane integrity as evidenced by the penetration of HRP to the cell interior. Further studies are needed to clarify the nature of these non-mitotic cells with leaky junctions.

As discussed above under Theoretical Analysis, using our value for the fraction of endothelial cells showing EBA leakage (4.6×10^{-4}) and the value for the fraction of endothelial cells that enter S phase over a 24-hr period as given by the thymidine index (3×10^{-3}),[24] we can make several estimates related to the duration of events in the endothelial cell cycle. Thus, the average lifetime of an endothelial cell is approximately 333 days, the average duration of EBA leakage is 3.7 hr, and the average duration of mitosis is 1.13 hr or 67 min. The partitioning of this duration of mitosis in its various stages is shown in Table III and also shown schematically in Fig. 13.

In our hypothesis that transiently open junctions exist in association with endothelial cell turnover, the junction becomes gradually widened with time as the cell enters the mitotic phase, and it gradually returns to normal dimensions with the regeneration of junctional complexes (Fig. 11). According to this concept, the duration of junctional leakage to macromolecules

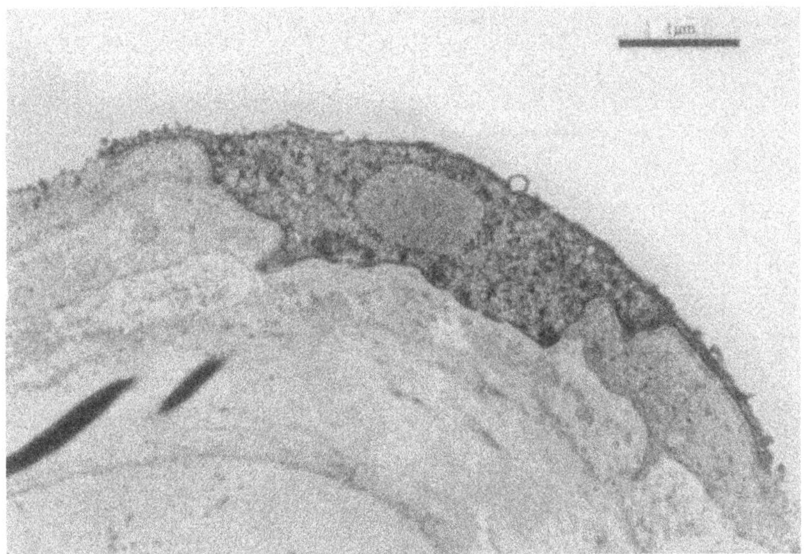

Fig. 12. Transmission electron micrograph showing a dying or dead endothelial cell which has lost the functional integrity of its plasmalemmal membrane, allowing the entry of HRP into the cell interior. Note that the endothelial junction is still intact, without allowing the leakage of HRP to subendothelial space.

would depend on the molecular size. A smaller macromolecule, such as HRP, would become leaky over a fairly long time, including time periods preceding and following mitosis. On the other hand, a large macromolecule, such as LDL, would be leaky through the junction only when is nearly maximally widened. Of course, besides the macromolecular size, factors such as electrical charge may also play a role in determining the duration of leakage.

SUMMARY

The present experiments were performed on twelve male Wistar rats to study the quantitative, topographic correlation between transendothelial permeability of Evans Blue-albumin (EBA)

Table 3. Estimated Time Periods in Endothelial Cell Cycle

Events in a Cell Cycle	Duration
Total Cycle Length	333 days
Albumin Leakage	3.7 hr
Mitosis	67 min
Prophase	21 min
Metaphase	14 min
Anaphase	10 min
Telophase	22 min

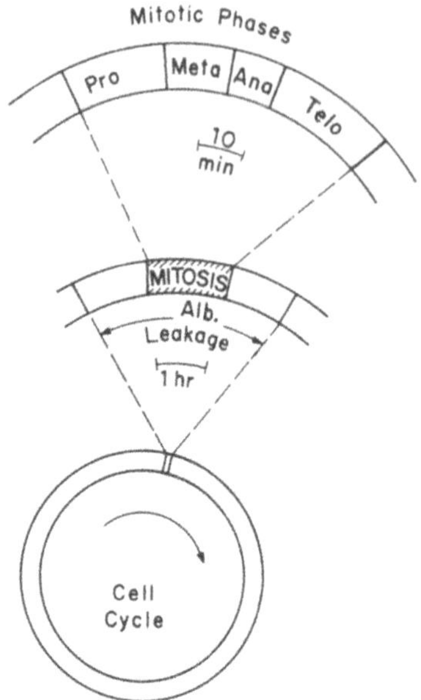

Fig. 13. Schematic drawing showing the mitotic phases in a cell cycle of the endothelial cell.

conjugate and endothelial cell replication at the single-cell level. En face preparations of the thoracic aorta were examined by fluorescence microscopy. We found a high degree of correlation between endothelial cell mitosis and EBA leaky spots. Although endothelial cell mitosis is very rare in occurrence, nearly all junctions around the dividing cells were leaky (99%), in contrast to only 0.03% of the non-mitotic cells. In addition, electron microscopic observations showed that the junction around a dividing endothelial cell is leaky, whereas that around a dying cell is not. With the aid of our theoretical model, we were able to analyze the dynamics of macromolecular passage through leaky endothelial junctions. The duration of endothelial cell mitosis was estimated to be 67 min, which constituted 0.01% of the duration of the total cell cycle. The time-dependent change in junctional geometry during endothelial cell turnover leads to an inverse relationship between macromolecular size and duration of junctional leakage. For albumin the duration of leakiness across aortic endothelial cell is approximately 3.7 hr. The present findings lend support to our hypothesis that transiently open junctions surrounding the dividing endothelial cells provide the major pathway through which macromolecules enter the subendothelial space to result in lipid accumulation.

ACKNOWLEDGMENTS

This work was supported by research grant HL 19454 from the National Heart, Lung and Blood Institute, N.I.H., and "Creativity" Grant Award CPE8500301 from N.S.F., U.S.A., and NSC-76-0412-B001-09 from the National Science Council, R.O.C. The authors wish to thank Mr. Jerry Norwich and Miss Honor O'Sullivan for their excellent technical assistance and Mrs. Micheline Faublas for secretarial help.

REFERENCES

1. S Glagov, Hemodyamic risk factors: Mechanical stress, mural architecture, medial nutrition and the vulnerability of arteries to atherosclerosis, *In*: "The pathogenesis of athrosclerosis," R.W. Wissler and J.C. Geer, ed., Baltimore, Williams and Wilkins Press, (1972).

2. M.A. Packham, H.C. Rowsell, L. Jorgensen and J.F. Mustard, Localized protein accumulation in the wall of the aorta, *Exptl Molec Pathol* **7**:214-232 (1967).

3. B.A. Caplan and C.J. Schwartz, Increased endothelial cell turnover in areas of in vivo Evans Blue uptake in the pig aorta, *Atherosclerosis* **17**:401-417 (1973).

4. R.G. Gerrity, M. Richardson, J.B. Somer, F.P. Bell and C.J. Schwartz, Endothelial cell morphology in area of in vivo Evans Blue uptake in the aorta of young pigs. II. Ultrastructure of the intima in area of differing permeability to proteins, *Am J Pathol* **89**:313-334 (1977).

5. S.M. Schwartz, E.P. Benditt, Clustering of replicating cells in aortic endothelium, *Proc Natl Acad Sci USA* **73**:651-653 (1976).

6. C.J. Schwartz, E.A. Sprague, S.R. Fowler and J.L. Kelley, Cellular participation in atherogenesis: selected facets of endothelium, smooth muscle and the periheral blood monocyte, *In*: "Fluid Dynamics as a Localizing Factor for Atherosclerosis," G. Schettler ed., Springer-Verlag Press, Berlin (1983)

7. H.S. Kruth, Subendothelial accumulation of unesterified cholesterol. An early event in atherosclerotic lesion development, *Atherosclerosis* **57**:337-341 (1985).

8. D. Steinberg, Lipoproteins and atherosclerosis. A look back and a look ahead, *Arteriosclerosis* **3**:283-301 (1983).

9. M.A. Reidy and S.M. Schwartz, Developments in the study of endothelial cells by scanning electron microscopy, *Artery* **8**:236-243 (1980).

10. C.K. Zarins, K.E. Taylor, R.A. Bomberger and S. Glagov, Endothelial integrity at aortic ostial flow dividers, *Scan Electron Microsc* **3**:249-254 (1980).

11. R.M. Nerem, M.J. Levesque and J.F. Cornhill, Vascular endothelial morphology as an indicator of the pattern of blood flow, *ASME J. Biomech Eng* **103**:172-176 (1981).

12. W.E. Stehbens, Endothelial cell mitosis and permeability, *Q J Exp Physiol* **50**:90-92 (1965).

13. S. Weinbaum, G. Tzeghai, P. Ganatos, R. Pfeffer and S. Chien, Effect of cell turnover and leaky junctions on arterial macromolecular transport, *Am J Physiol* **248**:H945-H960 (1985).

14. S. Weinbaum, G.B. Wen, P. Ganatos, R. Pfeffer, M. Lee and S. Chien, On the transient diffusion of macromolecules through leaky junctions and their subendothelial spread; Part I. Short time model for cleft exit region, *J Theor Biol,* in press (1988).

15. G.B. Wen, S. Weinbaum, P. Ganatos, R. Pfeffer and S. Chien, On the transient diffusion of macromolecules through leaky junctions and their subendothelial spread; Part II. Long time model for interaction between leakage sites, *J. Theor Biol,* in press (1988).

16. S.J. Lin, K.M. Jan S. Weinbaum and S. Chien, Enhanced macromolecular permeability of aortic endothelial cells in association with mitosis, *Atherosclerosis,* in press (1988).

17. T. Zand, J.M. Underwood, J.J. Nunnari, G. Majno and I. Joris, Endothelium and "silver lines". An electron microscopic study, *Virchows Arch* [Pathol Ana] **395**:133-144 (1982).

18. M. Bundgaard, The three dimensional organisation of tight junctions in a capillary with continuous endothelium revealed by serial section electron microscopy, *J Ultrastruct Res* **88**:1-17 (1984).

19. S.H. Song and M.R. Roach, Qauntitative changes in the size of fenestrations of the elastic laminae of sheep thoracic aorta studied with SEM, *Blood Vessels* **20**:145-153 (1983).

20. E.B. Smith and E.M. Staples, Plasma protein concentrations in interstitial fluid from human aortas, *Proc Roy Soc London* **B217**:59-75 (1982).

21. D. Fry, Mass transport, atherogenesis and risk, *Arteriosclerosis* **7**:88-100 (1987).

22. M.J. Karnovasky, The ultrastructural basis of capillary permeability studies with peroxidase as a tracer, *J Cell Biol* **35**:213-236 (1967).

23. M.B. Stemerman, E.M. Morrel, K.R. Burke, C.K. Colton, K.A. Smith and R.S. Lees, Local variation in arterial wall permeability to low density lipoprotein in normal rabbit aorta, *Arteriosclerosis,* **6**:64-69 (1986).

24. S.M. Schwartz and E.P. Benditt, Cell replication in the aortic endothelium: A new method for study of the problem, *Lab Invest* **28**:699-707 (1973).

25. G.E. White, M.A. Gimbrone and K. Fujiwara, Factors influencing the expression of stress fibers in vascular endothelial cells in site, *J Cell Biol* **97**:14-24 (1983).

26. I. Huttner, C. Walker and G. Gabbiani, Aortic endothelial cell during regeneration. Remodeling of cell junctions, stress fibers, and stress fiber-membrane attachment domains, *Lab Invest* **53**:287-302 (1985).

LEUKOCYTE-ENDOTHELIUM INTERACTIONS

THE ULTRASTRUCTURAL BASIS OF INTERACTIONS BETWEEN LEUKOCYTES AND ENDOTHELIUM

F. Hammersen*, A. Unterberg** and E. Hammersen*

*Department of Anatomy
Technical University Munich, FRG
**Institute for Surgical Research
Ludwig-Maximilians-University
Munich, FRG

INTRODUCTION

The emigration of white blood cells, mainly polymorphonuclear granulocytes (PMNs), is one of the most striking events occurring in the microcirculation under the influence of a variety of noxious stimuli. It has, therefore, attracted the early interest of electron microscopists in order to elucidate the structural events of this longknown phenomenon in more detail.[1,2,3,4] Already at that time it had been recognized that the escape of PMNs occurred either through or near the endothelial junctions, 'but that the PMNs may also be able to penetrate the endothelial cytoplasm at other points'.[4] In 1967 Welsch and Caesar[5] repeating the classic experiment of Cohnheim[6] by inducing an inflammatory reaction in the frog's tongue, provided compelling ultrastructural evidence that, at least in this model, the emigration of PMNs occurs exclusively transcellularly. Since this essential report remained uncited world-wide,[7] Faustman and Dermietzel[8] 'rediscovered' the trans-endothelial passage of PMNs following topical application of α-bungarotoxin to pial microvessels. In addition, a transcellular route of migration has been described for lymphocytes not only passing through specialized high endothelial venules,[9,10,11,12] although this has been questioned by some investigators (e.g., Schoefl 1972, Wenk et al. 1974),[13,14] the same mechanism, namely emperipolesis, should also be effective for lymphocytes extravasating through cerebral vessels.[15]

Irrespective of all these findings the tacit assumption generally hold is, that PMNs leave the postcapillary venules via an intercellular route.[16,17,18] This has become an unanimously accepted dogma, with merely 'few observers now consider neutrophils to pass through individual endothelial cells'.[19] This surprising unanimity is also reflected by the fact that, although there exists a number of most recent reports on the morphology of the interaction between leukocytes and the endothelium (e.g., Movat 1985, 1987, Movat and Burrowes 1985, Perkett et al. 1986, Thureson-Klein et al. 1984, 1986),[18,20,21,22,23,24] the emigration itself has experienced little or no attention at all.[23,24] The phenomenon 'leukodiapedesis' is obviously unanimously accepted as being definitely settled and therefore, most monographs and review articles published during the past few years illustrate leukocyte emigration with electron micrographs prepared 25 years ago (e.g., MacGregor 1980, Movat 1985).[18,25]

To clarify this controversial issue a little further we want to add some new informations on the morphological events occurring during the emigration of PMNs.

RESULTS AND DISCUSSION

Over the past decade we have collected specimens from various tissues and laboratory animals that were exposed to a wide spectrum of irritants (for details see legends of the respective Figures). Although our main interest was focussed at that time on the possible mechanisms of edema formation and structural alterations of the endothelial cells, we already noticed that closed endothelial junctions were often closely adjacent to the emigrating cells (Figs. 1-8)

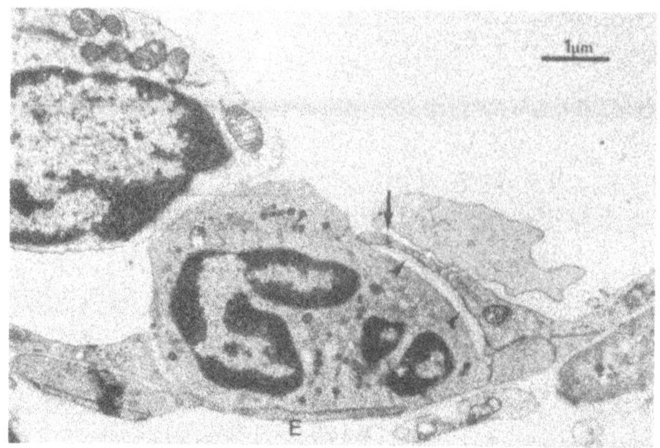

Fig. 1. Small segment of a larger venule from an ischemic (4 hrs) dorsal skinfold chamber of a syrian hamster. Partly extravasated PMN with closely attached endothelium (E) to its abluminal surface. Notice immediately adjacent closed endothelial junction (➡) and the intact basal lamina (➤).

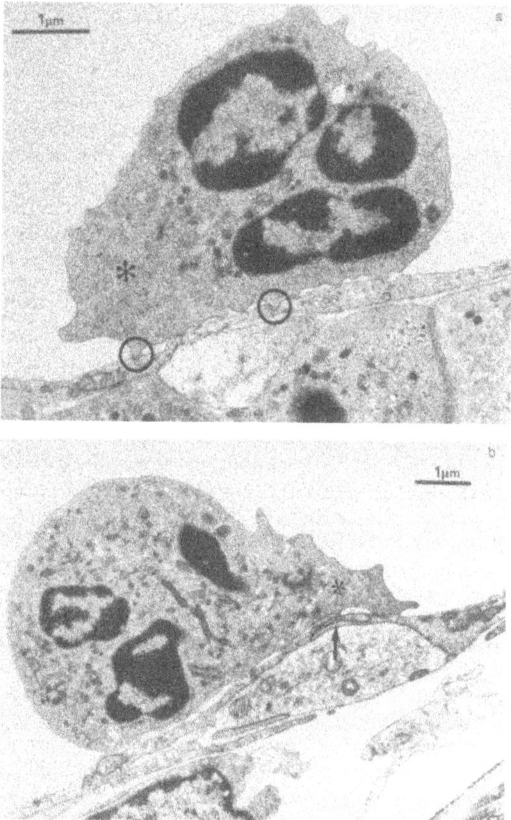

Fig. 2. Segments of small veins from hamster skinfold chamber after challenge of LTB$_4$. a) PMN projecting numerous spiny processes towards the endothelial surface, two of which (○) virtually indent the luminal cell membrane. Notice organelle-free stout process (✱) pointing in the direction of migration. b) PMN mainly flattened against the endothelial surface and in this case showing an elongated process (✱) pointing in the direction of migration. Notice closed endothelial junction (➡) beneath this migrating PMN.

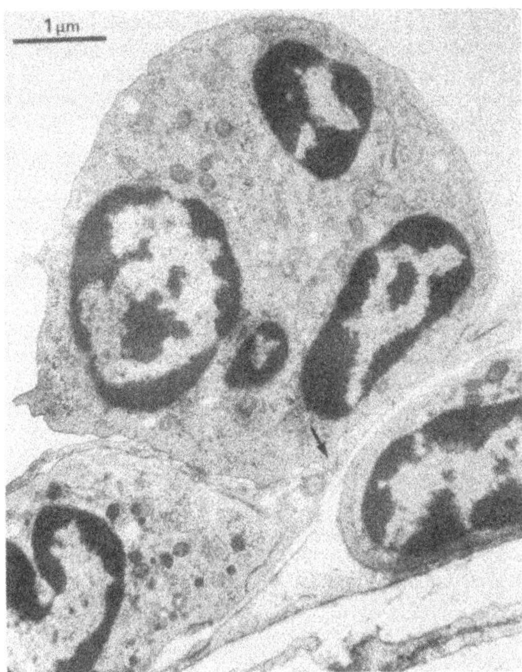

Fig. 3. PMN which has almost pierced with a single process (➤) the extremely thin endothelium of a larger venule (from mouse ear subjected to 4 hrs of ischemia and 30 min reperfusion).

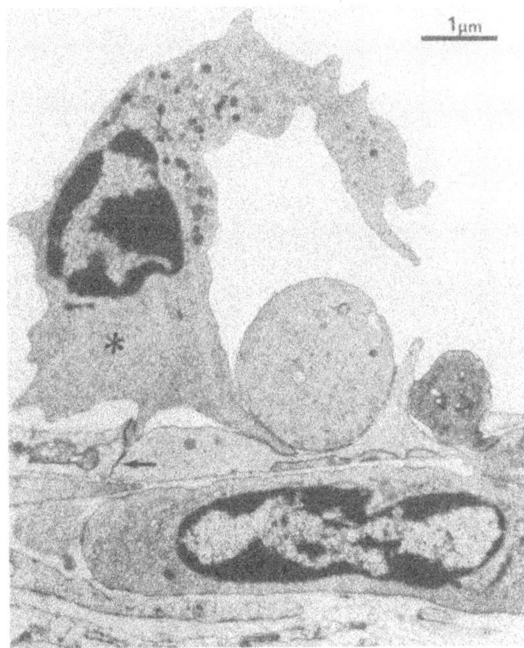

Fig. 4. Segment of a larger pial venule from a cat exposed to topically applied arachidonic acid. From the plumpish, organelle-free pseudopod (✻) a tiny process projects into the endothelium directly adjacent to a closed junction (➤). This may represent the first step of a combined trans- and intercellular passage of this PMN.

and this obviously did not fit into the concept of an intercellular passage of PMNs. When looking more closely into the structural events occurring during PMN extravasation, it became apparent that this process consisted of a sequence of consecutive steps. The first are margination and sticking, two well-known phenomena from vital microscopy, which are characterized by PMNs not only making close contact with the endothelial surface (Figs. 2a,b;3) but also projecting tiny, spicular processes towards the luminal plasmalemma (Figs. 2a;3). In case of 'sticking' these minute cellular feet indent the endothelial cell membrane with the PMN cell body either retaining its globular shape or becoming elongated and flattened against the endothelium over variant distances (Figs. 2a,b;3). Such cells invaginate the endothelial surface quite often with several such processes and develop, in addition, a single projection at one cellular pole (Figs. 2a,b), which is usually free of organelles. Such cells give the impression as if creeping along the surface like a caterpillar probing with its leading edge for the appropriate site for emigration (Fig. 2b).

In a second step only one of these PMN processes establishes firmer attachment and then penetrates further into the endothelial cytoplasm (Fig. 3) thereby pushing the luminal endothelial cell membrane continuously towards its basal counterpart until both membranes fuse and finally give way under the constant pressure of the leukocyte (cf. Figs. 3,6b). Once having forced its way through the endothelium, an increasing amount of cytoplasm streams into this now expanding leukocytic process which concomitantly broadens the initially small endothelial perforation, occasionally by simply turning the thin endothelium inside out (Figs. 5a,b).

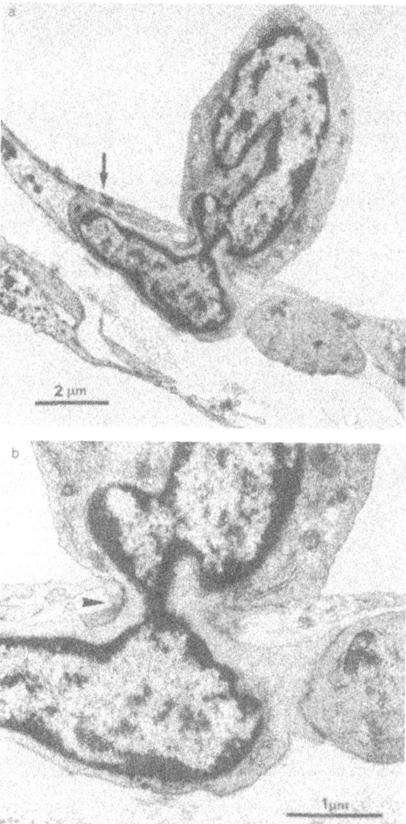

Fig. 5. Emigrating PMN through thin endothelium of a subcutaneous vein from hamster skinfold chamber exposed to hypothermia (5° C) for 1 hr. a) Notice closed junction (⟶) near the extravasating cell. b) A close-up of the preceding micrograph demonstrates the close apposition of endothelium and emigrating PMN. Notice the endothelial flap (▶) which has been turned inside out by the extravasating cell.

Quite often leukocytic pseudopods do not project perpendicularly and directly into the extravascular space, but they extend instead, obliquely or parallel to the surface into an endothelial cell thereby creating enormous endothelial outpocketings whose extremely thin walls do not show any remnants of a former endothelial junction (Figs. 6a,b). This phenomenon may give rise to electron micrographs illustrating PMNs in a truely intraendothelial location,[8] which are completely invested by a continuous, yet extremely thin sheath of endothelial cytoplasm (Fig. 8). Finally the basal part of this cytoplasmic sheath is perforated by smaller leukocytic processes to accomplish extravasation (Fig. 6b).

In this context it should be emphasized that in most cases the plasmalemmata of both the emigrating PMN and the abutting endothelial cell run strictly parallel to each other, leaving an intervening space of constant width of only 10-15 nm (Figs. 5a,b;6b). This explains why very high molecular tracers like carbon particles, often used to demonstrate venular leakages, do not escape concomitantly with the emigrating PMNs, except migration occurs via large inflammatory gaps, e.g., those induced by endotoxins or hyperimmunreactions.[18] If, however, a smaller probe molecule like ferritin is employed this will extravasate together with the emigrating PMN (Figs. 7a,b). In addition, the opposite is also true, i.e. the existence of endothelial gaps does not automatically imply extravasation of leukocytes and/or sticking of platelets at these sites.[7]

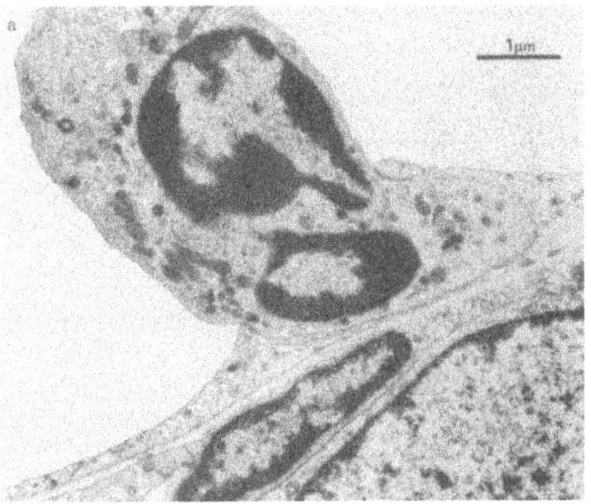

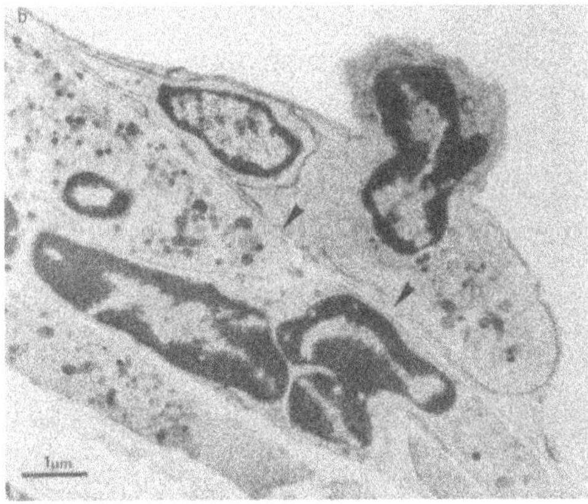

Fig. 6. a) Leukocyte projecting a clumsy pseudopod into the endothelium which becomes extremely attenuated. Notice absence of any signs of a possible endothelial junction. b) In an advanced stage a large proportion of the PMN is completely engulfed by a thin endothelial sheath the abluminal part of which is pierced by two leukocytic processes (➤). From feline pial veins exposed to topically applied arachidonic acid.

In summary we want to emphasize that, contrary to the general belief, the emigration of PMNs often occurs via a transcellular route, because (1) in many cases a closed endothelial junction or at least parts of it can be identified in the immediate vicinity of the emigrating cell. This very simple fact was consistently neglected by almost all investigators, because they were obvisouly preoccupied by the apparent plausibility that the endothelial junctions represent the most likely candidate for leukocyte emigration. The essential adverse argument resides in the distance between consecutive endothelial junctions in cross-sectioned postcapillary venules or other types of microvessels: Endothelial cells are predominantly two-dimensional elements with a considerable length (of up to < 100 μm), a lesser width (between several microns at their tapering ends and some 10-20 μm or more at their nucleated parts) and a comparably neglectable height of 0.2-0.5 μm (cf. Fig.6, p.67 in Majno 1964).[26] Therefore, in all those situations where a closed junction lies very close (distance approx. < 0.1 μm) to an emigrating PMN, it is extremely improbable that the extravasation occurs via a second, yet opened intercellular cleft, because the distance between these two consecutive junctions would be far too small (see Figs. 1,8). This also applies to a figure (Fig. F 22, p. 192) illustrated by Movat (1985)[18] which would imply that at least four junctions occur within a distance of 6.3 μm.

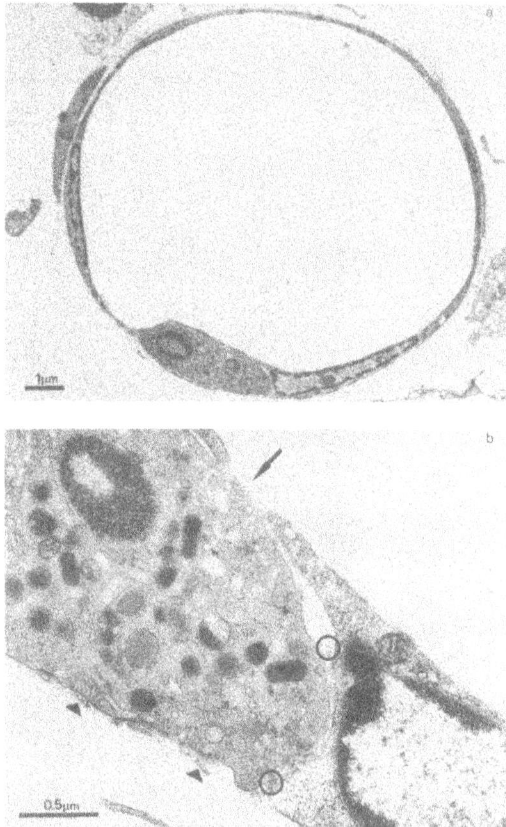

Fig. 7. a) Cross sectioned venule (inn.diam.: 20 μm) with extravasated granulocyte (PMN) from subcutaneous tissue of mouse ear fixed after 6 hrs ischemia and 15 min reperfusion. Notice that the endothelium appears normal except for that part that covers the PMN. b) High power of the right half of the emigrated PMN illustrates endothelial gap (⟶) together with the passage of ferritin (encircled) between PMN and adjoining endothelium. Clusters of ferritin (▲) are also seen between PMN and basal lamina.

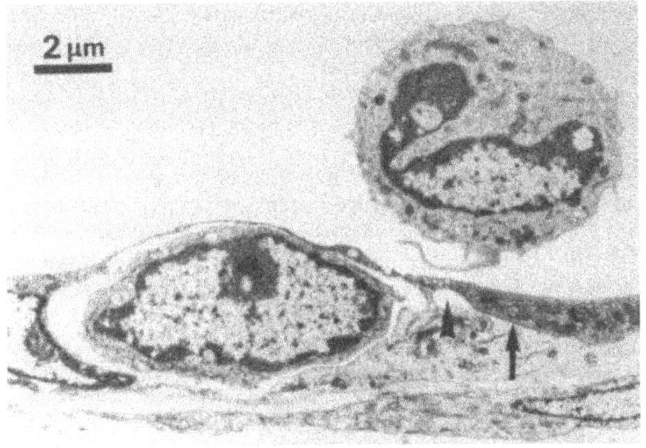

Fig. 8. Nucleated part of a leukocyte, probably a mono- or lymphocyte, completely encompassed by an extremely attenuated, yet continuous endothelial sheath. Notice close proximity of an endothelial junction (▶) which shows a focal distention (⟶). From hamster skinfold chamber exposed to hypothermia (5° C) for 1 hr.[7]

An additional and rarely addressed problem (see, however, Fig. 11 from Marchesi and Florey 1960)[4] resides in the difficulty to identify an 'opened' endothelial junction as such and discriminate it beyond any doubts from a transcellular perforation (cf. Figs. 5b;6b). The only conceivable structural criterion would be the demonstration of the halved endothelial adhesive devices along the cell membranes bordering the gap. However, postcapillary venular endothelial cells are usually said to be equipped with poorly differentiated attachment sites[27] which, therefore, are difficult to be clearly illustrated in electron micrographs. The second argument in favor of a transendothelial passage of PMNs is the fact, that quite often larger portions of the emigrating cells containing all kinds of organelles and even parts of the nucleus are found engulfed by correspondingly large outpocketings of the endothelium, which becomes attenuated to a closely attached, extremely thin sheath which does not contain any remnants of a former endothelial junction (Figs. 6a,b). Penetration of the endothelium is completed by smaller leukocytic processes perforating the basal part of the endothelial sheath. The third argument resides in the fact that early phases of a true interendothelial migration, namely PMNs extending a process just into the luminal portion of a junction with the rest of which remaining closed, are very rarely found.

However, a third pathway for emigration appears to be also operative, namely a combination of a trans- with an intercellular route, as it has been described by Cho and De Bruyn (1986)[10] for high endothelial venules. This assumption is supported by our findings that spicular leukocytic processes pierce the endothelium directly adjacent to the luminal portion of a closed junction (Fig. 4), which might explain the not infrequent observation that only the adluminal parts of a closed junction are lying near the emigrating cell. This process is possibly necessary to circumvent the interendothelial adhesive devises by a transcellular penetration that continues intercellularly into the deeper parts of the junctions which are usually void of attachment sites.

REFERENCES

1. H.W. Florey and L.H. Grant, Leucocyte migration from small blood vessels stimulated with ultraviolet light: an electron-microscope study, *J. Path. Bact.* **82**:13 (1961).
2. V.T. Marchesi, The site of leukocyte emigration during inflammation, *Q. Jl. exp. Physiol.* **46**:115 (1961).
3. V.T. Marchesi, Some electron microscopic observations on interactions between leukocytes, platelets and endothelial cells in acute inflammation, *Ann. N.Y. Acad. Sci.* **116**:774 (1964).
4. V.T. Marchesi and H.W. Florey, Electron microscopic observations on the emigration of leukocytes, *Q. Jl. exp. Physiol.* **45**:343 (1960).
5. U. Welsch and R. Caesar, Transendotheliale Granulocytenemigration in der Zunge des Frosches bei der Entzündung, *Beitr. path. Anat. allg. Pathol.* **135**:235 (1967).

6. J. Cohnheim, Über Entzündung und Eiterung, *Virchows Arch. Path. Anat.* **40**:1 (1867).

7. F. Hammersen and E. Hammersen, The ultrastructure of endothelial gap formation and leukocyte emigration, *Progr. appl. Microcirc.* **12**:1 (1987).

8. P.M. Faustmann and R. Dermietzel, Extravasation of polymorphonuclear leukocytes from the cerebral microvasculature. Inflammatory response induced by alpha-bungarotoxin, *Cell Tiss. Res.* **242**:399 (1985).

9. Y. Cho and P.P.H. De Bruyn, Transcellular migration of lymphocytes through the walls of the smooth-surfaced squamous endothelial venules in the lymph node: evidence for the direct entry of lymphocytes into the blood circulation of the lymph node, *J. Ultrastruct. Res.* **74**:259 (1981).

10. Y. Cho and P.P.H. De Bruyn, Internal structure of the postcapillary high-endothelial venules of rodent lymph nodes and Peyer's patches and the transendothelial lymphocyte passage, *Amer. J. Anat.* **177**:481 (1986).

11. A.G. Farr, Y. Cho and P.P.H. De Bruyn, The structure of the sinus wall of the lymph node relative to its endocytic properties and transmural cell passage, *Am. J. Anat.* **157**:265 (1980).

12. G. Kraal, A.M. Duijvestijn and H.H. Hendriks, The endothelium of the high endothelial venule: A specialized endothelium with unique properties, *Exp. Cell Biol.* **55**:1 (1987).

13. G.I. Schoefl, The emigration of lymphocytes across the vascular endothelium in lymphoid tissue, *J. exp. Med.* **136**:568 (1972).

14. E.J. Wenk, D. Orlic, E.J. Reith and J.A.G. Rhodin, The ultrastructure of mouse lymph node venules and the passage of lymphocytes across their walls, *J. Ultrastruct. Res.* **47**:214 (1974).

15. K.E. Aström, H.F. de Webster and B.G. Arnason, The initial lesion in experimental allergic neuritis, *J. exp. Med.* **128**:469 (1968).

16. I.G. Colditz, Margination and emigration of leucocytes, *Surv. Synth. Path. Res.* **4**:44 (1985).

17. B. Heymer, Causative agents, mediators and histomorphology of inflammation, *Path. Res. Pract.* **180**:143 (1985).

18. H.Z. Movat, "The inflammatory reaction," Elsevier Science Publishers B.V. Biomed. Division, Amsterdam, New York, Oxford (1985).

19. T.J. Williams, P.J. Jose, M.J. Forrest, C.V. Wedmore and G.F. Clough, Interactions between neutrophils and microvascular endothelial cells leading to cell emigration and plasma protein leakage, *in:* "White cell mechanics: Basic science and clinical aspects," M.A. Meiselman, P.L. Lightman, and P.L. LaCelle, eds., Liss. Publ., Inc., New York (1984).

20. H.Z. Movat ed., "Leükocyte emigration and its seqüelae," Karger, Basel, München, Paris, London, New York, New Delhi, Singapore, Tokyo, Sydney (1987).

21. H.Z. Movat and C.E. Burrowes, The local Shwartzman reaction: endotoxin-mediated inflammatory and thrombo-hemorrhagic lesions, *in:* "Handbook of endotoxins", vol. 3, Cellular biology of endotoxins, L.J. Berry, ed., Elsevier Science Publ., Amsterdam, New York, Oxford (1985).

22. E.A. Perkett, G. Disabato, K.L. Brigham and B. Meyrick, Lymphocyte and granulocyte migration across the endothelial layer of bovine pulmonary artery intimal explants towards lymphocyte conditioned medium, *Tissue & Cell* **18**:839 (1986).

23. A. Thureson-Klein, P. Hedqvist and L. Lindbom, Ultrastructure of polymorpho-nuclear leukocytes in postcapillary venules after exposure to leukotriene B_4 in vivo, *Acta physiol. scand.* **122**:221 (1984).

24. A. Thureson-Klein, P. Hedqvist and L. Lindbom, Leukocyte diapedesis and plasma extravasation after leukotriene B_4: Lack of structural injury to the endothelium, *Tissue & Cell* **18**:1 (1986).

25. P.R. MacGregor, Granulocyte adherence, *in:* "Handbook of inflammation," vol. 2, The cell biology of inflammation, G. Weissmann, ed., Elsevier/North-Holland Biomedical Press, Amsterdam, New York, Oxford (1980).

26. G. Majno, Mechanisms of abnormal vascular permeability in acute inflammation, *in:* "Injury, inflammation and immunity," L. Thomas, I.W. Uhr, and L. Grant, eds., Williams & Wilkens, Baltimore (1964).

27. M. Simionescu, N. Simionescu and G.E. Palade, Segmental differentiations of cell junctions in the vascular endothelium. The microvasculature, *J. Cell Biol.* **67**:863 (1975).

LEUKOCYTE ENDOTHELIUM ADHESION AND MICROVASCULAR HEMODYNAMICS

Herbert H. Lipowsky, Steven D. House and John C. Firrell

Department of Physiology and Cellular Biophysics
College of Physicians and Surgeons
Columbia University
New York, NY 10032, USA

INTRODUCTION

The effectiveness of the inflammatory response hinges upon the interaction between hemodynamic transport of white blood cells (WBCs) to a focus of adhesion on the endothelium and the shearing forces exerted by the blood stream which tend to dislodge them prior to emigration through the vascular wall.[1,2] Within the microvasculature, the preferential margination of WBCs along the venular endothelium predisposes leukocyte endothelium adhesion (LEA) when activation of adhesion complexes on the WBC and endothelial cell are initiated by an appropriate stimulus. Several mechanisms may promote the enhancement of venular WBC saltation, which may arise from either the kinematics of red blood cell (RBC) and WBC interaction,[3] the hemodynamic influence of RBC aggregation at reduced shear rates,[4] or the inherent rigidity of WBCs compared to RBCs.[5,6]

Regardless of the precise mechanisms which promote increased frequency of WBC to endothelium contact, it is apparent that the elevation of LEA with reductions in blood shear rate,[7] may result in an unstable process which leads to extensive vaso-occlusion. As shown previously,[8] LEA may cause dramatic increases in the resistance to blood flow which, theoretically, may result in further reductions in shear rate with an attendant increase in LEA. Inasmuch as the obvious result of this hypothetical sequence of events could lead to disastrous degradation of microvascular blood flow, we have undertaken to examine the balance of those forces which promote and oppose LEA. Based upon *in vivo* observations of LEA in mesentery in response to either shear rate reductions or a chemoattractant stimulus, it is shown that the above hypothetical viscious cycle of flow degradation may be mitigated by the deformability characteristics of the WBC and the inherent ability of the microvasculature to redistribute blood flow during vaso-occlusive events.

METHODS

The present study summarizes measurements of the resistance to blood flow made previously and detailed in the studies of House and Lipowsky.[9] Techniques employed in the measurement of the force of adhesion between WBC and endothelium have been described previously.[8,10] In brief, LEA was induced in the mesentery of the cat by a topical application of the chemoattractant N- formyl- methionyl- leucyl- phenylalanine (FMLP) at a concentration of 10^{-7}M in Ringer's solution. Measurements of intravascular pressure and pressure drop in single unbranched venules were made with the servo-null technique. Simultaneous measurements of red cell velocity (two-slit photometric method), microvessel hematocrit (differential optical density) and vessel diameter (image shearing) were also made. With these basic hemodynamic and geometric data, calculation of the resistance to blood flow were made during the course of LEA. The average force exerted to dislodge a WBC from the endothelium by the flow of blood in each microvessel was estimated by application of the principle of conservation of momentum to the measured pressure drops and flows prior to and during LEA, as described earlier by Lipowsky et al.[8]

To gain insight into the deformation of individual leukocytes for a specific level of wall shear stress exerted by the blood stream, high magnification observations were performed in the mesentery of the rat. In these studies, video recordings of the shape changes of adherent WBCs were made while manipulating intravascular shear rates by a proximal occlusion of the micro-vessel with a blunted microprobe.[11] Various indices of the shape and state of WBC deformation were derived from frame by frame analysis of these video recordings, as described in the following.

RESULTS AND ANALYSIS

Response to FMLP

To illustrate the shear rate dependency of LEA, presented in Fig. 1 is the number of WBCs sticking to the endothelium per 100 μm of vessel length for 16 venules ranging in diameter from 25 to 49 μm. Shown on the ordinate are values obtained prior to (control) and following suffusion of the mesentery with FMLP. Wall shear rate was estimated from the measured RBC velocity ($8V_{mean}/D$) and shear stress derived from the product of apparent viscosity (η) and $\dot{\gamma}$, where η was determined from measurements of microvessel hematocrit and *in vitro* correlations. Clearly, the result of reduced shearing forces is a three-fold rise in the numbers of WBC adhered to the endothelium, as shear rates fall from 1000 to 200 sec[-1]. These trends were obtained during the reduction of microvascular blood flow by the adhesion process. No significant correlation between the number of WBCs adhered and the vessel diameter was found, although in general, greater red cell velocities, and hence wall shear stresses, were found in the larger venules, as reported previously.[12] The apparent upper limit of the number of adhered WBCs at low shear probably arises from limitations in the rate at which WBCs are transported to specific adhesion sites due to reductions in bulk flow. Other limiting factors may include the saturation of receptor sites on the endothelium itself and the finite amount

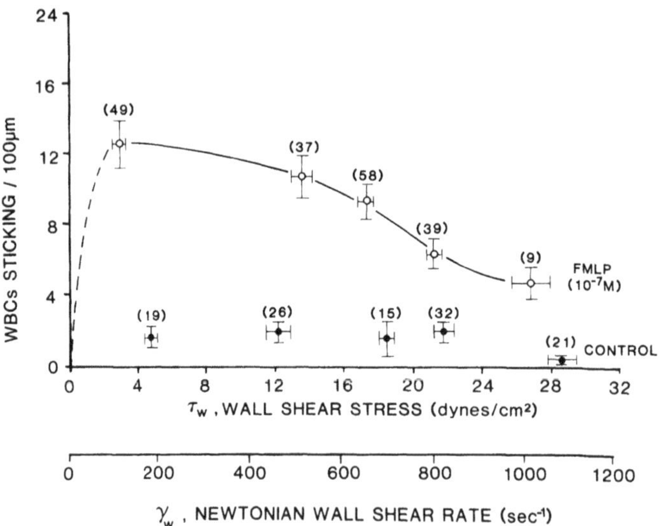

Fig. 1. Number of WBCs sticking to the endothelium vs. wall shear rates (γ_w) and shear stress (τ_w) following suffusion of the mesentery of the cat with Ringer's solution containing the chemoattractant FMLP. Control conditions correspond to suffusion with Ringer's solution only. From House and Lipowsky[9] with permission of Academic Press.

itself and the finite amount of time allowed for the observation, typically 180 sec.

The impact of LEA on hemodynamics within individual venules is typified in Fig. 2, where the time course of the measurements of upstream intravascular pressure, pressure drop, pressure gradient, bulk flow, microvessel hematocrit and intravascular resistance is presented for 16 venules during exposure to FMLP. The 10-fold increase in the number of adherent WBCs is accompanied by a 20% reduction in proximal perfusion pressure and bulk flow while intravascular resistance increases about 80%. The reduction in proximal (upstream) pressure is suggestive of a slight increase in arteriolar tone, due to a myogenic constriction (or arteriovenous reflex) in response to the increased venous resistance. The key point here is that although resistance increases almost two-fold, flow rate itself diminishes only by about 30%, due to redistribution of flow throughout the network. Measurements of pressures and flow in proximal arterioles of comparable diameter and devoid of LEA, demonstrate a small degree of vasoconstriction with attendant reductions in intravascular pressure. Thus, flow redistribution throughout the mesentery occurs in both arteriolar and venular portions of the network to attenutate the effect of increased venous resistance on microvascular blood flow.

To evaluate the hemodynamic forces which tend to counter the LEA process, the force (F) exerted on an average WBC was estimated from the loss of momentum calculated from the measured pressure drops and flows during adhesion. Shown in Fig. 3 are force vs. wall shear stress for three venules ranging in size from 25 to 49 μm with reductions in τ_w during exposure to the FMLP. Interestingly, F varies inversely with τ_w. While the precise magnitude of this inverse relationship may be subject to question, the statistically significant negative slopes of all but one venule lend credence to this departure from direct proportionality between force and wall shear stress. The mechanism whereby greater dispersal forces are imposed upon an adhered WBC at lower shear stress most likely arises from the deformability properties of the WBC itself.

White Blood Cell Deformation Under Shear

The deformability characteristics of individual WBCs were evaluated from video recordings at high magnification (40 $\times$ water immersion objective) during reductions in flow imposed by a proximal micro-occlusion of the venule. Presented in Fig. 4 are summary curves of three indicies of the shapes of individual WBCs measured under various levels of wall shear rate (estimated from RBC velocity). Measurements of the height (h) of a WBC and its overall

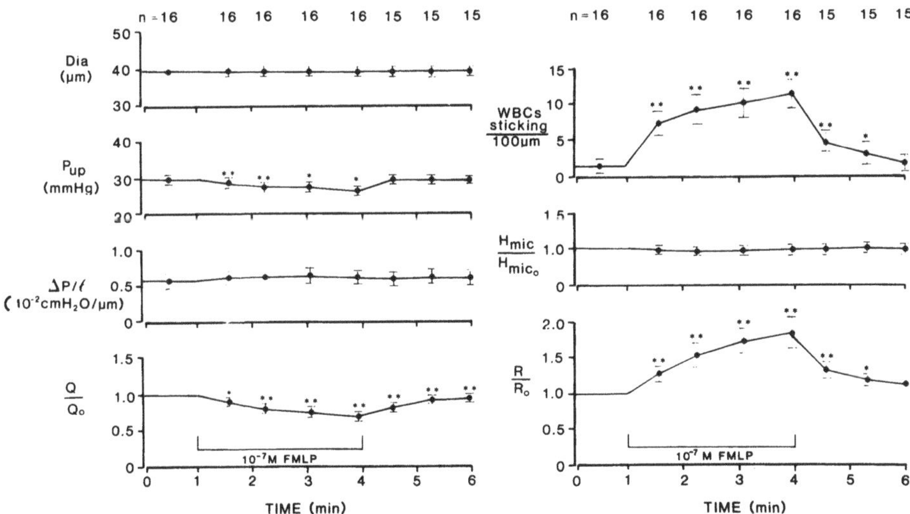

Fig. 2. Resultant changes in hemodynamic parameters in 16 venules following suffusion of mesentery with 10^{-7}M FMLP. Shown is the time course of the average diameter (DIA), upstream intravascular pressure (P_{up}) and pressure gradient ($\Delta P/1$), bulk flow, microvessel hematocrit (H_{mic}) and intravascular resistance (R). Subscript o denotes control conditions prior to exposure to FMLP. Asterisks denote significant departures from control at levels of $p < .05$ (*) and .01 (**). From House and Lipowsky,[9] with permission of Academic Press.

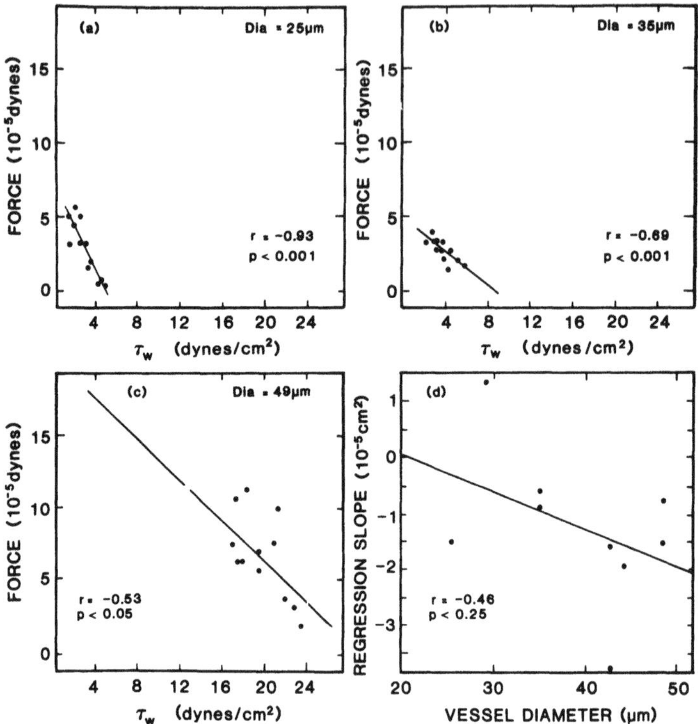

Fig. 3. Representative variations of the force acting on an adhered WBC (F) vs. estimated wall shear stress (τ_w) in the vicinity of the white cell, for three vessels of the indicated diameters. The slopes of such regressions for 9 venules are shown in panel d. From House and Lipowsky,[10] with permission.

length (L), permitted computation of a deformation index (Fig. 4a), by first, calculating the volume of a prolate spheroid with dimensions h and L, and second, computing the diameter of a sphere with equivalent volume. Assuming that the WBC volume does not change appreciably during deformation, the original length of the cell (L_o) was assumed to be that of the calculated spherical diameter. The deformation index was then calculated as the fractional departure from the original length, $(L_o - L)/L_o$. Additional indices of deformation were estimated from the contact length between WBC and endothelium (Fig. 4b) and the corresponding circular area of contact attendant to this length, Fig. 4c.

It is evident that as wall shear stresses increase the WBC tends to undergo an almost 60% elongation over the entire range of shear. Considering that the volume of a prolate spheroid is equal to $(\pi/6)Lh^2$, then a 60% elongation of a WBC is accompanied by a 21% reduction in its height (h) to maintain a constant volume. Such reductions in height, or the extent to which the WBC enchroaches upon the lumen of a microvessel, may directly affect the level of shear stress acting upon the WBC surface by increasing the effective diameter of the vessel. Shear rates and forces may thus be diminished as the cells deform (either passively or actively) and retract from the lumen. As indicated in Fig. 4b, as shear rates are increased, the length of the contact zone between WBC and endothelium also tends to increase, with an apparent increase in the area of contact (Fig. 4c) as estimated from the corresponding circular area.

Force Balance During Deformation

In the case of a nondeformable body attached to a wall in a shearing stream, it is intuitively obvious that the forces which aim to dislodge it must be proportional to the wall shear stresses in the vicinity of the adhesion site. The observation that F may actually decrease with increasing τ_w suggests that the shape and dimensions of the WBC tend to affect the hydrodynamic flow field around the WBC, thus influencing the shearing stresses which act on the cell surface and contribute to the dispersal force. A complete analytical solution of the intimate

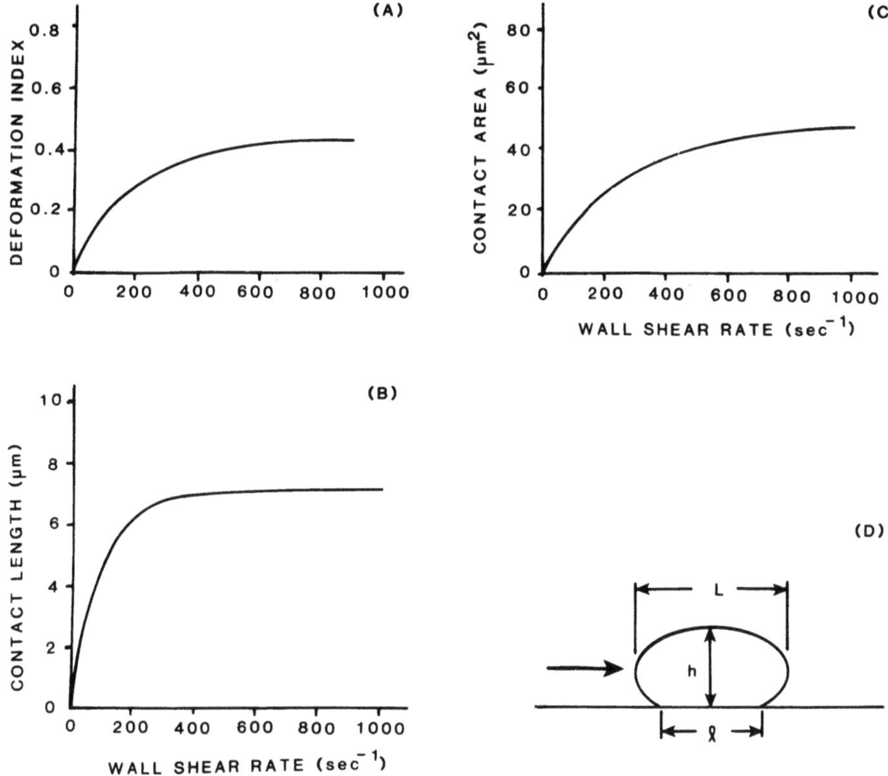

Fig. 4. Summary curves of the deformation characteristics of individual WBCs adhered to the endothelium under the indicated shearing conditions. Each curve represents a non-linear regression of the measured data. (A) Deformation index, calculated from the measured in vivo length and height of the WBC (see text), (B) the contact length (1), (C) the corresponding contact area and (D) schematic indicating the nomenclature used in the text. Modified from Firrell and Lipowsky.[11]

balance between the flow field and resultant WBC shape is a formidible task which requires detailed descriptions of the mechanical properties of the WBC. Even with such information, the task of computing the flow dynamics and resultant shear forces for a realistic three dimensional flow field is not trivial. However, to examine the possibilities for such hydrodynamic and mechanical interaction one may construct a simplified model of the flow field to examine the effect of shape changes on the hemodynamics and shearing forces. Presented in Fig. 5 is a simple "pill box" model of a WBC attached to the wall of a vessel visualized as a plane channel of height D. Based upon the assumption of one-dimensional flow, the mean velocity (V_m) on the surface of the cell may be calculated as a function of the mean velocity in the free stream (V_m) and the height (h) of the cell. By assuming a fully developed channel flow along the surface of the "pill box" of length s, the surface shear rates ($\dot{\gamma}$) and shear stresses (τ) may be calculated for Newtonian fluid behavior. Given that the volume of the cell is constant (vol = sh), the force of adhesion under static equilibrium may be computed in terms of the value of $\xi = h/D$, taken as an indicator of the extent of deformation of the cell between one state and another.

As indicated in Fig. 5, the force F is a parabolic function of ξ, with a minimum at $\xi = 1/3$. As the cell deforms from shape 1 to 2 with h approaching 0, F increases dramatically due to the relative increase in the surface area exposed to the surrounding flow field. Conversely, as the cell relaxes to fill the lumen ($\xi \rightarrow 1.0$), F increases concomitant to increased shear stresses on the surface of the cell. The range of variations in ξ for the analogous *in vivo* measurements obtained here presumably corresponds to $1/3 < \xi < 1$. Thus it is plausible that *in vivo*, as τ_w increases, the WBCs elongate (cf Fig. 4a) and ξ decreases, resulting in a diminished

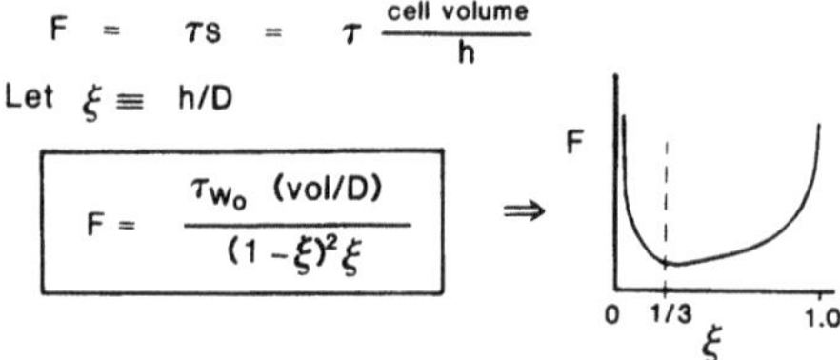

Conservation of Mass Flow:

$$V_m = V_{m_0} \frac{D}{(D-h)}$$

$$\dot{\gamma} = \frac{kV_m}{D-h} = \frac{kV_{m_0}D}{(D-h)^2}$$

Newtonian Fluid – Surface Shear Stress:

$$\tau = \eta \dot{\gamma}$$

$$\tau = \frac{\tau_{w_0} D^2}{(D-h)^2}$$

Forces Acting on "Cell":

$$F = \tau S = \tau \frac{cell\ volume}{h}$$

Let $\xi \equiv h/D$

$$F = \frac{\tau_{w_0}\ (vol/D)}{(1-\xi)^2\xi} \Rightarrow$$

Fig. 5. Simplified one-dimensional flow calculation of the force (F) of adhesion for a "pill box" shaped leukocyte adhered to the wall of a two-dimensional channel. By conservation of mass and the assumption of a fully developed flow at each point, F is found to vary as a parabolic function with the fractional height of the cell, $\xi = h/D$.

net force acting to dislodge the cell. It should be noted that the exact applicability of these simple estimates of the relationship between cell shape and shear force remains to be determined. In the three dimensional case of a spherical WBC attached to the wall of a circular tube, the potential for lateral or azimuthal relief of hydrodynamic shearing stresses as the cell fills more of the lumen would tend to strongly counter the hypothetical increase in shear stresses on the cell surface. Nonetheless, the trends of the simplified one-dimensional flow model and the *in vivo* measurements are in agreement, although the precise magnitude of force variations with cell deformation remains to be determined.

DISCUSSION

In the present study we have attempted to tie together several observations on the adjustments in network hemodynamics during LEA, the forces exerted upon an adhered cell and the possible role of WBC shape changes as a determinant of the force of adhesion. In retrospect, it appears that the most difficult of these tasks is to put into quantitative terms the relationship between alterations in pressure and flow throughout the microvascular network during regional increases in intravascular resistance. For a hypothetical network comprised of a purely serial succession of microvessels of various diameters, the effect of increased resistance in distal segments is readily discernible and can be quantitated by analogy to the simple voltage divider network. However, the complexities of the *in vivo* network preclude the applicability of such simplified models. The observations that reductions in venular flow are disproportionately

90

less than changes in venular resistance supports the hypothesis of flow redistribution throughout the network during increased LEA. In addition, the extent of redistribution is clouded by an apparent arteriolar vasoconstriction (on the order of 12%) in response to suffusion with FMLP. Evaluation of the precise extent to which an elevation in either arteriolar or venular vessel resistance may affect flow throughout the mesenteric network would require more detailed hemodynamic studies than those performed to date as well as more sophisticated analytical techniques. With regard to the latter, the micro-occlusion method introduced by Nellis and Zweifach[13] would appear to have the greatest potential for providing an interpretation of the relationship between flow and resistance changes. As shown there, analysis of the proportionality between changes in flow with intravascular pressure during obstruction of a single microvessel may be taken as a measure of the hemodynamic impedance between a specific network site and proximal or distal portions of the network. Specifically, complete occlusion of one true capillary vessel would reveal a comparatively small change of intravascular pressure with flow, since there are numerous alternate pathways for a redirection of flow around an occluded capillary. On the other hand, considerably greater changes in pressure with flow during vaso-occlusion occur in the larger arterioles and venules due to their greater impact on the total throughput of the network.

By taking vessel diameter as an index of position in the overall hierarchy of microvessels, some inferences may be made on the effect of occlusion by LEA on large compared to small venules. In general, vaso-occlusion of larger venules would tend to cause an increase in the local perfusion pressures, which would in turn provide an increase in intravascular shear stresses which would counter LEA by tending to disperse the adherent leukocytes. In the smaller venules, flow degradation can occur without substantial increases in local pressure gradients due to redistribution of flow. Hence, the propensity for LEA to occur in the immediate post-capillary venules is enhanced by virtue of the network branching pattern, i.e. the greater number of small compared to large venules. This behavior, in concert with the demargination of WBCs as small venules converge and their flows eventually mix, most likely are the major hydrodynamic factors for the initiation of LEA in the smallest venous vessels.

Estimates of the forces of adhesion between WBC and endothelium also give additional insight into the mechanics of how the adhesion process affects flow. It is evident that the correlation of adhesion force with vessel diameter is overshadowed by the prevailing level of wall shear stress, as indicated in Fig. 3 by the lack of significant trends of the slope of F vs. τ_w with luminal diameter. However, similar plots of F/τ_w vs. τ_w reveal a slope which becomes significantly more negative with diminishing vessel diameter.[10] This behavior would suggest that reductions in the effective lumen of the smaller venules give rise to greater shearing stresses acting upon the surface of the adhered WBC, compared to larger venules. This situation is schematized by the solid line in the upper panel of Fig. 6, where a hypothetical increase in shear stresses (τ) on the surface of an adhered WBC is shown. Hence, while smaller venules have lower values of τ_w due to the lesser pressure gradients in their network division, much greater forces may be generated to oppose the adhesion process. Thus, venules with diameters smaller than 30 μm would tend to have fewer numbers of adherent WBCs compared to those with diameters between 30 and 50 μm, thus promoting enhanced adhesion in these larger venules.

The role of WBC deformation has been addressed by both the force measurements and direct measurement of WBC shape under various levels of wall shear stress (rates). It is hypothesized that the effect of WBC deformation is to diminsh fluid shear stresses on the WBC surface, with this effect being greatest in smaller venules as depicted in Fig. 6 (upper panel). Also, shown in Fig. 6 is a hypothetical family of parametric F vs. τ_w curves which summarizes the effect of WBC shape change on force blance. In general, for a given state of deformation (shape), the force of adhesion (F) is linearly related to the wall shear stresses acting in the vicinity of the WBC. As cell deformation occurs, the F vs. τ_w relationship shifts to a line of lesser slope, and the net force decreases along the locus of points indicated in Fig. 6 and as measured *in vivo* (Fig. 3). These trends would continue to hold until a maximum degree of deformation is achieved, following which force would increase with τ_w. The fact that we do not observe this upswing in F vs. τ_w is most likely due to a progressive detachment of the WBC with an attendant increase in the adhesive stress between WBC and endothelium, as depicted in the lower panel of Fig. 6. Adhesive stresses presumably increase with τ_w until the maximum tolerable level is achieved, at which the cell is swept away. The direct observations of cell deformation are consistent with this hypothesis. As indicated in Fig. 4a, a maximum WBC deformation will be achieved at wall shear rates of about 600-800 sec^{-1}. From the number of cells adhered vs. shear rate and shear stress (Fig. 1) it is evident that as $\dot{\gamma}_w$ exceeds 600 sec^{-1}, the number of adhered cells declines rapidly.

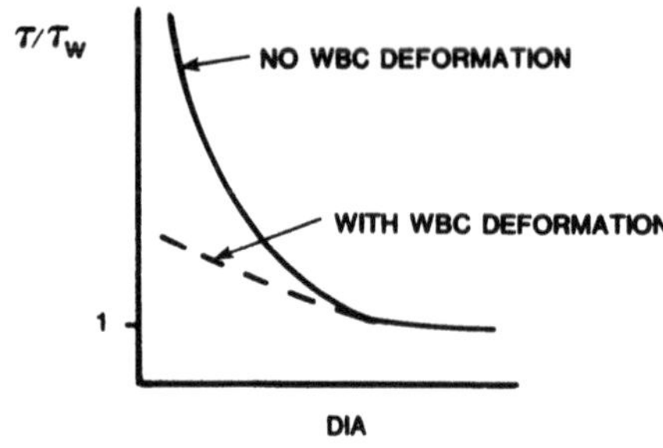

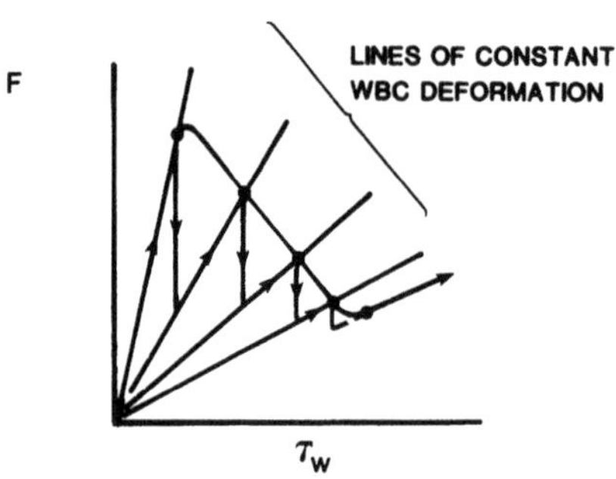

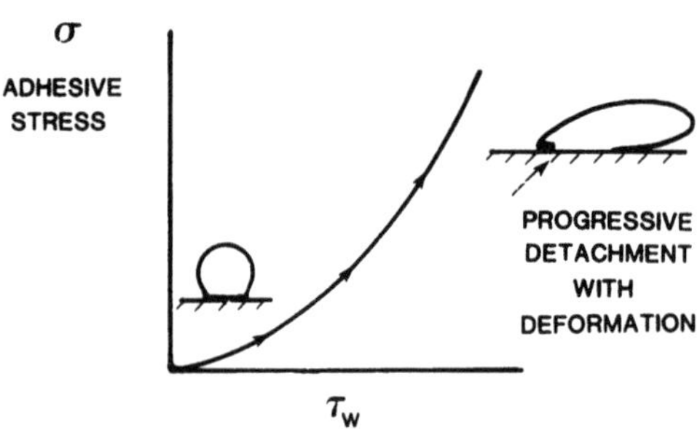

Fig. 6. Schema of the hypothetical dependency of adhesion force upon WBC deformability. In the top panel, shear stresses on the surface of a non-deformable WBC are envisioned to increase dramatically as vessel diameter is diminished, relative to the size of the WBC (solid line). These stresses, which contribute to formation of the net force (F) which tends to dislodge the WBC, are greatly attenuated by cell deformation under shear (dashed line). The relationship between F and τ_w is depicted as a proportional one for conditions of constant deformation (shape). Due to WBC deformation, F diminshes along the locus of points indicated by the arrows, to yield an inverse relationship between F and τ_w. This condition persists until the maximum tolerable adhesive stress is exceeded during a progressive detachment of the WBC attendant to its deformation, as schematized in the lower panel.

SUMARY AND CONCLUSIONS

In the present study we have attempted to provide quantitative details of hemodynamic determinants of leukocyte to endothelium adhesion in the microvasculature. To this end, several hypotheses have been advanced to suggest that the preferential adhesion of leukocytes in the larger venules (30-50 μm diameter) rests upon the inherent ability of the microvasculature to compensate for small perturbations in resistance and that WBC deformability may play a significant role in this process. Flow redistribution and attendant arteriolar vasomotor adjustments may forestall LEA in the larger collecting venules of the network, where venous obstruction may be countered by bringing the full weight of the arteriovous pressure gradient to oppose WBC adhesion. Direct measurements of the force of adhesion suggest that with diminishing vessel diameter, as for example in the immediate post-capillary venules, WBC dispersal forces will be greatest due to dramatic increases in the proportionality between force and wall shear stress. This event would tend to preclude adhesion in the smallest venular microvessels. It has also been shown that there is a strong potential for WBC deformability to affect the adhesion process by modification of the shear stresses acting on the WBC surface, as evidenced by an inverse relationship between force and wall shear stress and direct observations of WBC shape changes with increasing shear.

ACKNOWLEDGMENTS

The authors are indebted to Ms. Silvia Rofe for technical assistance in the experiments and preparation of the Figures. This work was supported in part by NIH research grants HL-28381, HL-16851 and HL-39286.

REFERENCES

1. A. Atherton and G.V.R. Born, Relationship between the velocity of rolling granulocytes and that of the blood flow in venules, *J. Physiol. London* **233**:157-165 (1972).
2. L. Grant, The sticking and emigration of white blood cells in inflammation, *in*: "The Inflammatroy Process," B.W. Zweifach, L. Grant and L. McClusky, eds., San Diego, CA, Academic Press, Inc, pp 205-249 (1973).
3. G.W. Schmid-Schoenbein, S. Usami, R. Skalak, and S. Chien, The interaction of erythrocytes and leukocytes in capillaries and post-capillary venules, *Microvasc. Res.* **19**:45-70 (1980).
4. U. Nobis, A.R. Pries, G.R. Cokelet and P. Gaehtgens, Radial distribution of white cells during blood flow in small tubes, *Microvasc. Res.* **29**:295-304 (1985).
5. H.L. Goldsmith, The microrheology of red blood cell suspensions, *J. Gen. Physiol.* **52**:5s-28s (1968).
6. H.L. Goldsmith and H.L. Spain, Margination of leukocytes in blood flow through small tubes, *Microvasc. Res.* **27**:204-222 (1984).
7. H.N. Mayrovitz, M.P. Wiedeman and R.R. Tuma, Experimental and clinical thrombosis. Factors influencing leukocyte adherence in microvessels, *Thromb, Haemostas.* (Stuttg.) **38**:823-830 (1977).
8. H.H. Lipowsky, S. Usami and S. Chien, *In vivo* measurements of "apparent viscosity" and microvessel hematocrit in the mesentery of the cat, *Microvasc. Res.* **19**:297-319 (1980).
9. S.D. House and H.H. Lipowsky, Leukocyte endothelium adhesion: Microhemodynamics in mesentery of the cat, *Microvasc. Res.* **34**:363-379 (1987).
10. S.D. House and H.H. Lipowsky, *In vivo* determination of the force of leukocyte-endothelium adhesion in the mesenteric microvasculature of the cat, *Circ. Res.* in press (1988).
11. J.C. Firrell and H.H. Lipowsky, Leukocyte Margination in Mesenteric venules of the rat, *In J. Micro.:Clin. and Exp.* (1988). submitted
12. H.H. Lipowsky, S. Kovalcheck and B.W. Zweifach, The distribution of blood rheological parameters in the microvasculature of cat mesentery, *Circ. Res.* **43**:738-749 (1978).
13. S.H. Nellis and B.W. Zweifach, A method for determining the segmental resistances in the microcirculation from pressure flow measurements, *Circ. Res.* **40**:546-556 (1977).

WHITE CELL-ENDOTHELIUM INTERACTION DURING POSTISCHEMIC REPERFUSION OF SKIN AND SKELETAL MUSCLE

K. Messmer, F.U. Sack, M.D. Menger, R. Bartlett,
J.H. Barker and F. Hammersen*

Dept. of Experimental Surgery
University of Heidelberg
Heidelberg, F.R.G.
*Dept. of Anatomy
Technical University of Munich
Munich, F.R.G.

Reperfusion failure after prolonged ischemia is characterized by sequestration of granulocytes within the microvasculature of the ischemic organs and tissues. Leukocytes, activated by tissue trauma, complement factor C5 and/or endotoxin interact with the endothelium surface and eventually emigrate through the vessel wall into the perivascular tissue. Sticking and emigration of polymorphonuclear granulocytes (PMN) is associated with formation of oxygen derived radicals and leakage of plasma through the microvascular walls indicating disturbance of the endothelial barrier function.[1,2]

While granulocyte-endothelium interaction and granulocyte capillary plugging has been analysed in various tissues,[3] this phenomenon has not been studied in greater detail in the skin tissue. The skin is, however, beside the skeletal muscle the target organ in ischemia from peripheral arterial occlusive disease (PAOD). In Fontaine stages III and IV of PAOD skin leasons and ischemic gangrene often require amputation of the leg which per se is a lifethreatening procedure, particularly in elderly people.

With the aim to beneficially influence skin and muscle ischemia we have therefore investigated the postischemic reperfusion phase with special emphasis on granulocyte-endothelium interaction.

METHODS

In hairless mice (4 - 6 weeks old, body weight 20 g) a venous catheter was implanted for drug administration. Following a 24 hours recovery period total ischemia was induced by applying a noncrushing clamp over the entire base of the ear for 6 hrs. 3 min prior to the opening of the clamp superoxide dismutase (SOD) (50 mg/kg) or 0.1 cc of normal saline solution were injected as a bolus, followed by a continuous infusion of 5 mg/kg SOD for a period of 30 min.[4,5]

Our second model consisted of syrian hamsters (6 - 8 weeks old, body weight 60-80 g) which were equipped with a dorsal skin fold chamber to allow intravital microscopic analysis of the microcirculation in skeletal muscle and skin tissue of the awake animal. This preparation as well as the techniques used for microcirculatory analysis has been described in detail previously.[6,7] In addition to the chamber two permanent catheters were implanted in the carotid artery and the jugular vein. Ischemia was induced in the lower part of the chamber by means of a transparent stamp fixed to the skin fold chamber.[8] Under microscopic control an external pressure of 40 - 50 mmHg was applied to 50% of the tissue within the observation window by means of an adjustable screw clamp so as to empty the vessels within the tissue. The noncompressed tissue (upper half of the observation window) served as nonischemic control tissue.[8,9] After a recovery period of 48 hours had elapsed, the control animals were subjected to ischemia of 4 hours followed by observation of the postischemic changes for up to 4 and 24 hours respectively.[9]

In the animals assigned to evaluate effects of prophylactic measures the systemic hematocrit was decreased from its initial control level of 45.0 ± 2.4 to $30.4 \pm 1.8\%$ by isovolemic hemodilution using 6% dextran 60 (Schiwa, Glandorf / FRG). During the exchange procedure mean arterial pressure and heart rate were monitored. When the hematocrit of 30% was reached 4 hours of ischemia were induced as in control animals with observaton periods of 4 and 24 hours respectively.

Vital microscopy was performed in the ear of the awake hairless mouse with long working distance objectives ($\times$ 60-460) over a 30 min observation period and recorded on video tape for assessment of PMN endothelial interaction: The white cells were stained with 0.2 mg of Acridin Orange administered intravenously. Macromolecular leakage was assessed by analysis of the extravasation of FITC Dextran (MW 150,000) by means of the computer assisted microcirculation analysis system (CAMAS) developped in our laboratory. Macromolecular leakage was quantified by densitometry and expressed as incremental changes in fluorescence intensity over time.

In the mouse ear the PMN-endothelium interaction was evaluated by observing the PMNs within a 100 μm section of venules (20 μm diameter) and classification as stickers and rollers.[5] RBC velocity was measured by means of photometric analyser and the dual window technique. All data were statistically analysed using the Mann-Whitney-test.

In the hamster skin fold preparation the quality of reperfusion was assessed by measurements of capillary density, RBC velocity and vessel diameters. For assessment of microvascular permeability contrast enhancement was obtained prior to ischemia by means of TRITC-labelled Dextran 70 (MW 70.000), while after ischemia FITC-Dextran 150 (MW 150.000) was used. As in the mice, the white cells were stained with Arcidine Orange given to the hamster intravenously. Statistical analysis in the hamster experiments included analysis of variance with t-test or Mann-Whitney-test, respectively.

RESULTS

Ischemia of 6 hours applied to the skin and to the skeletal muscle for a period of 4 hours resulted in severe reperfusion failure in both species.

Comparing the changes prior and 30 min after release of ischemia in the mouse ear, it became apparent, that the number of sticking PMNs as well as the number of rolling PMNs was significantly reduced as result of the treatment with superoxide dismutase while there was no significant difference in macromolecular leakage of FITC Dextran between the SOD and the saline-treated group (Tab. 1). RBC velocities were identical in both groups, differences in shear rates can therefore be excluded as factors contributing to the differences observed in PMN accumulation. Electron microscopy revealed platelet aggregates and a marked increase in the number of PMNs adhering to and emigrating through the venular walls. These phenomena were rarely encountered after treatment with SOD.[4,5]

REPERFUSION AFTER 4 HOURS OF ISCHEMIA TO SKELETAL MUSCLE

In the nontreated hamsters functional capillary density was found reduced to 30% of the initial values after 4 hours of ischemia. Only 50% of the capillaries initially perfused with red blood cells presented with RBC-flow 24 hours after reperfusion (Fig. 1). Furthermore the degree of heterogeneity of functional capillary densities had increased significantly after ischemia. Red blood cell velocity was markedly reduced in the early reperfusion phase and never recovered during the 24 hours observation time.[9]

In contrast, when 4 hours ischemia was induced after prophylactic hemodilution with dextran to a systemic hematocrit of 30% reperfusion failure of mild degree was observed. Functional capillary density was only slightly reduced after 4 hours of ischemia, and after reperfusion for 24 hours 90% of all initially perfused capillaries were reperfused. Capillary RBC velocity was slightly reduced in the early reperfusion phase but normalized within 24 hours. Light microscopic histology sections revealed severe leucocyte sticking and leucocyte plugging in the postcapillary venules of the untreated animals; in contrast, in the animals which had been hemodiluted prior to ischemia leucocyte sticking and plugging was virtually absent.

Table 1. Effects of 6 hrs of ischemia of the hairless mouse ear on macromolecular leakage and PMN-endothelium interaction.

Macromolecular Leakage				PMN-Endothelium Interaction		
Max intensity Increment	T_{50} (min)	T_{max} (min)		Stickers (n/100 μm)	Rollers (n/min)	RBC vel (mm/sec)
SOD (n = 8)	2.9 ± 0.9	2.5 ± 1.7	9.9 ± 4.1	SOD (n = 9)	4.2 ± 1.7	19.2 ± 7.5	0.4 ± 0.2
NaCl (n = 10)	3.0 ± 0.9	1.4 ± 0.6	9.4 ± 3.2	NaCl (n = 8)	8.8 ± 3.1	35.4 ± 14.7	0.4 ± 0.2
p value	n.s	< 0.001	n.s.	p value	< 0.001	< 0.001	n.s.

T_{50} and T_{max} and the tinks to reach 50% and maximum increments in fluorscence intensity.

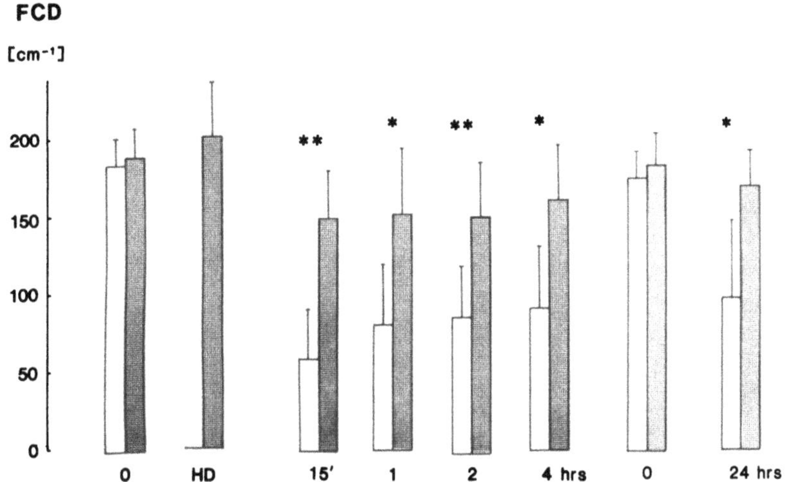

Fig. 1. Functional capillary density (FCD) prior and at different times after 4 hrs of ischemia of skeletal muscle. Control: white columns, hemodilution: filled columns (Mean ± SD, *p < 0.01, **p < 0.001)

CONCLUSIONS

Both models, the ear of the hairless mouse and the hamster dorsal skin fold chamber, are suitable for quantitative analysis of microvascular reperfusion following ischemia of skin and skeletal muscle tissue. Both models allow for the assessment of prophylactic and treatment modalities in order to prevent or to reduce postischemic reperfusion failure. The results obtained in the hairless mouse ear suggest that the beneficial effects of SOD at time of reperfusion of ischemic skin are due to a reduced accumulation of PMNs in the microvasculature. These PMNs are known to be one of the sources of oxygen derived free radicals;[1,2] it is likely that SOD prevents the effects of free radicals by its scavenging property and by inhibition of PMN recruitment allowing microvessel plugging. Since macromolecular leakage was not influenced by the SOD treatment, it appears that the endothelium damages and permeability changes are due to mechanisms other than oxygen free radical formation; however, it is also possible that with higher doses of SOD a more pronounced decrease in PMN concentration and thereby a prevention of macromolecular leakage could have been obtained.

In the hamster dorsal skin fold model, we have also demonstrated that within the microcirculation the nutritive capillary bed is most susceptible to reperfusion failure. This was demonstrated by the highly significant and persistent decrease of functional capillary density as well as by the extremely heterogeneous distribution of the remaining capillary flow. It has been proposed that flow stoppage in capillaries might be due to endothelial cell swelling and increased tendency of PMNs to interact with the endothelial cell surface.[10] Accordingly in our experiments we found leucocyte sticking as the prominent feature in the reperfusion phase. Reperfusion, however, was greatly enhanced, when the ischemia had been induced with an initially low systemic hematocrit (30%). Hence prophylactic hemodilution resulted in a marked reduction of microvascular reperfusion failure in skeletal muscle. A hematocrit intentionally lower than normal means lower yield shear stresses in the microvasculature and thereby better flow conditions.[11] Most importantly PMN-endothelial interaction was virtually absent when prophylactic hemodilution had been performed with Dextran 60 prior to ischemia.

Both models allow the quantitative analysis of the PMN-endothelial interaction during reperfusion for a prolonged period of time. We have recently established a computer assisted method to quantitate sticking and rolling PMNs as well as PMN-endothelium adhesion coefficients within the microvascular network. At present we are investigating mechanisms involved in microvascular reperfusion failure as well as the role of prophylactic and therapeutic measures in the treatment of ischemia induced tissue damage.

REFERENCES

1. K.E. Arfors and G. Smedegård, Permeability of macromolecules as affected by inflammatory cells, *Prog appl Microcirc* vol 12, pp 90-96 (1987).
2. J.M. McCord, Oxygen-derived free radicals in postischemic tissue injury, *N Engl J Med* 312:159-163 (1985).
3. G.W. Schmid-Schönbein, Mechanisms of granulocyte-capillary plugging, *Prog Appl Microcirc* vol 12, pp 223-230 (1987).
4. R. Bartlett, W. Funk, F. Hammersen, K.E. Arfors, K. Messmer and P. Nemir, Effect of superoxide dismutase on skin microcirculation after ischemia and reperfusion, *Surg Forum* 37:599-601 (1986).
5. J.H. Barker, R. Bartlett, W. Funk, F. Hammersen and K. Messmer, The effect of superoxide dismutase on the skin microcirculation after ischemia and reperfusion, *Prog appl Microcirc* vol 12, pp 276-281 (1987).
6. B. Endrich, K. Asaishi, A. Götz and K. Messmer, Technical report — a new chamber technique for microvascular studies in unanesthetized hamsters, *Res Exp Med* 177:125-134 (1980).
7. B. Endrich and K. Messmer, Quantitative analysis of the microcirculation in the awake animal, *In:* "Handbook of Microsurgery," W. Olszewksi ed., CRC Press, Miami/USA, pp 79-105 (1984).
8. F.U. Sack, W. Funk, F. Hammersen and K. Messmer, Microvascular injury of skeletal muscle and skin after different periods of pressure induced ischemia, *Prog Appl Microcirc* vol 12, 282-288 (1987).
9. M.D. Menger, F.U. Sack, J.H. Barker, G. Feifel and K. Messmer, Quantitative analysis of microcirculatory disorders after prolonged ischemia in skeletal muscle: Therapeutic effects of prophylactic isovolemic hemodilution, *Res Exp Med.* i88 in press (1988).
10. F. Hammersen and E. Hammersen, The ultrastructure of endothelial gap-formation and leukocyte emigration, *Prog appl Microcirc* vol 12, pp 1-34 (1987).
11. K. Messmer, U. Kreimeier and M. Intaglietta, Present state of intentional hemodilution, *Eur Surg Res* 18:254-263 (1986).

MORPHOMETRIC STUDIES ON
HUMAN LEUKOCYTE GRANULES

Geert W. Schmid-Schönbein* and Shu Chien**

Institute of Biomedical Sicences
Academia Sinica, Taipei, Taiwan 11529, R.O.C.
*Department of Applied Mechanics and Engineering Sciences — Bioengineering
University of California
San Diego, La Jolla, CA 92093
**Department of Physiology and Cellular Biophysics
College of Physicians and Surgeons
Columbia University, New York, NY 10032, U.S.A.

INTRODUCTION

The lysosomal granules[1] play an important role in the inflammatory process,[2] and a rather detailed picture of their biochemistry, formation and physiology has been drawn.[3] The granules are carriers of histamine, heparin and serotonin in eosinophils and basophils and the source of lytic enzymes in neutrophils.[4] These granules serve an important function in phagocytosis by contributing to the enzymatic digestion of engulfed microorganisms, and they provide a source of preformed membrane area which may be recruited in certain forms of phagocytosis or during cell spreading on substrates. Although the granules and other cell organelles have been subjected to detailed ultrastructural investigations,[5-8] quantitative information on granule membrane area, size, and distribution are limited; quantitative granule studies have been applied only to cells other than the circulating leukocytes.[9]

Morphometric information regarding these organelles is needed for the analysis of physiological leukocyte functions. For example, in neutrophil phagocytosis we need to know how much membrane area can be made available by exocytosis of granules by the plasma membrane.[10] To analyze the proteolytic action of the lysosomal granules on a per cell basis, we need to know the number of size of granules in a cell.

In this report we present our recent results[11] on direct measurements of granule density, membrane area and membrane volume in circulating leukocytes. The distribution in neutrophilic leukocytes in the passive state and in the active state during pseudopod formation was investigated. These basic data are needed for quantitative studies of phagocytosis, endocytosis, lysosomal damage to tissue, and other problems.

METHODS

Stereology

The granules in neutrophilic leukocytes or monocytes have different sizes and shapes, and current stereological methods do not allow the derivation of morphological parameters from random sections of such a system of nonuniform particles.[12] In order to circumvent this problem, we used a technique of mild cytoplasmic swelling in a hypotonic medium which causes the majority of granules to become spherical, so that the algorithm of Fullman[13] for poly-dispersed spheres can be applied. Such a procedure is justified if the granule membrane is not stretched and if no granules are released during swelling. These conditions and probably met since leukocyte or erythrocyte membranes generally appear to have a high membrane area compressibility modulus,[14] and since the total surface area of the granules remains constant in mildly hypotonic suspension media.[15] In contrast to the granules of neutrophils or monocytes, the electron dense granules of eosinophils and lymphocytes may in first approximation be regarded as spherical so that no swelling procedure was applied for the investigation of these granules with are nonuniform only in size.

To list the basic stereological relationships, consider a system of randomly mixed spherical granules with a distribution of diameters. Let the diameter, D_i, of each granule within a cell be measured from midpoint to midpoint of the membrane in a 3-dimensional sense, then the population average values of diameter, $\bar{D}$, membrane surface area, $\bar{S}$, and volume, $\bar{V}$, and the number density N_v, of the granules, are given by Fullman's equations[12]

$$\bar{D} = \pi/2\bar{m} \tag{1}$$

$$\bar{S} = 2\pi N_\varrho/\bar{m}N_a \tag{2}$$

$$\bar{V} = \pi V_v/2\bar{m}N_a \tag{3}$$

$$\bar{N}_v = 2\bar{m}N_a/\pi \tag{4}$$

where $m = \dfrac{1}{n} \sum\limits_{i=1}^{n} (1/d_i)$, d_i being the section diameters as seen on the electron micrographs; N_a is the number of granule cross sections per unit area; N_ϱ is the number of intersections between the test lines and the granules, and V_v is the granule/cell volume ratio. The total number of granules per cell is equal to

$$N_t = N_v \, V_c \tag{5}$$

where V_c is the average cell volume as measured previously.[11] The volume ratio, V_v, for the granules can either be computed from equations (3) and (4), as $V_v = N_v \, \bar{V}$, or it can also be measured independently from random sections with the point counting technique[12] as

$$V_v = P_p \tag{6}$$

where P_p is the fraction of random test points over the cell sections that fall inside the granules. If the granule volume, membrane area and diameter are computed for swollen granules which have a spherical shape in a hypotonic medium, then the question arises what these values would be in an isotonic medium. Since in isotonic medium the granules assume various shapes, no single diameter can suffice to specify the geometry. Over the range of solution tonicities selected in this study, the volume ratio of granules to whole cell remains constant[15] so that

$$\left[(V_v)_G \right]_{200} = \left[\frac{N_t \, V}{V_c} \right]_{200} = \left[(V_v)_G \right]_{300} = \left[\frac{N_t \, V}{V_c} \right]_{300}$$

where the subscripts specify the tonicity of the respective suspending media in milliosmoles per kg H_2O (mOsm).

When leukocytes become activated and project pseudopodia, the granules become redistributed within the cytoplasm. The question arises whether the active cells in free suspension would start to degranulate and thereby gain plasma membrane area. In order to investigate this question the surface/volume ratio, $(S_v)_G$, between granule membrane area and cell volume were measured and compared on cells with and without pseudopods. S_v was measured according to the method described by Underwood.[12] This method is independent of the shape of the granules and merely requires random sections. Specifically, a testline system is placed on a random cell section and S_v is determined as

$$(S_v)_G = 4 \, \frac{n}{\ell_t} \, M$$

where n is the total number of testline intersections with the granules, ℓ_t is the total length of the testline within the cell plasma membrane, and M is a magnification factor (cm/μm) for the micrographs.

Cell Preparation

Fresh venous blood samples were drawn from healthy laboratory workers (age 27-39 years) by venipuncture using as anticoagulants EDTA for the studies on passive cells and heparin for those on active cells. The samples were allowed to sediment at room temperature for 25-40 min, at which time the supernatant plasma layer with leukocytes, platelets, and a few red cells were collected. Passive cells were suspended in 10 ml of NaCl solution with 0.1 gm/dl EDTA (pH adjusted to 7.4), and active cells were suspended in 10 ml of human Ringer's solution. To prevent sedimentation these suspensions were gently agitated. Both solutions were adjusted to a salt concentration of 305 mOsm. For hypotonic swelling of cells, the NaCl solution was diluted to 150 mOsm. The osmolality of each solution was measured by freezing point depression (Fiske Osmometer, Fiske Assoc., Bethel, CT). The active cells were observed under light microscopy (40× objective, 10× eyepiece) until the majority of granulocytes formed pseudopods (about 2-3 hr after phlebotomy).

The leukocytes were then fixed and gelled by dropwise addition of a 2% glutaraldehyde solution at the same salt concentration as the cell suspension and to a final concentration of 1%. After about 1 hr the cells were postfixed in fresh 2% glutaraldehyde (in 50 mM NaCl), followed by 1% OsO_4 (in distilled water), and rinsed in 0.1 M cacodylate buffer and distilled water. Thereafter, the cells were subjected to stepwise dehydration in ethanol, rinsed in 100% propylene oxide, and embedded in araldite resin (Polyscience, Warrington, PA).

Ultrathin sections with 10-80 nm thickness were stained on one side with 6% uranyl magnesium acetate (Polyscience, pH = 5) and lead Reynold citrate (Eastman Kodak, Rochester, NY), and examined and photographed on a transmission electron microscope (EM 10 and EM 9; Zeiss, West Germany) at magnifications between 5000 to 20000×. Care was taken that the sections were stained only on one side. Without the stain, most ultrastructural features were barely visible so that the structures within the section gave only a negligible contribution to the image. Furthermore, we noticed that with an unstained section one cannot focus on a single plane, whereas after staining the surface of the section becomes an easily detectable plane for focus. As discussed elsewhere,[11] the images derived in this fashion represent a plane of polish in the stereological sense with negligible thickness. All images were calibrated with a length caliper (54000 lines/inch; Polyscience). Print size was 8 × 10 inch at a final magnification of about 25,000× to 100,000×. In addition, from 12 cells large scale montages (120,000×) were prepared for detailed investigation of the granule population.

RESULTS

(a) Average Properties

Figure 1a shows the electron micrograph of a neutrophil in an isotonic medium (305 mOsm); the cell is in the passive state without pseudopods. Figure 1b shows an electron micrograph of a neutrophil in a hypotonic solution (200 mOsm); almost all granules are spherical so that equations (1) to (5) apply. Table I shows a summary of the morphometric data derived for each cell type from a number of random sections. All data are calculated so that they refer to the isotonic case. No values are listed for the diameter of the neutrophil's and monocyte's granules since they are not spherical in such a medium. Since the numbers for $\overline{V}$, N_v, and V_v, are obtained by independent measurements, they are consistent among each other only within error of the measurements, e.g. the identity, $N_v \cdot \overline{V} = V_v \cdot V_c$ is satisfied only in an approximate sense. All values listed in Table I are given in absolute units.

The values in Table I were derived from cells which were kept in the passive state by the use of EDTA as anticoagulant. To explore the question whether the choice of EDTA has a specific influence on the granules, the granule volume density, $(V_v)_G$, was compared with those obtained on neutrophils in heparin. In both cases the cells were kept in free suspension without adhesion to a substrate, and the cells in heparin were rapidly fixed after cell harvesting to avoid the initiation of pseudopod formation. The results derived from 10 random sections in each case show a mean volume $(V_v)_G = 16.4\%$ and 15.9% in EDTA and heparin, respectively. The two values are statistically not different, suggesting that no degranulation has occurred.

(b) Granule Distribution in Neutrophils

The neutrophil granules can be divided ultrastructurally into two classes, the specific (primary) light electron density granules and the secondary high electron density (azurophilic) granules.

Table I. Leukocyte Granule Morphometry*

Cell Type	$\bar{D}$ (μm)	$\bar{S}$ (μm²)	$\bar{V}$ (μm³)	N_v (μm⁻³)	V_v	N_t**	V_t** (μm³)	V_c** (μm³)
Neutrophil (n = 24)	—	0.25 ±0.11	0.010 ±0.010	19.6 ± 7.6	0.16 ±0.05	3724 (1900-6300)⁺	30	190
Lymphocyte (n = 38)	0.19 ±0.03	0.11 ±0.03	0.005 ±0.002	0.39 ± 0.71	0.0019 ±0.0039	45 (0-150)⁺	0.23	116
Monocyte (n = 14)	—	0.12 ±0.03	0.004 ±0.001	7.9 ± 3.6	0.027 ±0.016	1848 (1400-2702)⁺	6.3	234
Eosinophil (n = 22)	0.60 ±0.11	1.22 ±0.44	0.13 ±0.06	2.03 ± 0.77	0.24 ±0.05	418 (260-780)⁺	49	206

n = number of random sections

* mean ± standard deviation of n sections

** mean values

+ range of values as estimated from individual sections

N_t computed according to equation 5

V_t = total granule volume per cell ($= V_v \cdot V_c$)

V_c = average cell volume from Schmid-Schönbein et al[15]

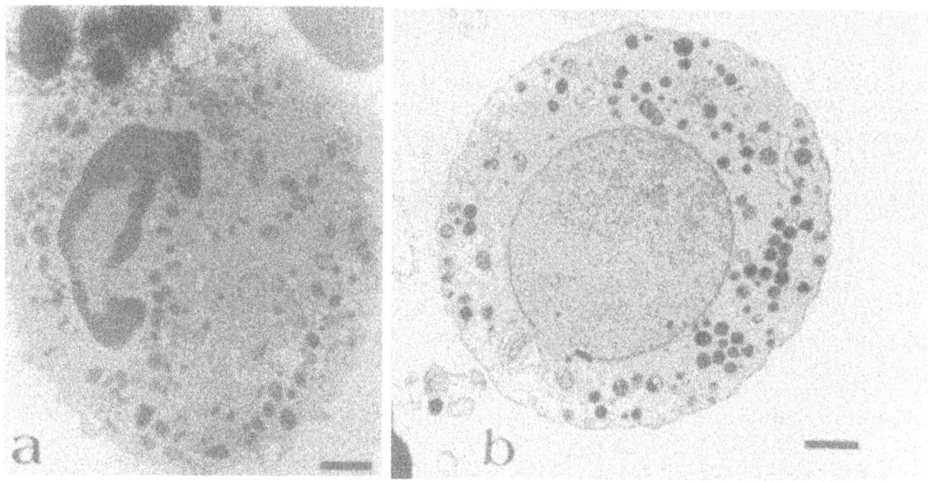

Fig. 1a. Transmission electron micrographs of a human neutrophil suspended in EDTA without pseudopods. The granules are irregular in shape. The insert shows individual granules at about 10-fold higher magnification. The length of the cross bars is 1 μm. 1b. Transmission electron micrograph of a human neutrophil in an hypotonic solution (200 mOsm). The granules exhibit almost uniformly circular cross sections. The length of the cross bar is 1 μm.

The primary granules are believed to be developed in the pregranulocyte stage,[5] whereas the secondary granules may develop as a result of pinocytosis, phagocytosis or autolytic events,[16] and may also be enzyme carriers. Figure 2 shows the radial distribution of these two types of granules as derived from neutrophil sections taken close to the center region of the cell, i.e. with cell section diameters greater than 8 μm. The data show a predominance of primary granules in the outer region of the cell, with the opposite trend for the secondary granules.

It has been suggested recently that there may exist a cortical shell made of actin in the

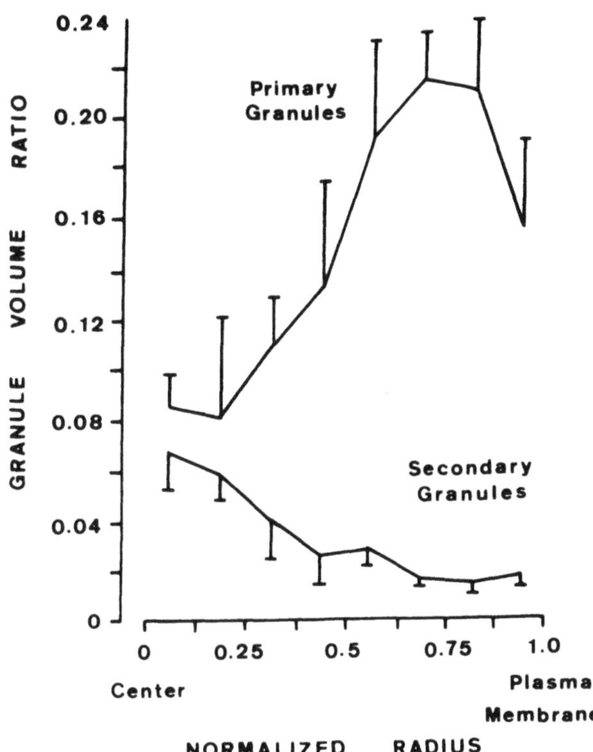

Fig. 2. Radial distribution of secondary and primary granules from five cell cross sections. Their cytoplasmic volume ratio, V_v, was measured in eight concentric ring regions from electron micrographs of cells transsected approximately through the center, as indicated by their large diameter (> 8 μm). The cells were suspended in heparin but were fixed before pseudopod formation was apparent. Mean values and standard deviations are shown for each type of granules.

submembrane space which provides in part the structural support for the cell.[17,18] If such a layer is made up of a cortical shell of fixed F-actin fibers, we expect an exclusion of granules in the shell. Figure 3 shows histograms of the closest approach between the immediate layer of subcortical primary and secondary granules and the plasma membrane. Both in heparin and EDTA the granules can approach the membrane to a distance of about 0.1 μm — 0.2 μm, but values less than this are observed less frequently. Mean values of closest approach position are of the order of 0.5 μm.

(c) Granule Exclusion of Pseudopods

One of the hallmarks of the initial phase of pseudopod formation is the exclusion of granules and other cell organelles. An example of this phenomenon in neutrophils and eosinophils is shown in Figure 4. During pseudopod projection the cells were kept in free suspension without adhesion to a substrate for a period of about 3 hr. Figure 5 shows the values for $(S_v)_G$ in passive and active states. The mean values for the two populations were the same within error of the measurement. Its uncertainty was estimated as the maximum possible error due to errors in the individual measurements and was found to be about 35%. Further confirmation for the absence of significant degranulation can also be obtained from measurements of the plasma membrane area/cell volume ratio, S_v. If a granule becomes incorporated into the plasma membrane and discharges its content into the cell exterior, S_v would increase due

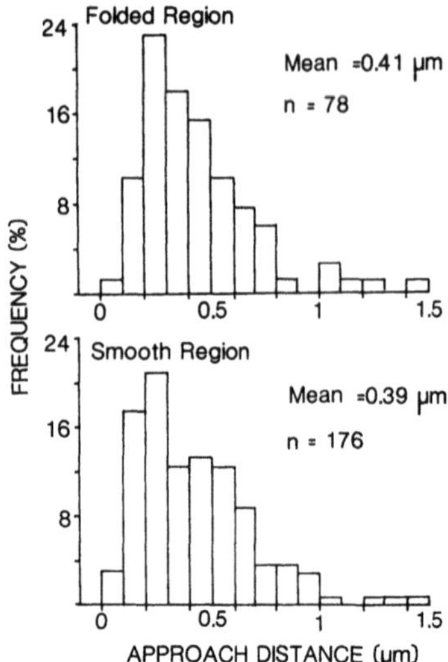

Fig. 3. The approach distance of cytoplasmic granules to the plasma membrane in neutrophils. The distance was measured as minimum length from the outer edge of the granule to the inner edge of the plasma membrane. Two cell regions were distinguished: (top) with the typical plasma membrane folds and (bottom) without folds. The cells were suspended and fixed in heparin with and without pseudopods. In these measurements only the outermost layer of granules adjacent to the plasma membrane was included. Similar measurements in EDTA gave the following results: in the region with folds the approach distance is 0.505 μm $\pm$ 0.231 μm (mean $\pm$ SD), in smooth regions without folds 0.450 μm $\pm$ 0.267μm.

to a gain in membrane area S and loss in volume $\overline{V}$. Measurement in passive cells gave a mean value of $S_v = 1.75$ μm^{-1} and in active cells $S_v = 1.70$ μm^{-1} (n = 50 random sections in each case) with a maximum measurement error estimated at 34%. Thus, the two values are also the same within error of measurment.

To demonstrate the redistribution of granules in the vicinity of the pseudopods, random sections of neutrophils, similar to that shown in Figure 4, were divided into three regions, (I) the pseudopod without any organelles, (II) the adjacent region about 2 μm in width where organelles are present, and (III) the inner region of the cell away from any pseudopods. The average granule density (volume of granules/volume of cytoplasm excluding the nucleus) were measured with the point counting technique. The results (Fig. 6) show that there is an enhancement of granule density in the cytoplasmic layer adjacent to the pseudopod (Region II). Similar observations were also made when the neutrophils under these conditions were in a more progressed active stage with more than one pseudopod present and without returning to the cell's original spherical configuration. Granule redistribution during pseudopod formation is also seen in monocytes and basophils. In lymphocytes no observations are available since they have a low granule density and are usually not activated under these circumstances.

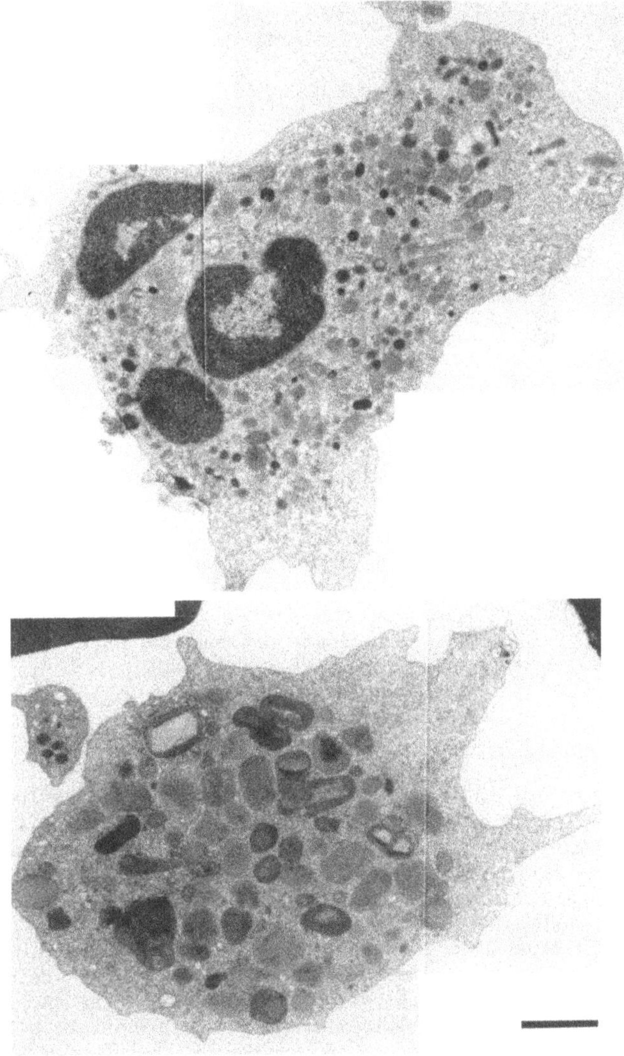

Fig. 4. Electron micrographic sections of eosinophil (top) and neutrophil (bottom) during pseudopod formation. The sections show the redistribution of the granules and exclusion from the tips of the pseudopods. The length of the cross bar is 1 μm.

DISCUSSION

The electron microscopic studies carried out in this and other studies have consistently confirmed the observation that after a conventional staining procedure of plastic resin sections, only a very thin layer of the stained surface of the sections is visible in the cytoplasm. In fact, if a conventional electron microscopic section after staining is re-embedded and sectioned at a right angle, a thin line is visible that coincides with the previously stained surface. Thus, in the current experiments no correction for section thickness was made. The data in the current study show striking differences in granule density, number, and size among the different types of leukocytes. Among the cells of a given kind the variation is small, and the standard deviations reported in Table I are in large part the result of measurement uncertainties. We have made several estimates of error by computing a total absolute differential of the measured quantity and thereby estimating the worst possible case. These values are different for each measurement and for each cell type, due to different visibilities on the sections. The magnitude

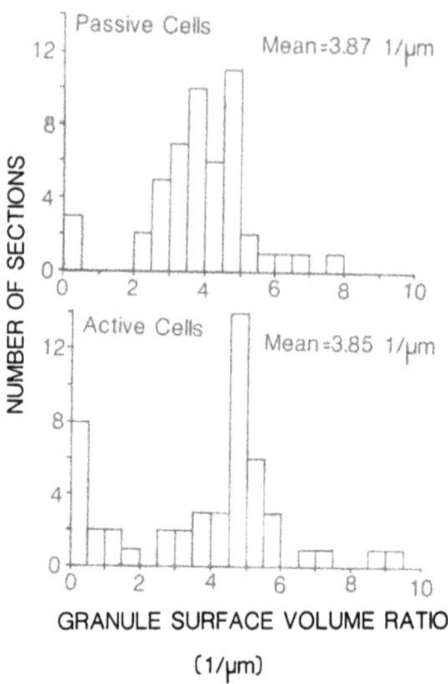

Fig. 5. Histogram of cytoplasmic granule membrane area per cell volume, $(S_v)_G$ in passive (top) and active neutrophils (bottom). Mean values and standard deviations are shown. The number of random electron microscopic sections analyzed in each case is n = 50.

of the maximum error for the data in Table I is generally less than 50% and typically 25% to 30%. The greatest error exists for the monocytes (about 40%) and is largely due to the problem that there exist cytoplasmic organelles whose identification and differentiation from the endoplasmic reticulum or membranes of the Golgi region is not always clear.

Our results suggest that the neutrophil has the largest number of granules with several thousand per cell. At first this was surprising since we had expected a lower number by just looking at single cell sections. Independent measurements of N_t by way of the ratio $V_t/\overline{V}$ and by way of the product $N_v \cdot V_c$, however, gave similar values. Our data do not include membrane structures in the vicinity of the Golgi region without an electron dense internal material.

The enzymatic content of the granules have in part been explored in the past. Bainton et al[19] have shown by means of a histochemical technique that the neutrophil's primary granules are the carrier of myeloperoxidase. Otherwise most of the current data on enzyme content has been derived from centrifugational fraction studies.[20,21] A summary of these enzymes is provided by Dewald et al.[22] These authors have described also the presence of a third type of granule, designated as C-particle. In our micrographs such a differentiation could not be made regularly, and the majority of these granules are probably lumped together with the secondary granules.

With the exception of the monocyte, the leukocytes probably have a low rate of lipid and protein synthesis while in the circulation. Thus, most of the lipid membranes are preformed in the cytoplasm and are therefore detectable by means of the electron microscope. It is possible to find several independent situations where membrane conservation has been documented. These include situations when the cells are swollen,[15] during micropipette aspiration,[23] during microsphere phagocytosis[10] and following cell compression on blood smears.[24] In light of the fact that there are other sources of membranes in the Golgi region, the endoplasmic reticulum, mitochondria and the nuclear envelope, the membrane of the granules seems to be specialized and the only one that is incorporated into the plasma membrane, e.g. during phagocytosis. This serves as further indication that the granules are not only subject to thermal motion, but are also controlled by specific interactions with the actin matrix and other organelles, a fact that is borne out also by granule specific exocytosis and the selective degranulation across the plasma membrane during microsphere phagocytosis versus degranulation into the phagosome after bacterial engulfment.[10] The underlying molecular mechanism is largely unexplored.

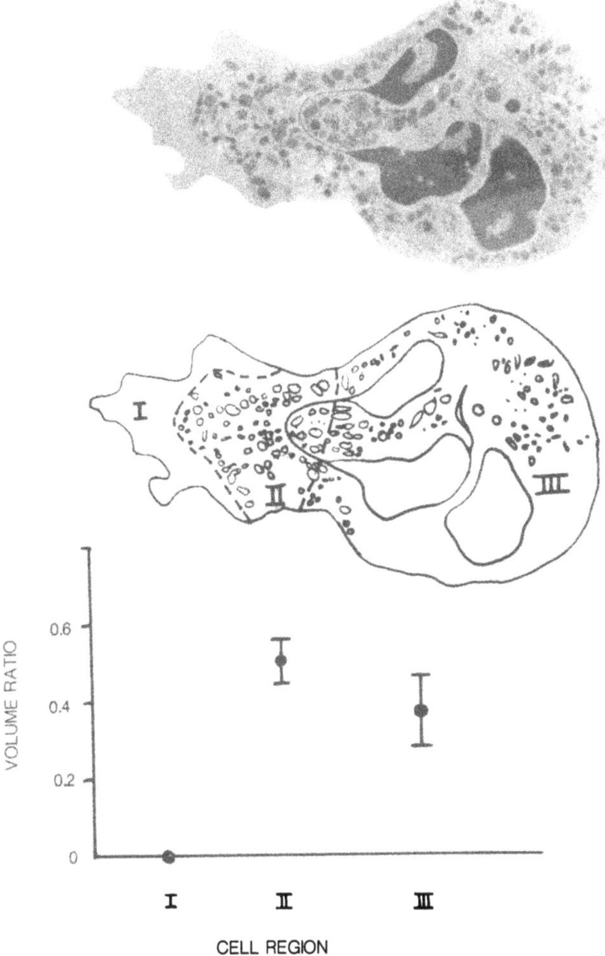

Fig. 6. The volume ratio, $(V_v)_G$, of granules and cell cytoplasm (without nucleus) in three adjacent regions in cells with pseudopods. The data are derived from 5 sections of different cells and the three regions were defined in each case as: (I) cytoplasm in the pseudopod without organelles; $(V_v)_G = 0$ by definition; (II) the adjacent region about 2 μm wide and (III) the region in the main cell body; in this region $(V_v)_G$ is about the same as in cells without pseudopods.

The current studies suggest that during the spontaneous activation of neutrophils in autologous plasma or in a reconstituted Ringer's-albumin solution, no morphologically detectable degranulation occurs. This is largely the result of the fact that we kept the cells in free suspension without any prolonged glass contact and adhesion. In contrast, if these cells were permitted to make contact with each other to form aggregates or with a solid substrate, exocytotic degranulation would occur. In this case pseudopod formation may project spontaneously and the granules can readily penetrate a cortical layer to fuse with the membrane.

As judged by the approach distance between the granule and plasma membranes, the thickness of the cortical layer, which was postulated largely from rheological studies, was found to be thin. No distinct morphological feature can be recognized with standard transmission electron microscopy. However, Boyles and Bainton[25] have been able to show, with a cell fracturing technique, the presence of an actin network in the submembrane space. They attached neutrophils firmly to a substrate and then sheared away the main cell body to leave in place the attached membrane and the adjacent cytoplasmic macromolecules. These observations suggest that there exists a firm attachment between the cell cytoplasm and membrane which may influence the fusion between granule and plasma membrane.

ACKNOWLEDGMENTS

This research was supported by USPHS Grants HL-16851 and HL-10881 from the National Heart, Lung and Blood Institute, U.S.A. and Research Grant NSC77-0412-B001-08 from the National Science Council, R.O.C. The authors would like to thank Brad Sargent and Marc Lacrampe for their excellent assistance with the stereological measurements.

REFERENCES

1. J. Berthet and C. Deduve, Tissue fractionation studies I. The existence of a mitochondria-linked, enzymatically inactive form of acid phosphatase in rat-liver tissue, *Biochem. J.* **50**:174 (1951).
2. R. Hirschhorn, Lysosomal mechanism in the inflammatory process, *in*: "The Inflammatory Process", B.W. Zweifach, L. Grant, R.T. McCluskey, eds., Academic Press, New York (1974).
3. J.G. Hirsch, Neutrophil leukocytes, *in*: "The Inflammatory Process", B.W. Zweifach, L. Grant, R.T. McCluskey, eds., Academic Press, New York (1974).
4. M. Baggiolini, The enzymes of the granules of polymorphonuclear leukocytes and their functions, *Enzyme,* **13**:131 (1972).
5. D.F. Bainton and M.G. Farquhar, Origin of granules in polymorphonuclear leukocytes. Two types derived from opposite faces of the Golgi complex in developing granulocytes, *J. Cell Biol.* **28**:277 (1966).
6. D.F. Bainton and M.G. Farquhar, Segregation and packing of granule enzymes in eosinophic leukocytes, *J. Cell Biol.* **45**:54 (1970).
7. F. Miller, E. Deharven and G.E. Palade, The structure of eosinophil leukocyte granules in rodents and in man, *J. Cell Biol.* **31**:349 (1966).
8. S.S. Spicer and J.H. Hardin, Ultrastructure, cytochemistry, and function of neutrophilic leukocyte granules, *Lob. Invest.* **20**:488 (1969).
9. M. Sato, M. Yonemaru and S. Sonoda, Quantitative analysis of secretory granules of the STH-cell in the rat hypophysis, *in*: "Recent Progress in Electron Microscopy of Cells and Tissues", E. Yamada V. Mizuhira, K. Kurosumi, T. Nagano, eds., University Park Press, Baltimore and London (1976).
10. S.I. Simon and G.W. Schmid-Schönbein, Biophysical aspects of microsphere engulfment by human neutrophils, *Biophys. J.* in press (1987).
11. G.W. Schmid-Schönbein and S. Chien, Morphornetry of human leukocyte granules, *Biorheology,* in press (1988).
12. E. Underwood, "Quantitative Stereology", Addison-Wesley, Reading, Massachusetts (1970).
13. R.L. Fullman, Measurement of particle sizes in opaque bodies, *J. Metals.* **197**:447 (1953).
14. G.W. Schmid-Schönbein, Rheology of leukkocytes, *in*: "Bioengineering", S. Chien, R. Skalak, eds., McGraw-Hill Book Co., New York (1987).
15. G.W. Schmid-Schönbein, Y.Y. Shih and S. Chien, Morphometry of human leukocytes, *Blood* **56**:866-875 (1980).
16. C. Deduve, The lysosome concept, *in*: "Ciba Foundation Symposium on Lysosomes", A.V.S. deReuck, M.P. Cameron, eds., Little Brown and Co., Boston (1963).
17. C. Dong, G.W. Schmid-Schönbein and R. Skalak, Rheological behavior of leukocytes, *in*: "Proc. 1985 Biomechanics Symposium", D. Bulter, T.K. Hung, R.E. Mates, eds., Joint ASCE/ASME Mechanics Conference, Albuquerque, New Mexico (1987).
18. E.A. Evans, Structural model for passive granulocyte behavior based on mechanical deformation and recovery after deformation tests, *in*: "White Cell Mechanics: Basic Science and Clinical Aspects", H.J. Meiselman, M.A. Lichtman, P.L. LaCelle, eds., Alan Liss, New York (1984).
19. D.F. Bainton, J.L. Ullyot and M.G. Farquhar, The development of neutrophilic polymorphonuclear leukocytes in human bone marrow. Origin and content of azurophil and specific granules, *J. Exp. Med.* **134**:907 (1971).
20. U. Bretz and M. Baggiolini, Biochemical and morphological characterization of asurophil and specific granules of human neutrophilic polymorphonuclear leukocytes, *J. Cell Biol.* **63**:251 (1974).
21. G. Murphy, U. Bretz, M. Baggiolini and J.J. Reynolds, The latent collagenase and gelatinase of

human polymorphonuclear neutrophil leukocytes, *Biochem. J.* **192**:517 (1980).

22. B. Dewald, U. Bretz and M. Baggiolini, Exocytosis induced in neutrophils by chemotactic agents and other stimuli, *in*: "Leukocyte Locomotion and Chemotaxis", Agents and Actions Supplements, H. Kellar, G.O. Till, eds., Birkhauser Verlag, Basel (1983).

23. K.L.P. Sung, G.W. Schmid-Schönbein, R. Skalak, G.B. Schuessler, S. Usami and S. Chien, Influence of physicochemical factors on rheology of human neutrophils, *Biophys. J.* **39**:101-106 (1982).

24. G.W. Schmid-Schönbein, K.-M. Jan, R. Skalak and S. Chien, Deformation of leukocytes on a hematological blood film, *Biorheology* **21**:767 (1984).

25. J. Boyle and D.F. Bainton, Changing patterns of plasma membrane-associated filaments during the initial phases of polymorphonuclear leukocyte adherence, *J. Cell Boil.* **82**:347 (1979).

PROSTAGLANDINS AND HEMOSTATIC FUNCTIONS OF VASCULAR ENDOTHELIUM

EFFECT OF VITAMIN E ON PROSTACYCLIN PRODUCTION FROM CULTURED AORTIC ENDOTHELIAL CELLS

Makoto Kunisaki, Fumio Umeda, Toyoshi Inoguchi, Hiroshi Ono
and Yasuhiro Sako

Third Department of Internal Medicine
Faculty of Medicine
Kyushu University
Fukuoka 812, Japan

INTRODUCTION

Vitamin E is known as a preventive agent against the development of atherosclerosis.[1] On the other hand, prostacyclin (PGI_2) generated by vascular endothelial cell is considered to play an important role to keep the homeostasis in vascular wall.[2-4] The reduction of PGI_2 production can be proposed as one of the possible causes of atherosclerosis. In our previous study, human plasma derived serum (PDS) showed a prostacyclin stimulatory activity (PSA) on cultured bovine aortic endothelial cells. Furthermore, the reduction of PSA in PDS was observed in diabetic rats and diabetic patients.[5,6] Since PSA can be one of the key modulators to the development of vascular lesions, the present study was done to evaluate the effect of vitamin E on PSA when stimulated by PDS.

MATERIAL AND METHODS

Preparation of plasma derived serum (PDS)

Ten healthy volunteers (age 45.0 ± 2.5 years, mean $\pm$ SEM) were chosen for the preparation. After overnight fasting, whole blood was collected from antecubital vein into a disposable syringe with 0.38% sodium citrate. Plasma was immediately separated by centrifugation. Then plasma was recalcified with 14mM $CaCl_2$, and allowed to clot at 37°C for 2 hours. After centrifugation, the supernatant was inactivated by heating at 56°C for 30 min. This specimen was used as PDS.

Endothelial cell culture

Endothelial cells were scraped off from thoracic aortic intima removed from young calves. The cells were cultured in Dulbecco's modified Eagle medium (DME) (Gibco Laboratories, Grand Island, New York) supplemented with 10% fetal calf serum (FCS) (Gibco Laboratories, Grand Island, New York) and 100μg/ml gentamycin (Schering Corporation, Kenilworth, New Jersey) at 37°C with 95% air and 5% CO_2. The medium was replaced twice weekly. Cells were identified as vascular endothelium by the morphological examination using a phase-contrast microscopy and the production of von Willebrand factor determined by a von Willebrand reagent (Behring Werk AG, Marburg, W. Germany). When the cells had reached monolayered confuluence, they were passaged with 0.05% trypsin solution. Then, the trypsinized cells were plated into 24-well cluster dishes (Flow Laboratories Inc., McLean, Virginia). The cells from the 5th to the 10th passage were used in the present experiment.

Determination of PSA

Confuluent cells were stimulated with DME containing 10% PDS for 1 hour with the addition or after the preincubation of vitamin E according to the experimental protocol. After the stimulation, the medium was removed and used for 6-keto-PGF$_{1\alpha}$ (a stable breakdown product of PGI$_2$) assay. PSA was expressed as the production of 6-keto-PGF$_{1\alpha}$ per 10^4 cells.

6-keto-PGF$_{1\alpha}$ assay

One-milliliter aliquot of the medium was acidified with 0.1 N HCl and extracted twice with 5ml of ethylacetate. The collected organic solvent was evaporated at 37°C and dissolved in 99.5% ethanol. The sample was kept at -20°C until assay. On the day of measurement, stock solution was again evaporated at 37°C and redissolved in 0.1 M phospate buffer (pH 7.2) with 1M NaCl and 0.1% gelatin. 6-keto-PGF$_{1\alpha}$ concentration was measured by radioimmunoassay using a kit obtained from New England Nuclear, Boston, Massachusetts. The bound and free ligands were separated with dextran-coated charcol, and the supernatant was counted in a LSC-700 liquid scintillation counter (Aloka, Tokyo, Japan).

Experimental protocol

At first, the effect of vitamin E on PGI$_2$ production was evaluated by the stimulation of DME containing 10% PDS with the simultaneous addition of vitamin E. When the endothelial cells reached monolayered confluence, they were washed twice with Dulbecco's phosphate buffered saline (PBS) (pH 7.2) without calcium and magnesium. Then, the cells were incubated with DME containing 10% PDS plus various concentrations of vitamin E. After 1 hour, the medium was removed and used for the measurement of PSA. Next, the effect of preincubation with vitamin E prior to the stimulation by 10% PDS was examined. After the preincubation with DME containing 10% FCS plus various concentrations of vitamin E, the cells were washed with PBS and stimulated by DME containing 10% PDS. PSA in these experiments were determined as mentioned above.

Data analyses

Student's *t* test was used for the differential analysis.

RESULTS

6-keto-PGF$_{1\alpha}$ production from cultured endothelial cells was stimulated by the addition of pooled PDS obtained from 10 healthy volunteers in a time and dose-dependent manner. It was confirmed that human PDS showed PSA on cultured bovine aortic endothelial cells. 6-keto-PGF$_{1\alpha}$ production reached a peak at 10min following the addition of DME containing 10% PDS. Then the maximal production of 6-keto-PGF$_{1\alpha}$ continued until 60min incubation. PDS stimulation of 6-keto-PGF$_{1\alpha}$ production showed the maximum with a final concentration of 10% (Fig. 1). Therefore, the stimulation by PDS was performed at 10% for 60min incubation.

Fig. 2. shows the effect of vitamin E addition when the cells were stimulated by DME containing 10% PDS plus vitamin E. It was demonstrated that vitamin E addition significantly enhanced 6-keto-PGF$_{1\alpha}$ production compared with the stimulation by 10% PDS alone. This additive enhancement of 6-keto-PGF$_{1\alpha}$ by vitamin E was observed in a dose dependent manner, and the maximal enhancement was observed at a dose of 4 μg/ml of vitamin E. However, vitamin E without 10% PDS did not affect 6-keto-PGF$_{1\alpha}$ production. There was no stimulation on 6-keto-PGF$_{1\alpha}$ production by any dose of vitamin E.

Fig. 3. shows the time effect of the preincubation with vitamin E prior to the 10% PDS stimulation. Endothelial cells were preincubated with DME containing 10% FCS plus 4μg/ml vitamin E. As shown in dotted bar, the production of 6-keto-PGF$_{1\alpha}$ stimulated by 10% PDS was significantly increased following the preincubation with vitamin E in a time dependent manner. The maximal enhancement was observed following 3 hour's preincubation prior to the 10% PDS stimulation. As shown in hatched bars, there was no effect of the preincubation without vitamin E on 6-keto-PGF$_{1\alpha}$ production by 10% PDS.

Fig. 4. shows the dose effect of the preincubation with vitamin E prior to the 10% PDS stimulation. The production of 6-keto-PGF$_{1\alpha}$ was significantly increased following 3 hour's

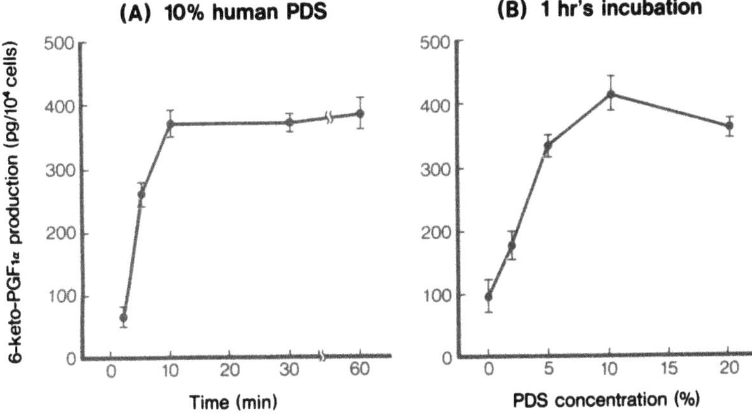

Fig. 1. Stimulation of 6-keto-PGF$_{1\alpha}$ production from cultured aortic endothelial cells by human plasma derived serum (PDS).

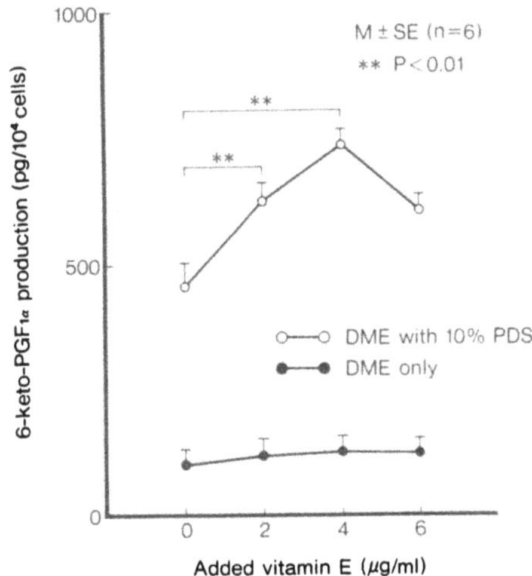

Fig. 2. Effect of 6-keto-PGF$_{1\alpha}$ production from cultured aortic endothelial cells by vitamin E.

preincubation with vitamin E in a dose dependent manner. The maximal enhancement was observed at a dose of 4μg/ml of vitamin E.

DISCUSSION

Vitamin E is known as an antioxidant which prevents the formation and accumulation of lipid peroxides in the vascular wall.[7] Therefore, it is considered that vitamin E is one of the effective agents against the development of atherosclerosis. However, the exact mechanism of its antiatherosclerogenecity has not been established yet. On the other hand, PGI$_2$ produced by vascular wall is an important factor to inhibit platelet aggregation and to protect the formation of thrombus and vascular lesions. Previous reports documented that vitamin E may affect the PGI$_2$ production in experimental animals.[8-12] Aorta obtained from animals supplemented with vitamin E generated greater amounts of PGI$_2$ than that from vitamin E deficiency.[11] It was suggested that the mechanisms of the increased PGI$_2$ production by vitamin E might be due to the activation of cyclooxygenase and/or the reduction of lipid peroxide formation which inhibits

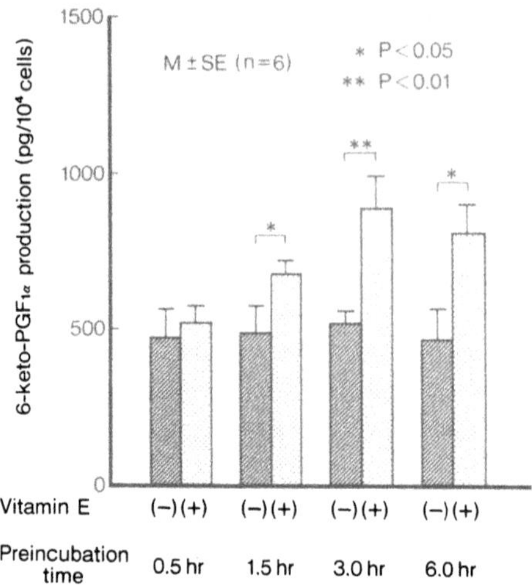

Fig. 3. Effect of 6-keto-PGF$_{1\alpha}$ production from cultured aortic endothelial cells by vitamin E (4µg/ml) following preincubation.

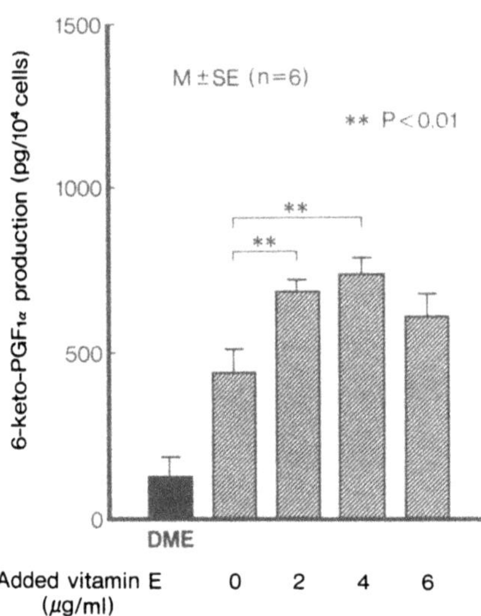

Fig. 4. Stimulation of 6-keto-PGF$_{1\alpha}$ production from cultured aortic endothelial cells by vitamin E following 3 hour's preincubation.

PGI$_2$ synthetase[13,14] However, the detail mechanism of its action remain unknown. Our previous study demonstrated that human plasma derived serum (PDS) has a prostacyclin stimulatory activity (PSA) on cultured bovine aortic endothelial cells.[5] In the present study, this PSA in PDS was used as the stimulator of PGI$_2$ production. It was evident that vitamin E in the presence of serum can enhance the PGI$_2$ production from cultured endothelial cells in a dose dependent manner, while vitamin E in the absence of serum showed no effect of PGI$_2$ production.

From these results, it was concluded that vitamin E with serum can be an effective agent for the PGI$_2$ production from vascular wall, leading to the prevention of development of vascular lesions such as atherosclerosis.

REFERENCES

1. G. Loewi, A lesion in the aorta of vitamin-E-deficient animals, *J. Path. Bact.* **50**:246 (1955).
2. S. Moncada, R.J. Gryglewski, S. Bunting and J.R. Vane, An enzyme isolated from arteries transforms prostaglandin endoperoxides to unstable substance that inhibits platelet aggregation, *Nature* **263**:663 (1976).
3. S. Moncada and J.R. Vane, Unstable metabolites of arachidonic acid and their role in haemostasis and thrombosis, *Br. Med. Bull.* **34**:129 (1978).
4. S. Moncada, E.A. Higgs and J.R. Vane, Human arterial and venous tissues generate prostacyclin (prostaglandin X), a potent inhibitor of platelet aggregation, *Lancet* **i**:18 (1977).
5. T. Inoguchi, F. Umeda, J. Watanabe and H. Ibayashi, Reduced serum stimulatory activity on prostacyclin production by cultured aortic endothelial cells in diabetes mellitus, *Haemostasis* **16**:447 (1986).
6. T. Inoguchi, F. Umeda, J. Watanabe and H. Ibayashi, Stimulatory activity on prostacyclin production decreases in sera from streptozotocin-induced diabetic rats, *Diab. Res. Clin. Pract.* **3**:243 (1987).
7. A.L. Tappel, Vitamin E and free radical peroxidation of lipids, *Ann. N.Y. Acad. Sci.* **203**:12 (1976).
8. A.C. Chan and M.K. Leith, Decreased prostacyclin synthesis in vitamin E-deficient rabbit aorta, *Am. J. Clin. Nutr.* **34**:2341 (1981).
9. M. Okuma, H. Takayama and H. Uchino, Generation of prostacyclin-like substance and lipid peroxidation in vitamin E-deficient rats, *Prostaglandins* **19**:527 (1980).
10. A.C. Chan and S. St-J. Hamelin, The effects of vitamin E and corn oil on prostacyclin and thromboxane B_2 synthesis in rats, *Ann. N.Y. Acad. Sci.* **393**:201 (1982).
11. C.W. Karpen, A.J. Melora, R.W. Trewyn, D.G. Cornwell and R.V. Panganamala, Modulation of platelet thromboxane A_2 and arterial prostacyclin by dietary vitamin E, *Prostaglandins* **22**:651 (1981).
12. C.W. Karpen, K.A. Pritchard Jr., J.H. Arnold, D.G. Cornwell and R.V. Panganamala, Restoration of prostacyclin/thromboxane A_2 balance in the diabetic rat. Infulence of dietary vitamin E, *Diabetes* **31**:947 (1982).
13. H. Sugumoto, M. Matumoto, T. Kimura and H. Ibayashi, The effect of vitamin E on the prostaglandin metabolism. Plasma lipoperoxide and aortic prostacyclin production in vitamin E deficient rats, *J. Jpn. Atheroscler. Soc.* **8**:575 (1980).
14. R.V. Panganamala and D.G. Cornwell, The effects of vitamin E on archidonic acid metabolism, *Ann. N.Y. Acad. Sci.* **393**:376 (1982).

PROSTACYCLIN PRODUCTION IN VASCULAR ENDOTHELIUM OF PATIENTS WITH BLACKFOOT DISEASE

Oi-Tong Mak

Department of Biology
National Cheng Kung University
Tainan 70101, Taiwan, Republic of China

INTRODUCTION

Blackfoot disease is an endemic disease of the peripheral vascular system reported more than fifty years ago in the southwest coast of Taiwan, Republic of China.[1] The symptoms are similar to those of the Buerger's disease or thromboangiitis obliterans.[2] It is characterized pathologically by intravascular clot formation and inflammation of the vascular wall, which lead to partial or complete occlusion of the vessels involved.[3] The area distributed by the diseased vessel then becomes discolored and gangrenous. The lesion often occurs on the lower extremities, hence the name Blackfoot disease.[4] Other findings include pigmentation, atherosclerosis and a high level of high density lipoprotein (HDL), but a low level of low density lipoprotein (LDL).[2,5] According to the statistics, 97% of Blackfoot disease patients will end up with either surgical amputation or natural disjointment due to gangrene.[6] After almost thirty years of investigations, no specific treatment has been found. The primary cause of Blackfoot disease still remains elusive despite some intensive studies.[7,8] Chen et al.[9] reported that the artesian well water of endemic areas contained high concentrations of arsenic (0.1 − 0.35 ppm). Lu and Ling[8] also found that ergotamine compounds were unusually high in level in the artesian well water. Both groups of investigators proposed that high concentrations of arsenic and ergotamine compounds in the drinking water in the endemic areas might be the main cause of Blackfoot disease. However, the installation of new water supply and drainage system since 1960 in the endemic areas has not eradicated or significantly reduced the incidence of the disease.[10] In the present report, study of prostaglandins, particularly on 6-keto $PGF_{1\alpha}$ and thromboxane B_2 (TXB_2), the stable natural metabolic intermediates of prostacyclin (PGI_2) and thromboxane A_2 (TXA_2) respectively, had been carried out among the patients. PGI_2 is an important factor in platelet anti-aggregation and blood vessel dilatation, and plays an important role in the prevention of atherosclerosis and arterial thrombosis.[11] TXA_2 exerts opposite physiological effects of PGI_2. The enzyme activities of prostacyclin synthase, the prime enzyme for the synthesis of PGI_2, and 15-hydroxyprostaglandin dehydrogenase (15-OH-PGDH), the enzyme involved in the conversion of PGI_2 to an inactive form 15-OH-PGI_2, were also studied. The aim is to determine whether there is any change in PGI_2 and TXA_2 metabolism in Blackfoot disease patients.

MATERIALS AND METHODS

Materials

All reagents and solvents used were of analytical grade supplied by Merck Chemical (Darmstadt, Federal Republic of Germany) unless otherwise stated. Glass distilled water was used throughout. Prostaglandin compounds were purchased from Upjohn Company (Kalamazoo,

Mich., U.S.A.). Radioactive prostaglandins and fatty acids were obtained from Amersham (Amersham, England). RIA kits for 6-keto-PGF$_{1a}$ and TXB$_2$ were purchased from New England Nuclear (Boston, Mass. U.S.A.). Scintillation cocktail was obtained from Lumac (Schaesberg, The Netherlands). Polypropylene test tubes and pipet tips were purchased from Gilson (Villiers-le-Bel, France). Arachidonic acid, NAD$^+$, heparin, aspirin (acetylsalicylic acid), and hematin were obtained from Sigma Chemical Company (St. Louis, Miss., U.S.A.). Sheep vesicular microsome was obtained from Hilran Biochemicals Ltd. (Tel-Aviv, Israel). TLC plates were purchased from Merck Chemical (Darmstadt, Federal Republic of Germany). Human arterial tissues were obtained from the Provincial Chiayi Hospital (Chiayi, Taiwan R.O.C.).

Preparation of human plasma

Fasting blood samples (2 ml) from 16 Blackfoot disease patients and 15 normal people were collected in polypropylene test tubes containing preweighed heparin (50 μg) and aspirin (acetylsalicyclic acid, 100 mg). Platelets and blood cells were removed immediately by centrifugation at 1,000 × g for 10 min. The supernatants were collected and kept in ice bath for testing of 6-keto-PGF$_{1a}$ and TXB$_2$ concentrations.

Radioimmunoassay

The levels of 6-keto-PGF$_{1a}$ and TXB$_a$ of the samples were determined by radioimmunoassay (RIA) as described by the manufacturer (NEN, Boston, Mass.). The concentrations of various 6-keto-PGF$_{1a}$ and TXB$_2$ standards used to construct the calibration curve were 50, 100, 250, 500, 1,000 and 2,500 pg/ml respectively. 100-μl of the standard or sample was added into RIA solution and mixed thoroughly, and the mixture was incubated overnight (16 hr) at 4°C. At the end of incubation, to all test tubes were added 500-μl pre-cooled charcoal suspension and the tubes were vortexed thoroughly. Suspensions were allowed to stand in ice bath for 15 min and centrifuged at 200 × g for 10 min. The supernatants were decanted without disturbing the charcoal residue, and the radioactivity measured in a LKB liquid scintillation counter.

Preparation of 15-OH-PGDH from human blood plasma

Human blood samples (2 ml) from Blackfoot disease patients and normal people were collected in polypropylene test tubes containing preweighed heparin (50 μg) and aspirin (acetyl-salicylic acid, 100 mg). Platelets and blood cells were removed immediately by centrifugation at 1,000 × g for 10 min and the platelet-poor plasma (PPP) were kept at 4°C. To the PPP was added ice-cold 1 M acetic acid, dropwise with stirring and cooling until the pH was 5.2. The precipitate was then spun for 1 hr at 10,000 r.p.m. (14,000 × g, Centrikon H-401, Kontron, Sweden) at 4°C. The supernatant was stored at 4°C and used for the assay of 15-OH-PGDH activity.

Enzyme assays of 15-OH-PGDH

Enzyme activity of 15-OH-PGDH in human blood plasma was measured spectrofluoro-metrically by the method of Mak and Chen[12] with excitation at 347 nm and emission at 468 nm in a Hitachi spectrofluorometer with prostaglandin E$_1$ (27 μM), NAD$^+$ (440 μM), glycerol (1.7%, v/v), ethanol (1.7%, v/v) and 50 mM potassium phosphate buffer, pH 7.4 at 37°C. One unit was defined as the transformation of 1 nmol of substrate in 1 min per ml of enzyme solution at 37°C.

Preparation of human arterial endothelial prostacyclin synthase

Samples of arterial vascular tissues from the Blackfoot disease patients or normal people were immediately kept in ice after amputation and brought to the laboratory for further study. The fat tissues were removed thoroughly from the artery, and the artery was washed with 100 mM Tris-HC1 buffer, pH 8.0. The tissues were rapidly frozen in liquid nitrogen and immediately homogenized into a fine powder by using a stainless steel blender. The powder was resuspended in 100 mM Tris-HC1 buffer, pH 8.0 (1:4, w/v) and homogenized at high speed by using a Potter-Elvehjem tissue grinder. The homogenate was then centrifuged at 10,000 X g for 30 min at 4°C. The supernatant was collected after centrifugation and used for the prostacyclin synthase assays.

Preparation of PGH₂

Preparation and purification of PGH_2 were carried out as described by Graff[14] using sheep vesicular microsome as enzyme source and $[1-{}^{14}C]$-arachidonic acid (5 µCi) as precursor.

Assay of prostacyclin synthase

Prostacyclin synthase activity was assayed by the modified method of Salmon and Flower.[13] Arterial tissue preparation (2 ml) was incubated with $[1-{}^{14}C]$-PGH_2 (0.2 µCi). After 3 min of incubation at 20°C, the protein in the mixture was precipitated with acetone (2 volumes). The mixture was centrifuged at 1,000 × g for 5 min and the aqueous phase was removed. To the aqueous phase, two volumes of petroleum ether was added and the mixture was vortexed thoroughly. The mixture was centrifuged at 1,000 × g for 5 min and the aqueous phase (lower layer) was removed. The pH of the aqueous phase was adjusted to between 4.0 and 4.5 with 1 M citric acid. Two volumes of chloroform was added to the aqueous solution and the mixture was vortexed thoroughly. Finally, the organic phase (lower layer) was removed and evaporated to dryness with nitrogen gas at 0°C. The residue was reconstituted in 100 µl of chloroform-methanol (2:1 v/v), and this solution was applied to TLC plate (50 µl each). The TLC plate was developed in the organic phase of ethyl acetate-2,2,4-trimethylpentane-acetic acid-water (110:50:20:100, v/v/v/v, upper phase). After development, the radioactive areas on the TLC plate were detected by radioisotopic TLC scanner and autoradiography. The relevent zones were then scraped off the plate, and the radioactivity in them was determined by liquid scintillation counting.

RESULTS

Radioimmunoassay of blood plasma

Results of the determination of the levels of 6-keto-PGF$_{1\alpha}$ and TXB_2 in the blood plasma of Blackfoot disease patients and normal individuals are summarized in Fig. 1. In the normal

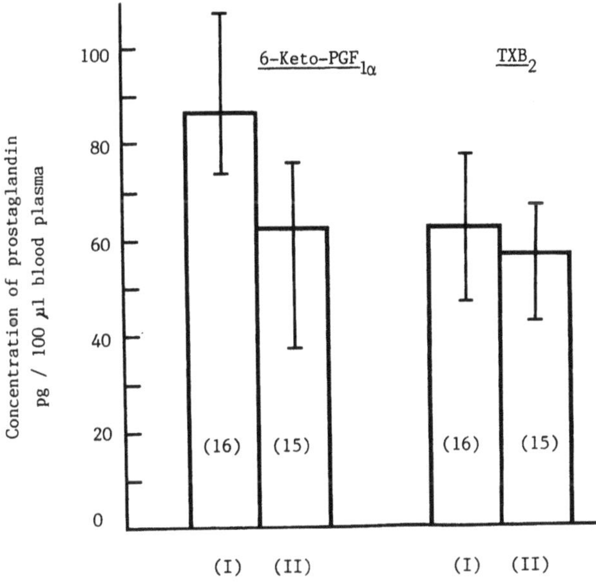

Fig. 1. Difference between normal people (I) and Blackfoot disease patients (II) of 6-keto-PGF$_{1\alpha}$ and TXB_2 concentration in blood plasma. Number of people tested are shown in brackets. TXB_2 and 6-keto-PGF$_{1\alpha}$ were measured by RIA method as described by the manufacturer (NEN, Mass., U.S.A.). For TXB_2 concentration, there is not any change between patients and normal people. For 6-keto-PGF$_{1\alpha}$ concentration, about 30% less among Blackfoot disease patients is observed.

controls, the average values of 6-keto-PGF$_{1\alpha}$ and TXB$_2$ in blood plasma were 870($\pm$81.6) and 608($\pm$99.5) pg/ml respectively, and in Blackfoot disease patients, they were 629($\pm$11.8) and 578($\pm$71.1) pg/ml respectively. No significant difference in the level of TXB$_2$ was observed between normal controls and Blackfoot disease patients. However, about 30% decrease in the level of 6-keto-PGF$_{1\alpha}$ is found in the patients. This result indicates either the rate of synthesis of PGI$_2$ by prostacyclin synthase in the endothelium is slower or the degradation of PGI$_2$ to 15-keto-PGI$_2$ by 15-OH-PGDH is enhanced.

Enzyme assay of 15-hydroxyprostaglandin dehydrogenase

The result of measuring 15-OH-PGDH activity in blood plasma shows less enzyme activity (29.8$\pm$1.6 nmol/min/ml) in Blackfoot disease patients than in normal controls (41.2$\pm$3.8 nmol/min/ml) (Fig. 2). These results suggest that the lower level of 6-keto-PGF$_{1\alpha}$ in blood plasma of Blackfoot disease patients is mainly caused by the slower rate of synthesis of PGI$_2$ in the endothelium.

Enzyme assay of prostacyclin synthase

Results of the assay of arterial prostacyclin synthase of Blackfoot disease patients and normal people control are shown in Fig. 3 and Table 1. 6-Keto-PGF$_{1\alpha}$ concentration was found to be lower after incubation of the arterial tissue of Blackfoot disease patients with PGH$_2$. This result suggests that prostacyclin synthase was either lacking or undetected in the endothelium of Blackfoot disease patients.

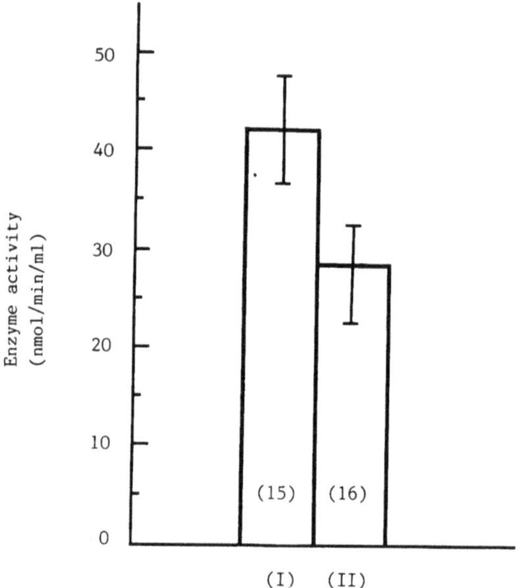

Fig. 2. Enzyme activity of 15-OH-PGDH in blood plasma among normal people (I) and Blackfoot disease patients (II). Number of people tested are shown in brackets. Assays of 15-OH-PGDH were carried out by measuring the rate of formation of NADH spectrofluorometrically with excitation at 347 nm and emission at 468 nm with PGE$_1$ (27 μM), NAD$^+$ (440 μM), glycerol (1.7%, v/v), ethanol (1.7%, v/v) and 50 mM potassium phosphate buffer, pH 7.4 at 37°C. One unit was defined as the transformation of 1 nmol of substrate in 1 min per ml of enzyme solution at 37°C. Blackfoot disease patients were found to have lower enzyme activity of 15-OH-PGDH (41.2$\pm$3.8 units) than normal controls (29.8$\pm$1.6 units).

Table 1. Radioactive countings (cpm) of the reaction products of prostacyclin synthase extracted from the arterial endothelium of Blackfoot disease patient (lane 1) and normal people (lane 2), and
prostaglandins standards (lane 3 and lane 4) respectively after
separating on TLC. Relevant zones were scraped off and the
radioactivity in them was determined by liquid scintillation counting. ND means not determined.

	Lane 1	Lane 2	Lane 3	Lane 4
^{14}C-AA	ND	86,548	ND	ND
^{14}C-PGH$_2$	3,576	ND	2,127	1,850
^{14}C-PGD$_2$	4,248	ND	7,037	7,246
^{14}C-PGD$_2$	6,741	ND	8,535	8,068
^{14}C-6-Keto-PGF$_{1\alpha}$	ND	ND	452	2,153

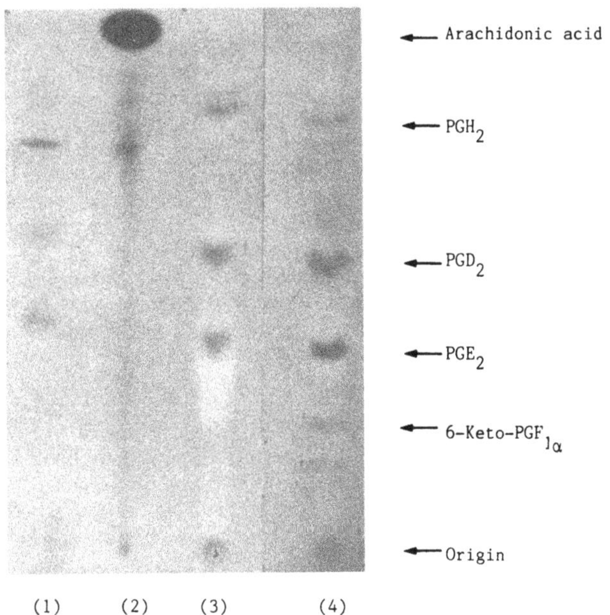

Fig. 3. Autoradiography of the production of prostacyclin among
the normal people (lane 4) and Blackfoot disease patients (land 3)
arterial endothelium by incubation with [1-^{14}C]-PGH$_2$. Radioactive
arachidonic acid, PGH$_2$, PGD$_2$ and PGE$_2$ are shown in lane 2 and
lane 1. Arterial endothelium prostacyclin synthase was prepared
as described in the text. [1-^{14}C]-PGH$_2$ was prepared by the method
of Graff.[14] Results showed that lower enzyme activity of prostacyclin synthase was present in Blackfoot disease patients. We
conclude that the lower concentration of 6-keto-PGF$_{1\alpha}$ obtained
in blood plasma among Blackfoot disease patients is directly
caused by the lower enzyme activity of prostacyclin synthase in
the endothelium.

DISCUSSION

It is well accepted that the balance between PGI_2 and TXA_2 production in the endothelium and platelets, respectively, is one of the crucial factors for the control of blood coagulation, vessel dilatation and vessel constriction.[15] Either lower PGI_2 production in endothelium or higher TXA_2 production in platelets will contribute to the formation of atherosclerosis or other peripheral vascular diseases.[11] As mentioned above, Blackfoot disease is reported to be an endemic disease of the peripheral vascular system in the southwest coast of Taiwan, Republic of China. For the past thirty years, Blackfoot disease is fatal because of lacking of effective drug or treatment for therapy. Moreover, the cause of this disease is still uncertain. Investigation on the concentrations of various prostaglandins in blood plasma will show their effects on the development of this disease. In this report, the concentration of PGI_2 in blood plasma of Blackfoot disease patients was found to be lower but the level of TXA_2 was normal compared to normal people. The concentration of PGI_2 in blood plasma is attributed to two metabolic pathways. They are the prostacyclin synthase and 15-OH-PGDH pathways. Either decreasing the enzyme activity of prostacyclin synthase or increasing the enzyme activity of 15-OH-PGDH will lower the concentration of PGI_2 in blood plasma. According to this study, 15-OH-PGDH enzyme activity was found to be lower in the blood plasma of Blackfoot patients. This indicates that the inactivation of PGI_2 by 15-OH-PGDH in patients should be lower than normal people, and the amount of PGI_2 present in blood plasma should be comparatively higher. However, the concentration of PGI_2 in blood plasma of patients was lower. Therefore, change of the enzyme activity of 15-OH-PGDH is not the cause for the lower concentration of PGI_2 found in blood plasma of Blackfoot disease patients. On the other hand, the enzyme activity of prostacyclin synthase was found to be undetectable in the arterial endothelium of Blackfoot disease patients after incubation with $[^{14}C]$-arachidonic acid. This is a very important discovery because PGI_2 is mainly synthesized in blood-vessel endothelium. If the enzyme activity of prostacyclin synthase in endothelium is lower, the rate of synthesis of PGI_2 will be slower and the balance between PGI_2 and TXA_2 will be disturbed. This disturbance will cause blood platelet aggregation and vasoconstriction which are the symptoms of Blackfoot disease. The low activity of prostacyclin synthase found might be related to the marked degeneration of the endothelial layer of the patient's ischaemic artery[16] which is unable to synthesize normal amount of PGI_2. All these results suggest that the cause of the pathological symptoms of Blackfoot disease might be contributed by the lower concentration of PGI_2 present in blood plasma which is caused by the lower enzyme activity of prostacyclin synthase in the endothelium. Forthermore, the inhibitory effects on PGI_2 production in cultured umbilical vein endothelium were related to the high concentration of ergotamine compounds, but not to the high concentration of arsenate.[17] Therefore, a higher concentration of arsenate present in the artesian well water of endemic areas might not be the main cause of Blackfoot disease. A careful survey of the endemic areas should be carried out. For the further study of Blackfoot disease, there will be two directions. The study of the inhibitions of prostacyclin synthase should be given first priority. Moreover, these results aim to provide the best treatment for Blackfoot disease. Due to the lower amount of PGI_2 in blood plasma of Blackfoot disease patients, treatment with infusion of PGI_2 or its analogs should be a proper trial to prevent this disease from further deterioration.

SUMMARY AND CONCLUSION

The levels of 6-keto-$PGF_{1\alpha}$ and TXB_2 were determined by the RIA method in Blackfoot disease which is an endemic disease of the peripheral vascular system found in the southwest coast of Taiwan. The level of TXB_2 was normal, but that of 6-keto-$PGF_{2\alpha}$ concentration was 30% lower than the normal. The activity of 15-hydroxyprostaglandin dehydrogenase was higher in patients' blood plasma than in the normal. Patient's vascular endothelium was also found to have lower prostacyclin synthase activity. These results suggest that the reduced prostacyclin production in vascular endothelium contributes to the pathogenesis of Blackfoot disease.

ACKNOWLEDGMENTS

I would like to thank Dr. M.Y. Wang from the Provincial Chiayi Hospital (Chiayi, Taiwan R.O.C.) for the free gifts of patients' and normal people' arterial tissues. I also want to thank Miss S.H. Chen for her assistance in the purification of 15-OH-PGDH and prostacyclin synthase. This work was supported by National Science Council, Republic of China (Grant NSC73-0412-B006-04 and NSC74-0204-B006-01).

REFERENCES

1. S. Yeh and S.W. How, A pathological study on the Blackfoot disease in Taiwan. *Reports, Institute of Pathology, Nat. Taiwan Univ.*, **14**:25 (1963).
2. W.P. Tseng, Outcome of patients with blackfoot disease, *J. Formosan Med. Asso.*, **74**:37 (1975).
3. F.J. Lu, Study on fluorescent compounds in drinking water of endemic areas for Blackfoot disease and re-investigation of the causes of Blackfoot disease, *National Science Council Monthly*, **6**:388 (1978).
4. K.P. Chen and H.Y. Wu, Epidemiologic studies on Blackfoot disease 2. A study of source of drinking water in relation to the disease, *J. Formosan Med. Asso.*, **81**:611 (1962).
5. F.L. Lee, Personal communication. Provincial Tainan Hospital, Taiwan, Republic of China (1985).
6. W.Y. Chen and E.P. Lien, Experimental studies on the drinking water of Blackfoot disease endemic areas 1. Studies on the changes of the limbs of experimental rats receiving repeated injections of drinking water of Blackfoot disease endemic area, *J. Formosan Med. Asso.*, **62**:794 (1963).
7. W.Y. Chen and W.P. Tseng, Experimental studies on the drinking water of Blackfoot disease endemic areas 3. Skin test with drinking water of Blackfoot disease endemic area, *J. Formosan Med. Asso.*, **63**:298 (1964).
8. F.J. Lu and K.H. Ling, Studies on fluorescent compounds in drinking water of Blackfoot disease endemic areas 6. A preliminary experimental study on peripheral vasculopathy, *J. Formosan Med. Asso.*, **78**:314 (1979).
9. K.P. Chen, H.Y. Wu and T.C. Wu, Epidemiologic studies on Blackfoot disease in Taiwan 3. Physiochemical characteristics of drinking water in endemic Blackfoot disease area, *Memoirs Coll. Med. Nat. Taiwan Univ.*, **8**:115 (1962).
10. O.T. Mak, S.J. Huang and S.H. Chen, Study of Blackfoot disease—sex, age, duration of disease, occupation and geographic distribution, *J. Cheng Kung Univ. Sci., Eng. & Med. Section*, **20**:119 (1985).
11. S. Moncada, Biology and therapeutic potential of prostacyclin, *Prog. Cerebrovascular Disease*, **14**:157 (1983).
12. O.T. Mak and S.H. Chen, Effects of two anti-depressant drugs—imipramine and amitriptyline—on the enzyme activity of 15-hydroxyprostaglandin dehydrogenase purified from brain, lung, liver and kidney from mouse, *Prog. Lipid Res.*, **25**:153 (1986).
13. J.A. Salmon and R.J. Flower, Preparation and assay of prostacyclin synthase, *Methods in Enzymol.*, **86**:91 (1982).
14. G. Graff, Preparation of PGG_2 and PGH_2, *Methods in Enzymol.*, **86**:376 (1982).
15. J.M. Bailey, Prostacyclins, thromboxanes and cardiovascular disease, *TIBS*, **4**:68 (1979).
16. Y.C. Ko, A critical review of epidemiologic studies on Blackfoot disease, *J. UOEH*, **8**:339-353 (1986).
17. O.T. Mak, S.H. Chen and M.H. Cheng, Effects of arsenate and ergot alkaloid compounds on prostacyclin synthesis in human umbilical endothelium, *Cell Biol. Int. Rep.*, **10**:287 (1986).

ENDOTHELIAL CELL FUNCTION IN HEMOSTASIS AND THROMBOSIS

Kenneth Kun-yu Wu, Karen Frasier-Scott and Helen Hatzakis

Division of Hematology-Oncology
Department of Internal Medicine
University of Texas, Health Science Center at Houston
Houston, TX 77225, USA

INTRODUCTION

The endothelium comprises a single layer of polygonal cells lining the entire length of blood vessels. It plays a pivotal role in modulating a number of physiologic and pathophysiologic processes including hemostasis, thrombosis, inflammation and immune responses.[1] This review will focus on the endothelial cell function in hemostasis and thrombosis. Hemostasis is a complex event involving multiple interactions between blood cells and the damaged vessel wall, the coagulation proteins and blood cell constituents and the cell-cell interactions. These complex biologic processes generally do not occur without endothelial damage. Intact endothelium appears to function not only as a physical barrier which blocks active interaction between the cellular and protein constituents of blood and the vessel wall but also as a biologically active tissue capable of synthesizing compounds that promote and control hemostatic function. Moreover, its surface possesses specific properties for modulating certain key reactions in the coagulation cascade.

Endothelial cells contribute significantly to the intricate balance and check system of hemostasis. For example, they produce molecules, i.e. von Willebrand factor (vWF), which promotes platelet adhesion to the subendothelium. They possess active membrane property for an alternative activation of the coagulation cascade. On the other hand, the endothelial cell surface exhibits unique properties to neutralize thrombin and to activate anticoagulant proteins such as protein C. They are capable of synthesizing the secreting plasminogen activators which facilitate lysis of blood clots. Further, when endothelial cells are activated, arachidonic acid is liberated and metablized to eicosanoids which possess potent action in regulating platelet aggregation and vascular reactivity. Hence, endothelial cells are an integral part of hemostatic and thrombotic reactions. Their contributions to various stages of hemostasis are summarized in Table 1 and will be discussed further with respect to their membrane properties, synthesis of coagulation and fibrinolysis proteins and eicosanoid formation.

ENDOTHELIAL CELL FUNCTION

1. Endothelial cell surface function. The endothelial cell membrane exhibits both procoagulant and anticoagulant properties. The procoagulant activity is triggered by the expression of tissue factor on its surface while the anticoagulant activity is initiated by binding of thrombin to a unique membrane receptor, thrombomodulin. Thrombomodulin is a specific thrombin receptor present in unstimulated endothelial cells.[2,3] Under stressful conditions, thrombin is generated and binds to thrombomodulin whereby protein C, a vitamin K dependent protein is activated and in the presence of its cofactor, protein S, it degrades factors V and VIII and hence limits the coagulation reaction.[4-6] In addition, activated protein C enhances fibrinolytic activity.[7] The bound thrombin is ultimately internalized and its activity is neutralized.[7] Furthermore, the endothelial cell membrane contains heparin-like molecules which enhance the neutralization

Table 1. Promotion and Inhibition of Hemostasis by endothelial Cells

	Endothelial Function	Key Activity
Coagulation:		
Pro-coagulant	(1) Expression of tissue factor on cell surface	↑ Thrombin
	(2) Binding of factor IX and IXa	↑ Thrombin
Anticoagulant	(1) Thrombomodulin-mediated thrombin activation of protein C	↓ fV and VIII
	(2) Internalization of thrombin	↓ Thrombin
	(3) Heparin-like molecules	↓ Thrombin
Platelet:		
Promoting	(1) vWF synthesis and secretion	platelet adhesion
	(2) Other adhesive glycoproteins	? platelet adhesion
Inhibiting	(1) Prostacyclin generation	↓ Platelet aggregation and secretion
Fibrinolysis:		
Promoting	(1) Tissue-type plasminogen activator (tPA)	↑ Plasmin
Inhibitors	(1) Plasminogen activator inhibitor	↓ tPA

of thrombin by antithrombin III.[8,9] It appears reasonable to assume that intact endothelium adjacent to vascular injury sites plays a critical role in down-regulating the hemostatic and/or thrombotic plug formation. Tissue factor (TF) is a complex of tissue factor apoprotein with phospholipid. TF is expressed following endothelial cell activation by physiologic agonists such as interleukin-1 (IL-1).[10,11] Once exposed, it serves as a co-factor for factor VII-initiated extrinsic coagulation pathway.[10] Recent studies have shown that factor VIIa may bind to endothelial cell surface and utilize TF expression as a cofactor to activate membrane bound factor IX to IXa[12-14] with the eventual generation of thrombin. The endothelial cell membrane hence functions as a bridge which links the extrinsic with the intrinsic coagulation cascade. This observation has generated great interest, but its relative physiologic role remains to be established. It seems possible that this coagulation activation process may have particular implications in certain pathophysiological condition initiated by direct endothelial insults such as endotoxin-induced disseminated intravascular coagulation.

2. von Willebrand factor and other glycoproteins. Platelets do not adhere to intact endothelium. However, once the endothelium is disrupted, they adhere to the subendothelial tissue. Adhesion of platelets to the subendothelium is mediated by von Willebrand factor (vWF), a multimeric protein synthesized by the endothelial cells as a 250 kD molecule.[15] It is cleaved into a 225 kD subunit and then processed into multimeric forms with molecular weight up to 20 million Da.[16,17] vWF appears to be stored in the Weibel-Palade body and released under physiologic stimulation.[18,19] Synthesis and release of vWF is highly regulated to maintain a tight circulating level among normal human subjects. The mechanism by which vWF mediates platelet adhesion to the subendothelial matrix is not entirely unclear. Recent studies suggest that vWF probably functions as a bivalent molecule which binds to platelets on one hand and to the subendothelial proteins on the other.[20] Circulating vWF also binds to coagulation factor VIII whereby the factor VIII activity is stabilized.[21] Immunochemical studies have shown that vWF is also released into the subendothelial matrix. Besides vWF, several other related glycoproteins such as fibronectin, thrombospondin and glycoaminoglycans as well as several subtypres of procollagen are produced by endothelial cells and released into the subendothelial matrix.[22,23] These cellular adhesive proteins probably play a role in regulating platelet vessel wall interaction and in maintaining vascular integrity.

3. Plasminogen activators (PA) and PA inhibitors. Fibrinolysis represents the ultimate defense mechanism against excessive fibrin formation. The reaction is triggered by the release of plasminogen activators (PA), which catalyze the conversion of plasminogen into plasmin. Plasmin is a potent serine protease which catalyzes the lysis of fibrin. Two types of PA's are identified, i.e. tissue-type (tPA) and urokinase (uPA).[24] Endothelial cells appear to be capable of synthesizing both types of plasminogen activators.[24,25] The relative physiologic role of these 2 types of PA's in catalyziing the fibrinolytic reaction remains to be established. It is further complicated by the recent demonstration of generation by endothelial cells of specific inhibitors

against plasminogen activator (PAI).[24,26] More than one type of PAI have been identified in various tissue and the PAI type produced by endothelial cells is categorized as type 1 (PAI-1). PAI-1 binds and inactivates tPA. As endothelial cells produce tPA and PAI concurrently under physiological stimulation, PAI probably plays a major role in controlling the fibrinolytic activity.

4. Eicosanoid production. Eicosanoids are metabolites of arachidonic acid which function as autacoids in modulating biological processes. Upon endothelial cell stimulation, arachidonic acid is liberated from membrane phospholipids and metabolized via 2 enzymatic pathways. In the so-called cyclooxygenase pathway, PGH synthase catalyzes the conversion of arachidonic acid to PGG_2 and then to PGH_2. PGH_2 is further converted to prostacyclin (PGI_2) by PGI synthase. PGH_2 may also be converted to PGE_2 and $PGF_{2\alpha}$. Lipoxygenase catalyzes the conversion of arachidonic acid to hydroperoxyeicosatetraenoic acid (HPETE) which is then hydrolyzed to hydroxyeicosatetraenoic acid (HETE). A number of lipoxygenase enzymes have been identified in various cells. The major lipoxygenase enzyme in endothelial cells is 15-liopxygenase which generates 15-HETE. In addition to the above eicosanoids, thromboxane as well as 12-HETE and 11-HETE are produced by endothelial cells in trace quantities. Although the eicosanoid productions differ due to species or vascular origin differences of endothelial cells, the major eicosanoid is prostacyclin (PGI_2).[27] PGI_2 is a potent vasodilator and inhibitor of platelet aggregation.[28] It plays a significant role in controlling platelet aggregate formation on the damaged vessel wall. The physiologic role of other eicosanoids from endothelial cells is less clear.

MODULATION OF ENDOTHELIAL FUNCTION

Endothelial cells are highly reactive. The membrane as well as the synthetic and secretory activities are highly regulated by a number of agents including thrombin, histamine, bradykinin, hypoxia and mechanical stress[28-33] (Table 2). Thrombin plays a key role in hemostasis. It is a potent serine protease which promotes hemostatic and thrombotic plug formation by catalysis of conversion of fibrinogen into fibrin and stimulation of platelet aggregation. Paradoxically, it also plays a major part in the control of hemostasis through its stimulation of prostacyclin production and activation of protein C as described earlier. Moreover, thrombin appears to stimulate tPA and PAI-1 production by endothelial cells with an overall effect of suppressing fibrinolytic activity.[34]

Recent studies have shown that cytokines exhibit diversified effects on endothelial cell function (Table 3). For example, interleukin-1 (IL-1) stimulates endothelial cell prostacyclin synthesis, induces tissue factor expression, regulates fibrinolytic activity and enhances the interaction between polymorphonuclear cells and endothelial cells.[35,36] Tumor necrosis factor exhibits overlapping property with IL-1 while interferon-gamma has little effects on endothelial cells except for causing distinct morphological changes. We have been interested in understanding how IL-2 modulates endothelial cell function. IL-2 is a 15 kD glycoprotein secreted by lymphoctyes. It was first described as a lymphokine capable of promoting the long term growth of activated T-lymphocytes in vitro.[37,38] It has subsequently been shown to modulate the functions of several subtypes of lymphocytes including cytotoxic T-cells,[30,40] natural killer cells,[41,42] activated B cells[43,44] and lymphokine activated killer cells.[45,46] We discovered that the biological activity of IL-2 is not entirely limited to lymphocytes. When purified natural IL-2 was added to freshly prepared bovine aorta, it caused endothelial cells to undergo dramatic shape change and contraction and perturbed the vascular permeability. Further, it stimulated endothelial cells to synthesize prostacyclin.[47] Similar stimulatory effect was observed when IL-2 was added to cultured human

Table 2. Modulators of endothelial cell function

1. Thrombin

2. Vasoactive amines
    Histamine, bradykinin

3. Blood cell products
    PMN: elastase
    Mononuclear cells: cytokines

4. Insults
    Hypoxia
    Mechanical
    Endotoxain

Table 3. Modulation of endothelial cell function by cytokines

	IL-1	TNF	IFN-γ	IL-2
Surface function				
TF Expression	↑	↑	N	
Synthetic Function				
PGI_2	↑		N	↑
vWF			N	N
tPA	↓		N	N
PAI				
Cell adhesion				
Granulocytes	↑	↑	N	
Monocytes	↑	↑	N	
Lymphocytes	↑	↑	N	
Morphologic Change		+	+	+

Abbreviations: TNF: Tumor necrosis factor
IFN-γ: Interferon-Gamma
IL-1 and IL-2: Interleukin 1 and 2

Symbols: ↑ elevation: N: No effect, ↓ Suppression
Blank: unknown   + Positive effect

umbilical vein endothelial cells (HUVECS) and bovine aorta endothelial cells (BAECS). The stimulation was dose- and time-related.[47] The steady rate of PGI_2 stimulation by IL-2 over a 24 hour period is interesting because previous studies have shown that PGI_2 stimulation by exogenous arachidonic acid is a self limited process due to autoinactivation of cyclooxygenase activity of PGH synthase.[48-50] That IL-2 stimulation is sustained over a prolonged period of time implies de novo synthesis of PGH synthase. To test this hypothesis, we have performed 3 different experiments. The first series of experiments involved pretreating cells with a specific protein inhibitor, cycloheximide, and a RNA synthesis inhibitor, actinomycin D, followed by stimulation of the cells with IL-2. Both inhibitors exerted a dose-related inhibition of IL-2 stimulated PGI_2 synthesis. Hence, IL-2 stimulation of PGI_2 synthesis depends on protein synthesis. We then treated the endothelial cells with aspirin which causes a permanent inactivation of PGH synthase. Following washing off free aspirin, the cells were treated with fresh medium in the presence and absence of IL-2. At various time periods, arachidonic acid was added and $6KPGF_{1\alpha}$ production was measured. In the absence of IL-2, aspirin-treated cells produced little $6KPGF_{1\alpha}$. By contrast, those cells incubated with IL-2 were able to synthesize $6KPGF_{1\alpha}$ after only 4 hrs of IL-2 stimulation. The generation of PGH synthase under IL-2 stimulation was further determined by Western blot using a polyclonal antibody directed against ram vesicle PGH synthase. This antibody cross-reacts with the endothelial cell enzyme. Preliminary data indicate that the 70 kD PGH synthase band was enhanced by IL-2 2 hrs after the addition of IL-2 to the cultured cells. We then carried out additional experiments to determine whether the IL-2 induced de novo synthesis of PGH synthase in endothelial cells is a selective process. Does IL-2 concurrently stimulate production of physiologically important proteins such as vWF and tPA? Cultured HUVECS were incubated with IL-2 and at various time periods, the medium was removed and its vWF, tPA and $6KPGF_{1\alpha}$ content was measured by immunoassays. Contrary to a time-related increase in 6-keto-$PGF_{1\alpha}$ level, there was no elevation of tPA or vWF concentrations. Hence, IL-2 appears to exert a rather specific stimulatory effect on de novo synthesis of PGH synthase to permit a sustained production of PGI_2. As PGI_2 is a potent autacoid with multiple biological activites including vasodilatation, vascular permeability, suppressing immune responses and inhibiting platelet aggregation, selective stimulation of PGI_2 production is likely to have important physiologic and pathophysiologic implications particularly at sites where there is an active contact between lymphocytes and vascular endothelium.

SUMMARY AND DISCUSSION

Endothelial cells play a pivotal role in hemostasis and thrombosis. They produce a myriad of factors either associated with the membrane or released into the blood stream and the subendothelial matrix which are involved in various steps of hemostasis. The endothelial cell function is modulated by a diversified group of biologically active molecules, notably thrombin, vasoactive amines and cytokines. Mechanism and selectivity of the effects of these molecules differ and the difference may have important physiolgoical implications. Most of the information is gathered through experiments performed in cultured endothelial cells. Availability of the cultured cells has greatly facilitated the understanding of endothelial cell biology. In vivo models, however, are still needed to understand how the endothelial cell function is modulated. Furthermore, as the cultured endothelial cells exhibit nor only species diferences but also vascular origin difference in behavior and function, these factors should be carefully considered when designing experiments involving the use of cultured endothelial cells.

ACKNOWLEDGMENTS

The authors wish to thank Dr. Elizabeth R. Hall for providing endothelial cells and Ms. Mary Morrison for excellent assistance in preparing the manuscript.

The work is supported by a Program Project Grant for U.S. Public Health Service, National Institute of Health (P50 NS-18494)

REFERENCES

1. M.A. Gimbrone, ed., "Vascular endothelium in Hemostasis and Thrombosis," Churchill Livingstone, Edinburgh (1986).
2. C.T. Esmon and W.G. Owen, Identification of an endothelial cell cofactor for thrombin catalyzed activation of protein, *C. Proc. Natl. Acad. Sci (USA)* **78**:2249-2252 (1981).
3. W.G. Owen and C.T. Esmon, Functional properties of an endothelial cell cofactor for thrombincatalyzed activation of protein, *C. J. Biol. Chem.* **256**:5532-5535 (1981).
4. F.J. Walker, P.W. Sexton and C.T. Esmon, The inhibition of blood coagulation by activated protein C through the selective inactivation of activated factor V, *Biochim. Biophys. Acta* **571**:333-342 (1979).
5. F.J. Walker, Regulation of activated protein C by protein S: The role of phospholipid in factor Va inactivation, *J. Biol. Chem.* **256**:11128-11131 (1981).
6. P.C. Comp and C.T. Esmon, Generation of fibrinolytic activity by infusion of activated protein C into dogs, *J. Clin. Invest.* **68**:1221-1228 (1981).
7. N. Savion, J.D. Issacs, D. Gospaclarowicz and M.A. Shuman, Internalization and degradation of thrombin and up regulation of thrombin binding sites in corneal endothelial cells, *J. Biol. Chem.* **256**:4514-4519 (1981).
8. J.A. Marcum and R.D. Rosenberg, Anticoagulantly active heparin-like molecules from vascular tissue, *Biochem.* **23**:1730-1737 (1984).
9. J.A. Marcum, L. Fritze, S.J. Galli, G. Karp and R.D. Rosenberg: Microvascular heparin-like species with anticoagulant activity, *Amer. J. Physiol.* **245**:H725-733 (1983).
10. Y. Nemerson and R. Bach: Tissue factor revisited, *Progress in Hemost. and Thromb.* **6**:237-261 (1982).
11. M.P. Bevilacqua, J.S. Pober, G.R. Majeau, R.S. Cotran and M.A. Gimbrone, Jr. Interleukin-1 (IL-1) induces biosynthesis and cell surface expression of procoagulant activity in human vascular endothelial cells, *J. Exp. Med.* **160**:618-623 (1984).
12. D.M. Stern, M. Drillings, H.L. Nossel, A. Hurlet-Jensen, K. La Gamma and J. Owen, Binding of factor IX and IXa to cultured vascular endothelial cells, *Proc. Natl. Acad. Sci. (USA)* **80**:4119-4123 (1983).
13. P.P. Nawroth and D.M. Stern, An endothelial cell coagulant pathway, *J. Cellular Biochem* **28**:253-264 (1985).
14. D.M. Stern, P.P. Nawroth, W. Kisil, G. Vehar and C.T. Esmon, The binding of factor IXa to cultured bovine aortic endothelial cells, *J. Biol. Chem.* **260**:6717-6722 (1985).
15. T.S. Zimmerman, Z.M. Ruggeri and C.A. Fulcer, Factor VIII/VWF factor, *In* "Progress in Hematology," E.B. Brown, ed., Grune and Stratton, New York. Vol. 13, P. 279-309 (1983).
16. D.C. Lynch, R. Williams, T.S. Zimmerman, E.P. Kirby and D.M. Livingston, Biosynthesis of the subunit of factor VIIIR by bovine aortic endothelial cells, *Proc. Natl. Acad. Sci. (USA)* **180**: 2738-2742 (1983).
17. D.D. Wagner and V.G. Marder, Biosynthesis of vWF protein by human endothelial cells, *J. Biol. Chem.* **258**:2065-2067 (1983).
18. D.D. Wagner, J.B. Olmstead and V.J. Marder, Immunolocalization of vWF in Weibel-Palade bodies

of human endothelial cells, *J. Cell Biol.* **95**:355-360 (1982).

19. B.M. Ewenstein, M.J. Warhol, R.I. Handin and J.S. Pober, Composition of the vWF storage organelle (Weibel-Palde body) isolated from cultured human umbilical vein endothelial cells, *J. Cell Biol.* **104**:1423-1433 (1987).

20. J.J. Sixma, K.S. Sakariassen and P.A. Bohuis, The relationship between the multimeric structure of factor VIII/vWF and the facilitation of platelet adhesion to human subendothelium, *Thromb. and Haemost.* **46**:199 (1981).

21. L.W. Hoyer, The factor VIII complex: Structure cell function, *Blood* **58**:1-13 (1981).

22. D.F. Mosher, M.J. Doyle and E.A. Jaffe, Synthesis and secretion of thrombospondin by cultured human endothelial cells, *J. Cell Biol.* **93**:343-348 (1982).

23. H. Sage, Characterization and modulation of extracellular glycoproteins secreted by endothelial cells in culture in vascular endothelium, *in:* "Hemostasis and Thrombosis." M.A. Gimbrone Jr., ed. Livingstone, Edinburgh, pp. 187-208 (1986).

24. D. Collen, On the regulation and control of fibrinolysis, *Thromb. and Haemost.* **43**:77-89 (1980).

25. D.J. Loskutoff and T.S. Edgington, Synthesis of a fibrinolytic activator and inhibitor by endothelial cells, *Proc. Natl. Acad. Sci. (USA)* **74**:3903-3907 (1977).

26. D.J. Loskutoff, J.A. VanMourik, L.A. Erickson and D. Lawrence, Detection of an unusually stable fibrinolytic inhibitor produced by bovine endothelial cells, *Proc. Natl. Acad. Sci. (USA)* **80**:2956-2960 (1983).

27. S. Moncada, R. Gryglewski, S. Bunting and J.R. Vane, An enzyme isolated from arteries transform prostaglandin endoperoxides to an unstable substance that inhibits platelet aggregation, *Nature* **263**:663-665 (1974).

28. B.B. Weksler, Prostacyclin. *In:* "Progress in Hemostasis and Thrombosis," T.H. Spaet ed., Grune and Staton, New York. Vol. 6 113-138 (1982).

29. B.B. Weksler, C.W. Ley and E.A. Jaffe, Stimulation of endothelial cell prostacyclin production by thrombin, trypsin and ionophore A23187, *J. Clin. Invest.* **62**:923-930 (1978).

30. N.L. Baenziger, L.E. Force and P.R. Becherer, Histamine stimulates PGI_2 synthesis in cultured human umbilical vein endothelial cells, *Biochem. Biophys. Res. Comm.* **92**:1435-1440 (1980).

31. J.C. Goldsmith and J.J. McCormick, Immunologic injury to vascular endothelial cells: Effects on release of prostacyclin, *Blood* **63**:984-989 (1984).

32. F. Alhence-Gelas, S.J. Tsai, K.S. Callahan, W.B. Campbell and A.R. Johnson, Stimulation of prostaglandin formation by vasoactive cells, *Prostagl.* **24**:723-742 (1982).

33. D.K. Miller, S. Sadowski, D.D. Soderman and F.A. Kuehl, Endothelial prostacyclin production induced by activated neutrophils, *J. Biol. Chem.* **260**:1006-1014 (1985).

34. D.J. Loskutoff, Effect of thrombin on the fibrinolytic activity of cultured bovine endothelial cells, *J. Clin, Invest.* **64**:329-332 (1979).

35. M.P. Bevilacqua, J.S. Pober, M.E. Wheeler, R.S. Cotran and M.A. Gimbrone Jr., IL-1 activation of vascular endothelium: effects on procoagulant activity and leukocyte adhesion, *Am. J. Pathol.* **121**:394-403 (1985).

36. M.P. Bevilacque, R.R. Schleef, M.A. Jr., Gimbrone and D.J. Loskutoff, Regulation of fibrinolytic system of cultured human vascular endothelium by IL-1, *J. Clin. Invest* **78**:587-591 (1986).

37. D.A. Morgan, F.W. Ruscelli and R.C. Gallo, Selective in vitro growth of lymphocytes from normal human bone marrows, *Science* **193**:1007-1008 (1976).

38. F.W. Ruscetti, D.A. Morgan and R.C. Gallo, Functional and morphologic characterization of human T cell continuously growth in vitro, *J. Immunol.* **119**:131-138 (1977).

39. J.M. Zarling and F.H. Bach, Continuous culture of T cells cytotoxic for autologous human leukemia cells, *Nature* **280**:685-688 (1979).

40. S. Gillis, K.A. Smith and J. Watson, Biochemical and biologic characterization of lymphocyte regulatory molecules. II. Purification of a class of rat and human lymphokines, *J. Immunol.* **124**:1954-1962 (1980).

41. C.S. Henney, K. Kuribayashi, D.E. Kern and S. Gillis, Interleukin-2 augments natural killer cell activity, *Nature* **291**: 335-338 (1981).

42. J.R. Ortaldo, A.T. Mason, J.P. Gerard, L.E. Henderson, W. Farrar, R.F. Hopkins, R.B. Herberman and H. Rabin, Effect of natural and recombinant IL-2 on regulation of IFN-γ production and natural killer cell activity, *J. Immunol.* **133**:779-783 (1984).

43. M.C. Mingari, F. Gerora, G. Carra, R.S. Acold, A. Moretta, R.H. Zubler, T.A. Waldman and L. Moretta, Human interleukin-2 promotes proliferation of activated B cells via surface receptors similar to those of activated T cells, *Nature* **312**:641-643 (1984).

44. B.C. Pike, A. Raubitischets and G.J.V. Nossal, Human interleukin 2 can promote the growth and differentiation of single hapten-specific B cells in the presence of specific antigen, *Proc. Natl. Acad. Sci.* **81**:7917-7921 (1984).

45. E.A. Grimm, A. Mazumder, H. Zhang and S.A. Rosenber, Lymphokine-activated killer cell phenom-

enon: Lysis of natural killer resistant fresh solid tumor cells by interleukin 2 activated autologous human peripheral blood lymphocytes, *J. Exp. Med.* **155**:1823-1841 (1982).

46. A. Mazumder and S.A. Rosenberg, Successful immunotherapy of natural killer resistant established pulmonary melanoma metastases by the intravenous adoptive transfer of synegeneic lymphocytes activated in vitro by interleukin 2, *J. Exp. Med.* **159**:495-507 (1984).

47. E.R. Hall, A.C. Papp, W.E. Jr. Seifert and K.K. Wu, Stimulation of endothelial cell prostacyclin formation by IL-2, *Lymphokine Res.* **5**:87-96 (1986).

48. E.A. Hann, R.A. Egan, D.D. Soderman, P.H. Gale and F.A. Kuehl, Jr., Peroxidase-dependent deactivation of prostacyclin synthetase, *J. Biol. Chem.* **254**:2191-2194 (1979).

49. R.W. Egan, J. Paxton and F.A. Keuhl, Jr., Mechanism for irreversible self-deactivation of prostaglandin synthetase, *J. Biol. Chem.* **251**:7325-7335 (1976).

50. M.E. Hemler and W.E.M. Lands, Evidence for a peroxide-initiated free radical mechanism of prostaglandin biosynthesis, *J. Biol. Chem.* **255**:6253-6261 (1980).

MICROCIRCULATORY DISTURBANCES IN ENDOTOXIN-INDUCED DISSEMINATED INTRAVASCULAR COAGULATION

THE EFFECTS OF HEPARIN AND GABEXATE MESILATE ON LOCOMOTIVE AND METABOLIC CHANGES OF NEUTROPHILS

Masayuki Suzuki, Makoto Suematsu, Soichiro Miura, Chikara Oshio,
Masaya Oda and Masaharu Tsuchiya

Department of Internal Medicine
School of Medicine
Keio University
Tokyo 160, Japan

INTRODUCTION

It is well recognized that the intravenous administration of endotoxin causes a transient neutropenia followed by a systemic increase in neutrophils.[1] The initial depression of neutrophils is considered as the result of adhesive changes of neutrophils to the endothelium.[2]

Accumulation of neutrophils in microvasculature may play an important role in aggravation of endothelial damage because neutrophils produce a variety of vasoactive substances such as lysosomal enzymes[3] and active oxygen metabolites.[4] However, the mechanism by which endotoxin affects neutrophil behaviors in microvascular beds has not been fully investigated. In addition, the vasoactive substances which modulate locomotive and metabolic changes of neutrophils remain to be identified.

In this report, we show that endotoxin primarily affects the venular endothelial walls, which may promote the sticking phenomenon of neutrophils to the endothelium and the stimulation of oxyradical-generating ability. In addition, we compare the attenuation effects of heparin, which has been widely used for the treatment of DIC, with those of gabexate mesilate, a synthetic protease inhibitor, on the neutrophil behaviors by using an experimental model of endotoxemia.

MATERIALS AND METHODS

Animal preparation

Male Wistar rats weighing 250 g were anesthetized intraperitoneally with 30 mg/kg of pentobarbital sodium. Jugular and femoral veins were cannulated with polyethylene tubes for the infusion of endotoxin and other agents. The carotid artery was also cannulated to monitor the systemic blood pressure continuously. After the abdomen was opened via a midline incision, the ileocecal portion of the mesentery was exteriorized and placed gently on a plastic plate. The mesentery was kept warm and moist by continuous superfusion with saline at 37°C. The mesenteric microcirculation was observed under intravital microscopy assisted by TV-videotape recorder system (Olympus, Japan) according to the method of Chambers and Zweifach.[5]

The experimental model of endotoxin-induced disseminated intravascular coagulation (DIC) was designed by the method of Schoenderf and Rosenberg.[6] Endotoxin (*E coli*, O-111 B4, Difco, USA) was dissolved in the physiological saline at a concentration of 0.5 mg/ml and infused from the jugular vein at a rate of 2.0 mg/kg/hour.

In vivo visualization of leukocytes and endotoxin

The behaviors of leukocytes were visualized by using a fluorescent microscopy assisted by Silicon Intensifier Target Image Tube (SIT) camera with Contrast Enhance Unit (Hamamatsu Photonics, Shizuoka, Japan) and the fluorochrome, acridine orange (Sigma, USA). Acridine orange was dissolved in the physiological saline at a concentration of 10 μg/ml. The solution was subsequently filtered through 0.22 μm filter. A fresh solusion was prepared on the day of the experiment. The intravenous administration of acridine orange was performed to visualize the behaviors of leukocytes in the mesenteric microcirculation according to a modified method of Bagge and Karlson.[7]

The acridine orange solution (0.2 ml) was administered with a bolus injection into the femoral vein. Two minutes after the injection of acridin orange, the fluorescent illuminator was turned on for the excitation of the fluorochrome and leukocyte behaviors were recorded in the videorecorder for 60 seconds every 10 minutes. To evaluate sticking leukocytes to the venules, the number of illuminated cells in the area selected from umbranched straight venules (diameter = 50 μm, length = 200 μm) was obtained from the stored images in the videorecorder. To calculate the mean values of cells in each period, six still flames at 10-sec intervals were used. The density of sticking leukocytes in the venules was expressed as the ratio versus control (density index, DI) according to the following formula.

$$DI = Nt / Mo$$

Nt : The number of sticking leukocytes in each experiment.
Mo: The mean value of sticking leukocytes before the infusion of endotoxin.

The same dose of FITC-endotoxin conjugates (E coli, O-111 B4, Sigma, USA) was administered via a jugular vein to evaluate the distribution of endotoxin in the microvasculature of the rat mesentery. The fluorescence activity of FITC was observed by using the fluorescent microscopy.

Luminol-dependent chemiluminescence study

Metabolic changes of neutrophils during the infusion of endotoxin were also studied by measuring luminol-dependent chemiluminescence (ChL) activity. Three hundred microliters of whole blood sample was taken from the mesenteric venule using a microsyringe containing 10 units of heparin sodium (Kodama Chem. Co., Japan) before and 60 minutes after starting the infusion of endotoxin in each separate group. One hundred microliters of the sample were used for counting the number of neutrophils and lymphocytes after Türk and Giemsa staining. Two hundred microliters of the sample were incubated in 800 μl of minimum essential medium solution containing 20 μg/ml of luminol (Sigma, USA). The samples were transfered to a photomultiplier OX-7 (Tohoku Electric Industry, Japan) to determine the ChL activity of whole blood according to the method of Faden and Maciejewski.[8] The activities were displayed automatically on a scintillating counter every 30 seconds. After measuring a basal value of ChL for 5 minutes, 100 μl of opsonized zymosan (12.5 mg/ml) was added to the cuvette. The ChL activity was gradually increased and a maximum ChL value was obtained. Neutrophils are regarded as the major contributors to whole blood chemiluminescence;[9] therefore ChL activity of individual neutrophil was defined as follows:

$$\text{Individual ChL activity} = \frac{\text{Maximum ChL value} - \text{Basal ChL value}}{\text{Total number of neutrophils in the sample}}$$

Agents studied

We evaluated the effects of gabexate mesilate, a synthetic protease inhibitor (FOY, Ono Pharm. Co., Japan) and heparin sodium on the sticking phenomenon and the activation of ChL value of neutrophils caused by endotoxin. Gabexate mesilate and heparin sodium were dissolved with saline and infused continuously into the jugular vein at a rate of 10 mg/kg/hour and 20 U/kg/hour respectively during the experiment.

STATISTICAL ANALYSIS

The significance of the difference between the mean value of the groups was tested by

Student's t-test for unpaired values.

RESULTS

In vivo visualization of leukocytes

After starting the administration of endotoxin, rolling and sticking of leukocytes were remarkably increased along the endothelium of venules but not arterioles. The sticking leukocytes can be clearly demonstrated after the injection of acridine orange (Figure 1). The time-course of changes of the density index of sticking leukocytes along the venule is shown in Figure 2. The density index gradually increased progressively with the continuous infusion of endotoxin. Sixty minutes after starting the infusion of endotoxin, the density index was approximately three times higher than that of controls. Pretreatment with gabexate mesilate significantly attenuated the adhesive changes of leukocytes induced by endotoxin, but heparin sodium did not show any inhibitory effects.

Distribution of FITC-endotoxin

Fifteen minutes after starting the infusion of FITC-endotoxin, multiple fluorescent patches gradually appeared along the venular walls. In contrast, there was no fluorescent activity on the arteriolar side, which may suggest that endotoxin primarily affects the venular endothelium (Figure 3). We also detected fine leakage of FITC-endotoxin around the venule, which may be a reflection of venular endothelial damages and the leakage of intravascular components.

Changes of leukocyte counts and ChL activities of neutrophils

Figure 4 shows the alterations of peripheral neutrophil counts and luminol-dependent ChL activities 60 minutes after starting the endotoxin. The administration of endotoxin caused a significant neutropenia as compared with control value. Moreover, ChL activities of neutrophils were also elevated in endotoxin-treated group. This result may suggest that the ability of neutrophils to generate oxyradicals is primed by the intravenous administration of endotoxin. Both changes were significantly attenuated by the pretreatment with gabexate mesilate, whereas heparin sodium did not prevent these changes effectively.

These results show that gabexate mesilate may inhibit the neutrophil-mediated endothelial damage induced by endotoxin more effectively than heparin sodium.

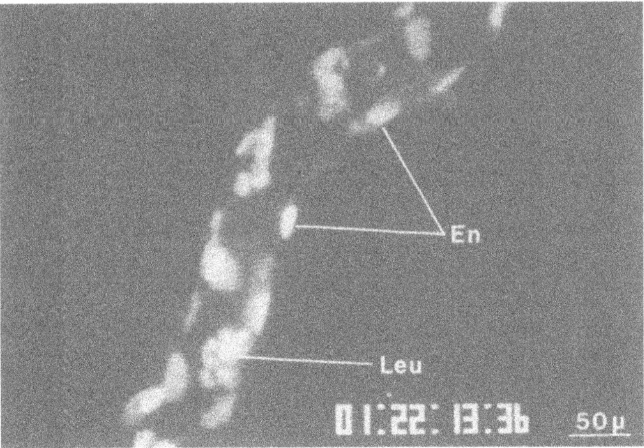

Fig. 1. Visualization of sticking leukocytes in the venules by the injection of acridine orange. Two types of illuminating cells are observed — spindle-shaped and spheriod-shaped. Spheroid-shaped fluorescent patches were counted as sticking leukocytes (Leu). Spindle-shaped patches were considered to be endothelial cells (En).

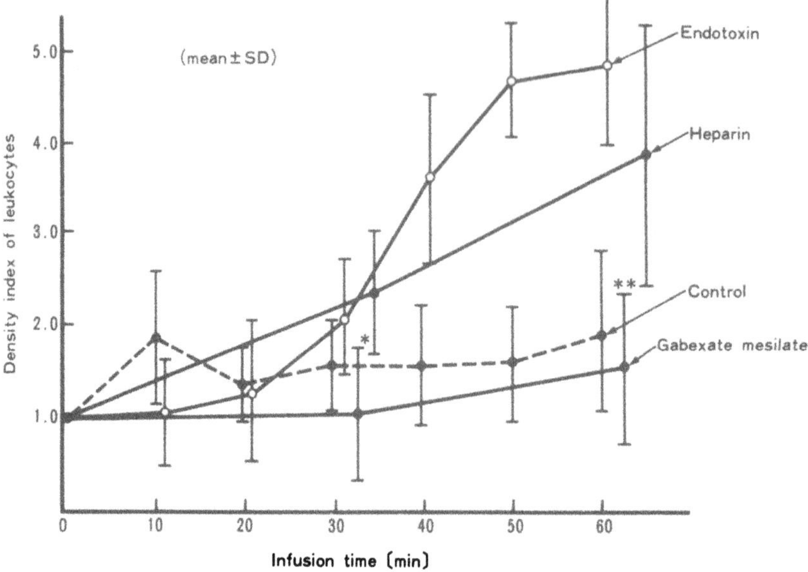

Fig. 2. The time-course changes of the density of sticking leukocytes along the venule and effects of gabexate mesilate and heparin sodium. The index was gradually increased after starting the infusion of endotoxin. Gabexate mesilate significantly inhibited this change, while heparin sodium did not. *P<0.05 and **P<0.001, compared with the group of endotoxin.

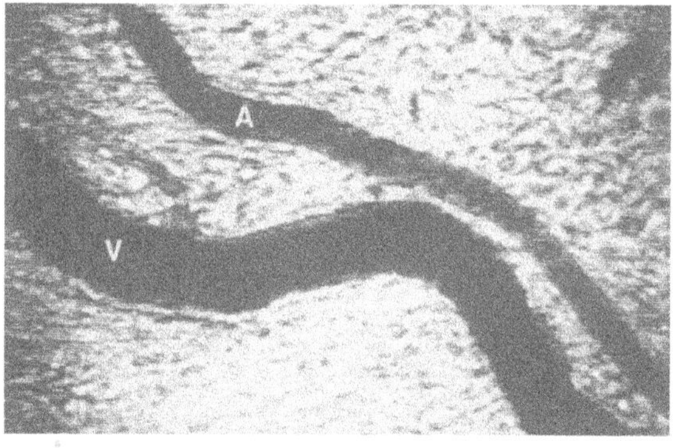

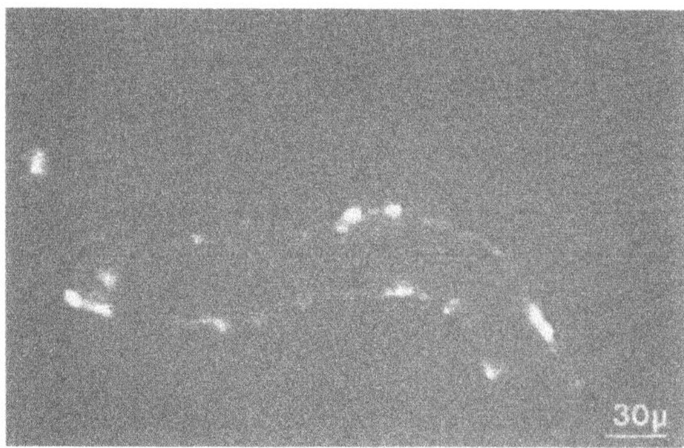

Fig 3. The distribution of FITC-labeled endotxin in the mesenteric vessels. The upper picture was obtained by transmission microscopy, the lower one by using the fluorescent microscopy. Multiple fluorescent patches were demonstrated along the venular walls, while there was no fluorescence on the arteriole.

138

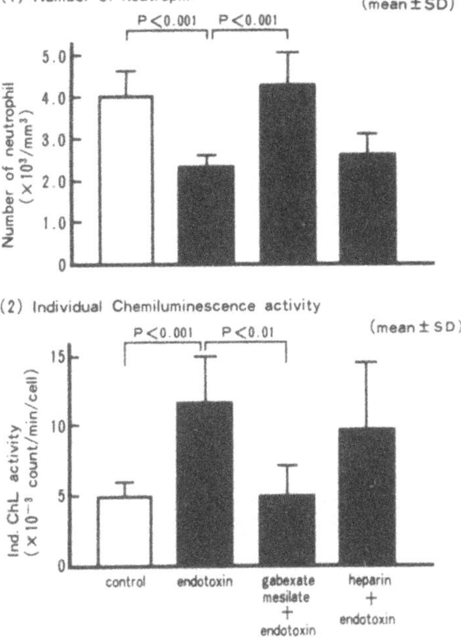

Fig. 4. Changes of the number of neutrophils, individual chemiluminescence (ChL) activity in endotoxemia and the effects of gabexate mesilate and heparin sodium. Sixty minutes after starting the endotoxin infusion, a remarkable neutropenia was observed. ChL activity of individual neutrophil was significantly elevated, which may imply the enhanced ability of neutrophils to generate oxyradicals in endotoxemia.

DISCUSSION

Neutrophils may play an important role in the acute microcirculatory response to various pathological states, including inflammation, endotoxin-induced disseminated intravascular coagulation or shock, etc. Recently, much attention has come to be paid to oxygen-dervied free radicals from neutrophils such as superoxide anion (O_2^-), hydroxyl radical ($\cdot OH$), or hypochlorous anion (ClO^-). Because of the high reactivity and short-livedness of these active oxygen molecules, the cell membrane of endothelial cells was believed to be the primary site of injury by neutrophil-derived oxyradicals.[10] To what extent the vascular endothelial cells are damaged by neutrophil-mediated oxidative stress is thought to depend on at least two factors, the number of sticking cells in microvasculature and the ability of an individual neutrophil to release oxyradicals. The present study showed that endotoxin can increase neutrophil-mediated oxidative stress on the surface of endothelial cells in the post-capillary venules.

What kinds of vasoactive mediators contribute to endotoxin-induced locomotive and metabolic changes in neutrophils has not been fully understood. However, we have reported that leukotriene B_4 may play an important role in neutrophil-mediated oxidative stress in endotoxemia in the same experiemental model by using a specific inhibitor of 5-lipoxygenase, AA-861.[11]

In the present study, gabexate mesilate also attenuated neutrophil-mediated oxidative stress induced by endotoxin. The agent is known as a serine protease inhibitor, especially an inhibitor of platelet aggregation caused by thrombin.[12] Since heparin did not show any improving effects on oxidative stress in endotoxemia, the attenuation effects of gabexate mesilate on neutrophil-mediated oxidative stress can not be explained by anti-thrombin effects.

Recently, it has been reported that serine proteases may play an important role in the modulation of respiratory burst of neutrophils.[13] The results show the possible role of a serine protease as a mediator of neutrophil-mediated oxidative stress in endotoxemia.

It is of interest that endotoxin affect the surface of venular endothelial cells in the early period of the administration of endotoxin, as shown in the study using FITC-endotoxin conjugates. The distribution of FITC did not correspond to that of sticking leukocytes. These results imply that the primary changes caused by endotoxin may be the damage of the venular endothelium which results in the exacerbation of sticking changes of leukocytes.

The role of platelets in endothelium-neutrophil interaction should be further examined in this experimental model of endotoxin-induced DIC. However, protease inhibitors may contribute to the reduction of neutrophil-mediated oxidative stress in microcirculatory disturbances caused by endotoxin. The present findings may provide a therapeutic effect of gabexate mesilate on endotoxin-induced circulating failure, which is not shared by heparin sodium.

SUMMARY AND CONCLUSION

Neutrophil-mediated oxidative stress on the rat mesenteric microcirculation was studied in the experimental model of endotoxin-induced disseminated intravascular coagulation (DIC) by using an intravital fluorescent technique and luminol-dependent chemiluminescence (ChL) analysis.

Leukocytes sticking to the venules were visualized by the injection of acridine orange, a fluorochrome tracer which shows high affinity to white cells. Endotoxin (E coli, O-111B4, Difco, USA) was infused intravenously at a dose of 2 mg/kg/hr. After starting the infusion of endotoxin, the number of sticking cells were gradually increased on the venular endothelium followed by a transient neutropenia. In order to investigate the distribution of infused endotoxin in the microvasculature, FITC-labeled endotoxin (Sigma, USA) was used. After administration of FITC-endotoxin, multiple patches of fluorescence along the venular walls were observed, while no fluorescent conjugates were found at the sticking neutrophils and along the arteriolar walls. ChL activities of neutrophils were also dramatically elevated, which may reflect the enhanced abitity to generate oxyradical species. To investigate the inhibitory effects of heparin sodium and gabexate mesilate which was a synthetic protease inhibitor on locomotive and metabolic changes of neutrophils induced by endotoxemia, both agents were administered prior to endotoxin infusion. Gabexate mesilate attenuated these changes, but heparin sodium did not show any improving effects. It was concluded that endotoxin primarily affects the venular endothelial cells, resulting in the activation of neutrophils. Gabexate mesilate was more likely to attenuate neutrophil-mediated oxidative stress on microvasculature in endotoxin-induced DIC than heparin sodium.

ACKNOWLEDGMENT

This work is supported by the Grant of Keio University, School of Medicine, Tokyo.

REFERENCES

1. C.A. Stetson, Jr., Studies on the mechanism of the Shwartzman phenomenon. Certain factors involved in the production of the local hemorrhagic necrosis, *J. Exp. Med.* **93**:489 (1951).

2. J.W. Athens, O.P. Haab, S.O. Raab, et al., Leukokinetic studies. IV. The total blood, circulating and marginal granulocyte pools and the granulocyte turnover rate in normal subjects, *J. Clin. Invest.* **40**:989 (1961).

3. D.C. Morrison and R.J. Ulevitch, The effects of bactrial endotoxin on host mediation system, *Am. J. Pathol.* **93**:527 (1978).

4. T. Yoshikawa, M. Murakami, Y. Furukawa, et al., Lipid peroxidation and experimental disseminated intravascular coagulation in rats induced by endotoxin, *Thromb. Haemostas.* **49**: 214 (1983).

5. R. Chambers and B.W. Zweifach, Topography and function of the mesentric circulation, *Am. J. Anat.* **75**:173 (1944).

6. T.H. Schoendorf, M. Rosenberg and F.W. Beller, Endotoxin-induced disseminated intravascular coagulation in nonpregnant rats, *Am. J. Pathol.* **65**:51 (1971).

7. U. Bagge and P. Karlson, Maintenance of white blood cell margination at the passage through small

venular junctions, *Microvasc. Res.* **20**:92 (1980).

8. H. Faden and N. Maciejewski, Whole blood luminol-dependent chemiluminescence, *J. Reticulo-endothelial Soc.* **30**(3):219 (1981).

9. A.L. Sagone, Jr., G.W. King and E.N. Metz, A comparison of the metabolic response to phagocytosis in human granulocytes and monocytes, *J. Clin. Invest.* **57**:1352 (1976).

10. M. Suematsu, C. Oshio, S. Miura and M. Tsuchiya, Real-time visualization of oxyradical burst from single neutrophil by using ultrasensitive video intensifier microscopy, *Biochem. Biophys. Res. Commun.* **149**(3):1106 (1987).

11. M. Suematsu, S. Miura, M. Suzuki, H. Nagata, T. Morishita, C. Oshio and M. Tsuchiya, 5-lipoxygenase inhibitor (AA-861) attenuates neutrophil-mediated oxidative stress on the venular endothelium in endotoxemia, *J. Clin. Lab. Immunol.* **25**:41-45 (1988).

12. Y. Tamura, M. Hirado, K. Okamura, Y. Minato and S. Fujii, Synthetic inhibitors of trypsin, plasmin, kallikrein, thrombin, C1F and C1 esterase, *Biochim. Biophys. Acta.* **484**:417-422 (1977).

13. M. Suematsu, H. Nagata, S. Miura, et al., Changes of respiratory burst of leukocytes and lipidperoxidation in microcirculatory disturbance, *Japanese Journal of Circulation Research* **Vol. 9**(2):119-125 (1986).

HISTAMINE AND ENDOTHELIUM

CHANGING SENSITIVITY TO H_1 AND H_2 RECEPTOR AGONISTS IN THE GROWING VASCULATURE

L.H. Smaje, N.M. Noor and G.F. Clough*

Departments of Physiology
Charing Cross and Westminster Medical School &
*St. Mary's Hospital Medical School
London, UK

INTRODUCTION

A number of reports in the literature indicate that young or newly-grown blood vessels fail to respond to inflammatory mediators in the same manner as mature adult vessels.[1,2]

Our own observations[3] on the growing micro-vasculature in implanted chambers in the rabbit ear indicate that neither histamine nor C5a induce visible macromolecular leakage from the vasculature of chambers implanted for less than ten weeks. From 10-12 weeks onwards, the vasculature responds in the expected way by forming post-capillary venular leaks. The arrangement and ultrastructure of vessels that respond to histamine and C5a differ from those of unresponsive vessels. There is a sinusoid-like arrangement of the immature, non-responding, vasculature which contrasts with the narrower straighter microvessels of the mature, responsive, vasculature. Ultrastructurally the young endothelium is thicker and contains an abundance of mitochondria, free ribosomes and a well developed endoplamic reticulum.[4] In our sections, junctions appeared to be well-formed. The mature, responding, vessels are similar to descriptions of normal adult tissue (eg. see Majno, 1965).[5]

In order to analyse this phenomenon more deeply we required a quantitative model and chose implanted polyvinyl sponges. Following implantation, blood vessels grow into the sponge and reach their final density within one week.[6] A major advantage of the sponge is that it is simple to distinguish accurately between newly formed and adjacent old tissue.

METHODS

CFY rats of either sex were anaesthetised and four polyvinyl sponges (Prosthex Ltd) $12 \times 12 \times 3$ mm were implanted aseptically in the subcutaneous tissue of the dorsum.[6] Incisions were then sutured and the animals allowed to recover. One week (immature vessels) or one month (mature vessels) later the rats were reanaesthetized and the trachea, the right external jugular vein, and in some experiments the right ventricle, were cannulated in order to measure albumin extraction or blood flow to the sponge in response to histamine.

Preliminary experiments showed that there was an approximately linear increase in extravascular albumin accumulation for about 1 hour and that the ^{51}Cr-EDTA space was not significantly different in the immature and mature vasculature. Accordingly, the extravascular albumin space 30 min after injection of saline or histamine was used as a measure of macromolecular permeability.

The experimental protocol was as follows: ^{125}I-human albumin (Amersham International plc) 10 μCi was injected iv and 0.1 ml of saline or histamine 10^{-6} to 10^{-4} mol/l injected into the sponge. Twenty-five minutes later ^{131}I-human albumin (New England Nuclear) 1 μCi was injected iv and 5 minutes later a blood sample was taken, the animal was killed and the sponges removed. In some experiments, 5 minutes after the histamine was given, blood flow was measured using the microsphere technique and approx 0.7 × 10⁶ ⁵⁷Co microspheres 15 μm diameter (3M) were given into the left ventricle and flow calculated using the reference organ technique.[7] A femoral arterial sample was taken starting 5 s before the microsphere injection and for 90 s after it was completed. Both kidneys were removed to check that injections had been uniform and the lungs were monitored to check for AV anastamoses. Counts were corrected for background and cross channel contamination and expressed per gram of sponge or plasma.

Extravascular albumin , expressed as equivalent plasma volume, was thus:

$$= \frac{^{125}\text{I sponge}}{^{125}\text{I plasma}} - \frac{^{131}\text{I sponge}}{^{131}\text{I plasma}}$$

Blood flow, Q, (ml min⁻¹ g⁻¹) was:-

$$Q = \frac{^{57}\text{Co sponge}}{^{57}\text{Co reference sample}} \times \text{flow rate of reference sample}$$

When appropriate, the animals were pretreated with either mepyramine (25 mg/kg iv) or cimetidine (125 mg/kg iv) 30 minutes before administration of the ¹²⁵I albumin.

RESULTS

Fig. 1 illustrates that the qualitative impression gained from previous studies was correct, namely that the immature vasculature is much less responsive to histamine than the mature vasculature. It also shows that the immature vasculature is more leaky in the control situation, or at least in response to saline, than is the case with mature vessels but that in the highest dose used, 10⁻⁴ mol/l, histamine does lead to an increased macromolecular leakage.

This was analyzed further by studying the effects of H_1 and H_2 antagonists. Fig. 2 shows that in the immature vasculature the H_2 antagonist has a significant effect in reducing both basal and histamine-induced macromolecular leakage, while the H_1 antagonist is less effective. In the mature vasculature, by contrast, it is the H_1 antagonist that is more effective (Fig. 3).

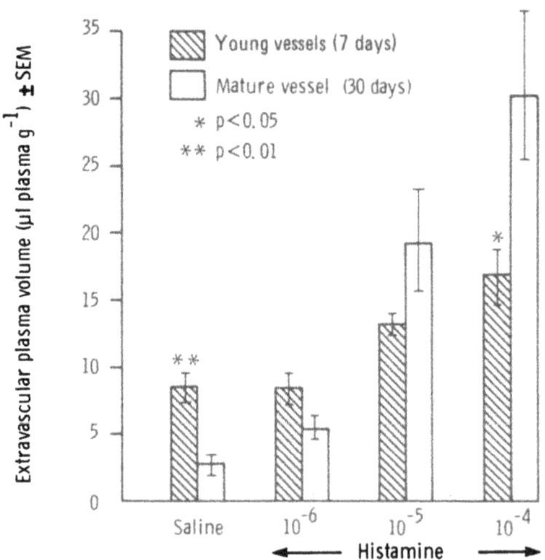

Fig. 1. Macromolecular leakage (extravascular equivalent plasma volume, μl g⁻¹) in sponges aged one week and one month in response to injections of saline or histamine (mol l⁻¹) into the sponge. Mean ± SEM, N = 5 in this and all subsequent figures.

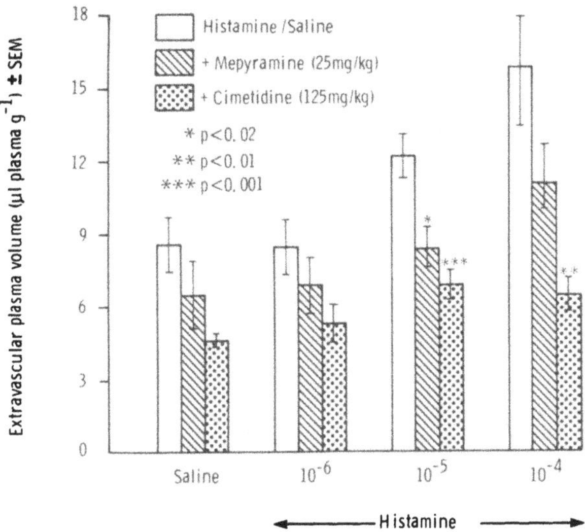

Fig. 2. Effect of H_1 and H_2 receptor antagonists on equivalent plasma volume following histamine in sponges one week after implantation.

MATURE VESSELS

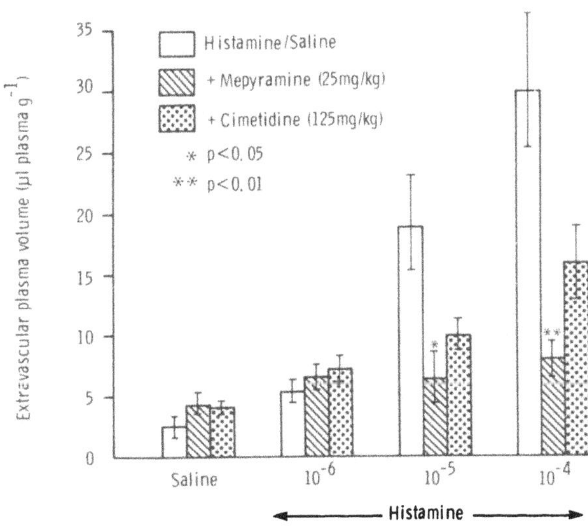

Fig. 3. Effect of H_1 and H_2 receptor antagonists on equivalent plasma volume following histamine one month after implantation. Note different scale from Fig. 2.

Since macromolecular leakage is heavily dependent on convection it was decided to measure blood flow in the sponges and the results are shown in Figs. 4 and 5. Resting flow in the immature vasculature is some ten times that in the mature bed and histamine increases both still further. H_2 antagonists reduce blood flow in the resting immature vasculature to that found in the mature vessels and have no significant effect on the latter. Following histamine, the H_2 antagonist reduces blood flow to control in both immature and mature vessels. The H_1 antagonist has insignificant effects on blood flow.

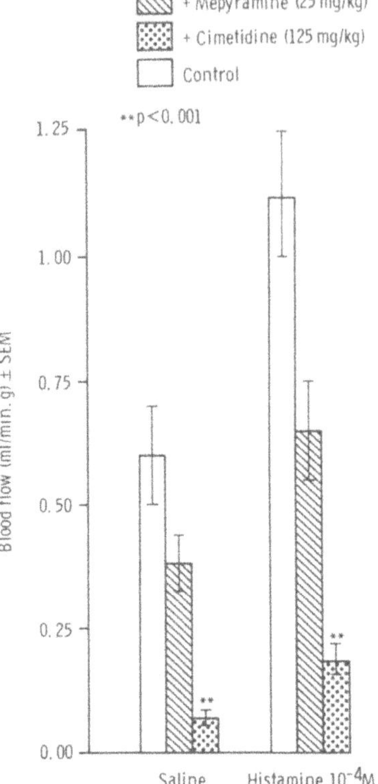

Fig. 4. Effect of H_1 and H_2 antagonists on blood flow to sponges one week after implantation in response to saline and histamine.

DISCUSSION

The results obtained in this study, while incomplete, allow some important inferences to be drawn.

Firstly they confirm that the immature vasculature is indeed less responsive to the inflammatory mediator histamine than is the mature vasculature, although they also show that the immature vessels do indeed leak protein in response to histamine. They also demonstrate that there is a higher basal macromolecular efflux from the immature vasculature than the mature vasculature. The use of H_1 and H_2 antagonists and the blood flow studies allow us to make some tentative interpretations of these basic findings.

Firstly, the basal leakage of the immature vasculature is probably not a response to the trauma of the injection as non-injected sponges show insignificantly different albumin spaces (saline: $8.3 \pm 1.5 \, \mu l \, g^{-1}$, non-injected sponge $5.5 \pm 1.9 \, \mu l \, g^{-1}$). They are moreover consistent with Chien, Jan & Lin's findings[8] that endothelial cells undergoing mitosis permit paracellular macromolecular leakage. The fact that the H_2 antagonist more or less abolishes the high blood flow and macromolecular leakage in this situation suggests that the leakage is largely convective in origin and suggests that permeability *per se* may not be different in the two situations. This is consistent with our observation that FITC-dextran 150 and FITC-albumin do not leak out of immature vessels in the rabbit ear chamber[3] and that junctions in the immature microvasculature closely resemble the mature structures. They do, however, rather conflict with the observations of Schoefl, 1961.

The responses to exogenous histamine are a little more complex but nonetheless fit into a consistent explanation. Histamine increases blood flow (and hence convection of proteins) in

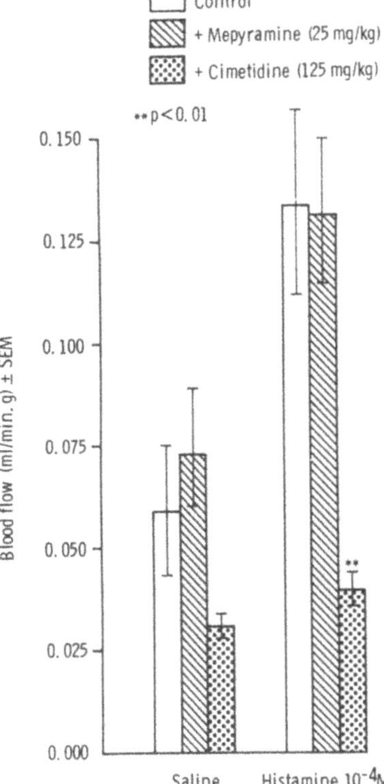

Fig. 5. Effect of H_1 and H_2 antagonists on blood flow to sponges one month after implantation in response to saline and histamine. Note different scale from Fig. 4.

both the immature and mature vasculature (Figs. 4 and 5) and this effect is mediated largely by H_2 receptors.

In the mature vasculature H_1 receptor activation leads to an increased permeability, presumably by gap formation,[9] which combined with the increased convection leads to a massive protein efflux. H_2 receptor blockade reduces the convective component but does not abolish macromolecular leakage altogether. H_1 receptor blockage seems to prevent the leak formation in the first place and the small increased convection is insufficient to produce significant effects.

In the immature vasculature by contrast, H_1 receptor activation does not occur or at least the effects of gap formation are absent.

Further analysis is necessary to elucidate whether the receptors are missing, or the cellular machinery necessary for gap formation (assuming this is the cause of the macromolecular leakage!) is in some way incomplete or faulty.

Currently we are exploring both possibilities and the responses of other inflammatory mediators. The phenomenon would not appear to be an artefact and presumably has biological significance. What this is, remains in the realm of speculation.

SUMMARY AND CONCLUSIONS

1. Resting albumin efflux is greater from immature vessels than from mature and this is associated with a greater blood flow in immature vessels.
2. Both resting blood flow and albumin efflux in immature vessels are reduced by an H_2

antagonist.
3. Histamine produces a greater albumin efflux from mature vessels than from immature and the associated increase in blood flow in response to histamine was also greater in mature vessels.
4. Blood flow and permeability increase produced by histamine are separately mediated via H_2 and H_1 receptors respectively in mature vessels.
5. In immature vessels, H_2 receptors appear to mediate both responses.

REFERENCES

1. M.J. Angle, L.M. McManus and R.N. Pinckard, Age-Dependent Differential Development of Leukotactic and Vasoactive Responsiveness to Acute Inflammatory Mediators, *Lab Invest,* Vol 55, No 6, 616-621 (1986).
2. J.V. Hurley, B. Edwards and K.N. Ham, The response of newly formed blood vessels in healing wounds to histamine and other permeability factors, *Pathology,* 2, 133-145 (1970).
3. G. Clough, N. Noor and L.H. Smaje, Effect of inflammatory mediators on the developing microcirculation of the rabbit ear chamber, *J. Physiol.,* 374, 17P (1986).
4. G.I. Schoefl, Studies on inflammation. III. Growing capillaries: their structure and permeability, *Virchows Arch. path. Anat.* 337, 97-141 (1963).
5. G. Majno, Ultrastructure of the vascular membrane, *In:* "Handbook of Physiology," W.F. Hamilton and P. Dow, editors. American Physiological Society, Washington, D.C. Section 2, Circulation Vol III, 2293-2375 (1965).
6. L.C. Edwards, L.N. Pernokas and J.E. Dunphy, The use of a plastic sponge to sample regenerating tissue in healing wounds, *Surgery, Gynecology and Obstetrics,* Vol 105, 303-309 (1957).
7. M.A. Heymann, B.D. Payne, J.I.E. Hoffman and A.M. Rudolph, Blood flow measurements with radionuclide-labelled particles, *Prog. Cardiovasc. Dis.* 20, 55-79 (1977).
8. S. Chien, K.M. Jan and S.J. Lin, Enhanced macromolecular transport through endothelial junctions around mitotic cells, *In*: "Vascular Endothelium in Health and Disease" S. Chien ed., Plenum Press, N.Y., pp. 59-74 (1988).
9. G. Majno and G.E. Palade, Studies on inflammation. I. Effect of histamine and serotonin on vascular permeability. An electron microscopic study, *J. Biophys. Biochem.,* 11, 571-605 (1961).

RADIOAUTOGRAPHIC CHARACTERIZATION OF H₁ AND H₂ RECEPTOR ANTAGONISTS

BINDING SITES IN RAT GASTRIC MUCOSAL MICROCIRCULATORY SYSTEM

Masahiko Nakamura, Masaya Oda, Kotaro Kaneko, Koya Honda,
Hirokazu Komatsu and Masaharu Tsuchiya

Department of Internal Medicine
School of Medicine
Keio University
Tokyo 160, Japan

INTRODUCTION

Histamine is thought to be one of the most important neuromodulators in the gastric mucosa, participating mainly in the regulation of hydrochloric acid secretion and blood flow. Pharmacological studies revealed that the action of histamine is mediated by two types of receptors: H_1 and non-H_1 receptors, i.e., H_2 receptors. The existence of non-H_1 receptors was initially revealed through evidence that certain effects of histamine, such as gastric acid secretion and cardiac chronotropism, are not antagonized by typical antihistamines.[1] The important derivation of a second class of histamine antagonists[2] defined this new class of receptors, the H_2 receptors, as being those which are unaffected by classical H_1 antihistamines like pyrilamine. The subsequent phenomenal success of this new H_2 receptor antagonist, cimetidine, in treating duodenal ulcers by suppression of acid secretion has confirmed the functional significance of histamine in the gastric mucosa.

From recent studies,[3,4] however, the H_2 receptor pathway is thought to mediate not only the stimulation of hydrochloric acid secretion, but also the relaxation of vascular smooth muscle. In the cat and the rabbit,[5] the H_1 receptor also takes part in the regulation of hydrochloric acid secretion. Thus, the categorization into H_1 and H_2 receptors is somewhat confusing because of its inability to clearly distiguish between the actions of each receptor. Consequently, a re-evaluation of H_1 and H_2 receptor distribution in the gastric mucosa is necessary to clarify the mechanism underlying the histamine-mediated regulation of gastric mucosal function and microcirculatory system.

The present study was thus designed to clarify the distribution of the H_1 and H_2 receptor antagonist-binding sites in the rat gastric mucosa *in vivo* and isolated gastric endothelial and epithelial cells *in vitro* via radioautography using the tritiated histamine H_1 receptor antagonist, pyrilamine, and the histamine H_2 receptor antagonist, cimetidine.

MATERIALS AND METHODS

In Vivo Study

Wistar strain male rats weighing 200-250 g were used in the present experiments. The rats were divided into ³H-cimetidine- and ³H-pyrilamine-treated groups. Each group was composed of control and cold-ligand-treated subgroups. Although only radiolabeled ligands were administered in the control group, 10^{-12}, 10^{-10}, 10^{-8} or 10^{-6} mol/kg body weight of cimetidine or pyrilamine were mixed with the radiolabeled ligand and administered in the cold ligand-treated group, through an intra-aortic catheter in the following manner.

Under light anesthesia administered by intraperitoneal injection of sodium pentobarbital, the abdomen was opened by a lower middle incision, and a polyethylene catheter was inserted into the abdominal aorta up to the bifurcation of the celiac artery. A dose of 0.7-ml aqueous solution of ^{3}H-cimetidine (1 mCi/kg b.w.; 1×10^{-7} mmol/kg; Amersham) or ^{3}H-pyrilamine (1 mCi/kg b.w.; 5×10^{-7} mmol/kg; Amersham) was infused for 15 min through the aortic catheter by an infusion pump at a constant rate of 2.8 ml/hr, followed by the infusion of physiological saline for 5 min to wash out the unbound ligands.

Immediately after the infusion, the stomach was removed and cut into small tissue blocks ($2 \times 2 \times 2$ mm^3). These were quickly frozen in isopentane cooled to its freezing point with liquid nitrogen. The stomach tissue blocks were freeze-dried for 48 hr in a vacuum apparatus (Oka Science OTD-ISF) cooled to -50°C and evacuated at 9×10^{-3} torr. The freeze-dried tissue blocks were then exposed to osmium vapor, followed by infiltration in Epon with a dripping unit evacuated by rotary pump. The tissue blocks were removed and embedded in freshly prepared Epon and polymerized at 60°C.[6]

In Vitro Study

Wistar strain male rats were anesthetized with pentobarbital, the stomach was removed and transformed into everted sacs, followed by incubation with Hanks BSS containing dispase (1000 PU/ml) at 37°C for 15 min. The mucosal layer was stripped off and incubated with the same dispase solution for 15 min. The cell suspension obtained was passed through stainless meshes and was centrifuged. The pellet obtained was resuspended in Dulbecco MEM and incubated in a Petri dish using a CO_2 incubator. Most of the spindle-shaped cells were found to be immunoreactive to OK-M5 antibody, corresponding to capillary endothelial cells. On the other hand, most of the round-shaped cells were negative to OK-M5 immunoreactivity, probably coinciding with epithelial cells, most likely parietal cells. The radiolabeled ligands, ^{3}H-cimetidine or ^{3}H-pyrilaminie, were then added to the incubation medium in a concentration of 10 μCi/ml, incubated for 5 or 30 min, fixed with 1% osmium solution for 1 hr, and directly embedded in Epon. The specificity of the reaction was checked by adding a tenfold amount of cold ligands in some of the specimens to the incubation medium, mixed with the radiolabeled ligands and processed in the same way.

Radioautographic Procedure

Semithin (1 μm) or ultrathin (1000-2000 Å thick) sections were cut with an LKB ultramicrotome using ethylene glycol instead of water (6). Radioautographic emulsion (Sakura NR-H2 or M2) was diluted (1:2 or 1:3) with distilled water at 40°C in a dark room. According to the dry-mounting procedure,[8] emulsion films were created in the middle of vinyl-coated iron-wire loops by dipping the wire loops into a solution composed of 10 ml diluted emulsion and 4 ml 2% aqueous solution of di-2-ethylhexyl sodium sulfosuccinate, with the wire loops allowed to stand at room temperature until the films were almost dry. The films were then applied to glass plates or meshes on which the sections were mounted. The sections were kept refrigerated in the dark for exposure at 4°C for 4 to 8 weeks. After developing and fixing, they were examined by light and electron microscopy.

Analysis of Radioautogram

To verify the localization of silver grains corresponding to the ligand binding sites on the endothelial and parietal cells, the grains on these cells were checked by light microscopy using a histogram representing the distance from the basolateral membrane. This histogram was compared with the predicted grain distribution pattern determined from the half distance (HD),[9] in which it was assumed that the ligand-binding sites are located on the basolateral plasma membranes of these cells. An HD of 0.49 μm was determined by the line source method presented in our previous study.[10] Student's t test was used throughout the study.

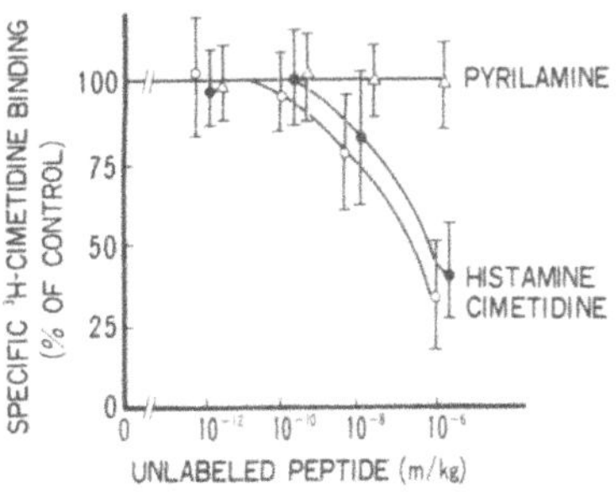

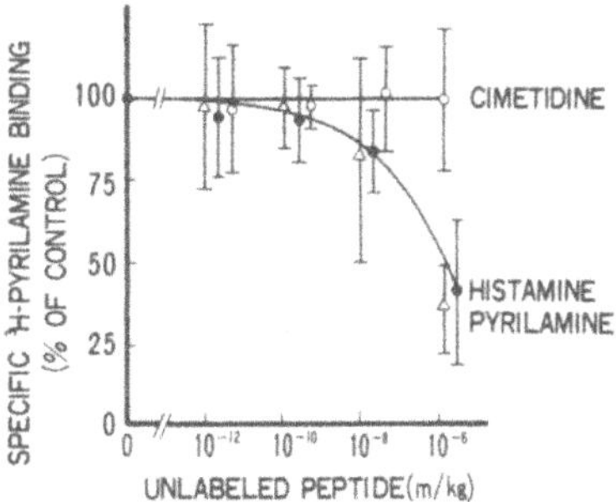

Fig. 1. Effects of unlabeled pyrilamine, cimetidine and histamine on the specific brinding of ³H-cimetidine to gastric mucosa.

Fig. 2. Effects of unlabeled cimitidine, pyrilamine and histamine on the specific brinding of ³H-pyrilamine to gastric mucosa.

RESULTS

Assay of ³H-Cimetidine and ³H-Pyrilamine Binding to Gastric Mucosa

As shown in Figs. 1 and 2, cimetidine and pyrilamine had an inhibitory effect on the binding of ³H-cimetidine and ³H-pyrilamine respectively, and that histamine exerted the inhibitory effect on both ligands.

Distribution of ³H-Cimetidine Binding Sites in the Gastric Mucosa

1. Light microscopic observation
Silver grains corresponding to the localization of ³H-cimetidine were found on the parietal cells (Fig. 3) and on the collecting venules (Fig. 4). By comparison with the cold cimetidine-treated group, the distribution of the grains on the parietal cells and the collecting venules was found to be specific for cimetidine (Table 1).

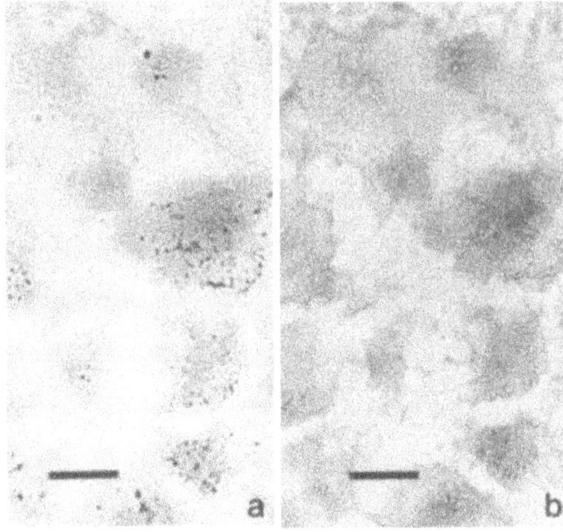

Fig. 3. Light microscopic radioautographs of the middle portion of the gastric mucosa of the ³H-cimetidine-infused rat. In the middle portion of the gastric mucosa, the grains are recognized on the large epithelial cells (bar = 10 μm), **b** focused on underlying tissue, and **a** focused on silver grains.

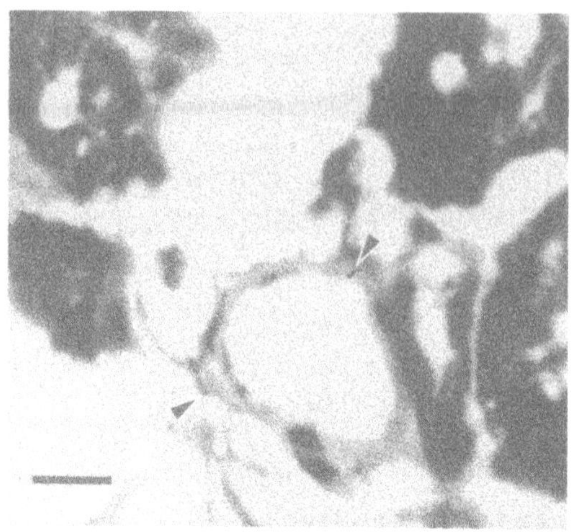

Fig. 4. Light microscopic radioautograph of the lower portion of the gastric mucosa of the ^{3}H-cimetidine-infused rat. In the basal portion of the gastric mucosa, the grains (arrowheads) are exclusively recognized on the collecting venules, with the chief cells having no grains (bar = 10 μm).

Table 1. Number of ^{3}H-cimetidine grains/cell

	^{3}H-Cimetidine alone	^{3}H-Cimetidine + cold Cimetidine	^{3}H-Cimetidine + cold Histamine	^{3}H-Cimetidine + cold Pyrilamine
Surface Mucous Cell	0.40 ± 0.20	0.40 ± 0.32	0.80 ± 0.42	0.40 ± 0.32
Mucous Neck Cell	0.40 ± 0.32	0.80 ± 0.40	0.40 ± 0.32	0.40 ± 0.32
Parietal Cell	10 ± 2.4	1.20 ± 0.40	2.0 ± 0.68	12 ± 3.2
Chief Cell	1.2 ± 0.80	1.0 ± 0.40	0.80 ± 0.40	1.0 ± 0.40
Collecting Venule	3.2 ± 0.80	0.42 ± 0.32	0.40 ± 0.24	2.8 ± 0.46
True Capillary	1.2 ± 0.80	0.48 ± 0.40	0.40 ± 0.24	0.40 ± 0.24

Values are means ± SD (n = 5).
*P < 0.001

2. Electron microscopic observation
   As indicated in Fig. 5, most of the grains on the collecting venules were found on the luminal side of the endothelium.

Distribution of ^{3}H-Pyrilamine Binding Sites in the Gastric Mucosa

   Silver grains corresponding to the localization of ^{3}H-pyrilamine were found on the post-capillary venules and capillaries draining into the collecting venules. Few grains were found on

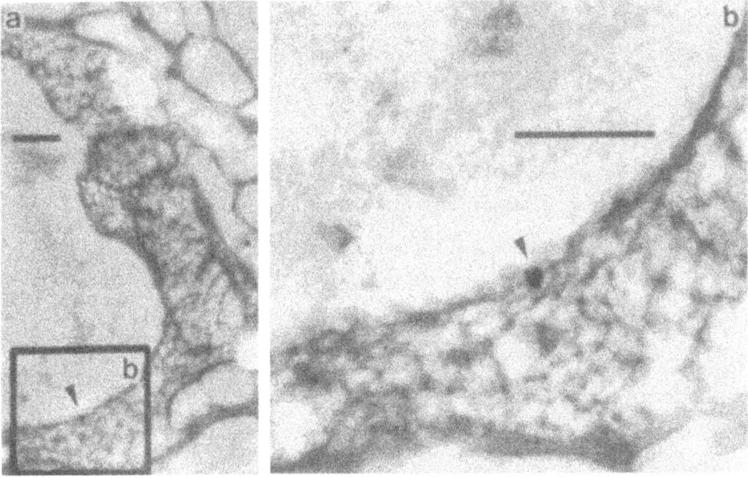

Fig. 5. Electron microscopic radioautograph of the lower portion of the gastric mucosa of the ³H-cimetidine-infused rat. Electron microscopically, the grains (arrowheads) are recognized on the luminal surface of the endothelium of the collecting venules (bars = 2 μm; **b** is a magnification of the square area in **a**).

the epithelia of the gastric mucosa (Fig. 6). Election microscopically, the pyrilamine-binding sites on the collecting venules were exclusively found on the abluminal surface of the endothelial cells (Fig. 7). By comparison with the cold pyrilamine-treated group, the distribution of the grains on the collecting venules and capillaries in the upper half of the fundic mucosa was found to be specific for pyrilamine (Table 2).

Localization of ³H-Cimetidine Binding Sites on the Isolated Endothelial Cells

The localization of the ³H-cimetidine binding sites was found on both the epithelial and endothelial cells (Fig. 8). The distribution of the silver grains on the endothelial cells were seen near the plasma membrane, while those on the epithelial cells were dispersed in the cytoplasm (Fig. 9).

Localization of ³H-Pyrilamine Binding Sites on the Isolated Endothelial Cells

The spindle-shaped endothelial cells had specific binding sites of pyrilamine on the endothelial cells, while few binding sites were found on the epithelial cells (Fig. 10).

DISCUSSION

As to the interaction of histamine with the gastric microcirculatory system, arterioles and venules are thought to be their target organs. Both H_1 and H_2 receptors have been demonstrated to be associated with the gastric blood flow and vascular permeability by pharmacological studies.[3,4,11] In this study, the collecting venules are found to have both of the specific cimetidine- and pyrilamine-binding sites. This clearly indicates the existence of H_1 and H_2 receptors on the non-muscular or pericytic venules in the gastric mucosa.

The existence of H_2 receptors on the non-muscular venule has been shown in the diaphragm using a histamine-ferritin conjugate,[12] especially on the luminal side of the endothelium. Since ferritin has a molecular weight of 460,000 and presents difficulty in permeating the cytoplasm of the endothelium, H_2 receptors have been concluded as not being localized on the vascular endothelium. In this study, electron microscopic radioautographs have clarified the exclusive localization of H_2 receptors on the luminal surface, and H_1 receptors on the abluminal surface of the endothelium. In addition, the H_1 receptors were found on the cytoplasm-rich area of the endothelium, which may suggest the interaction of histamine more with the micropinocytosis pro-

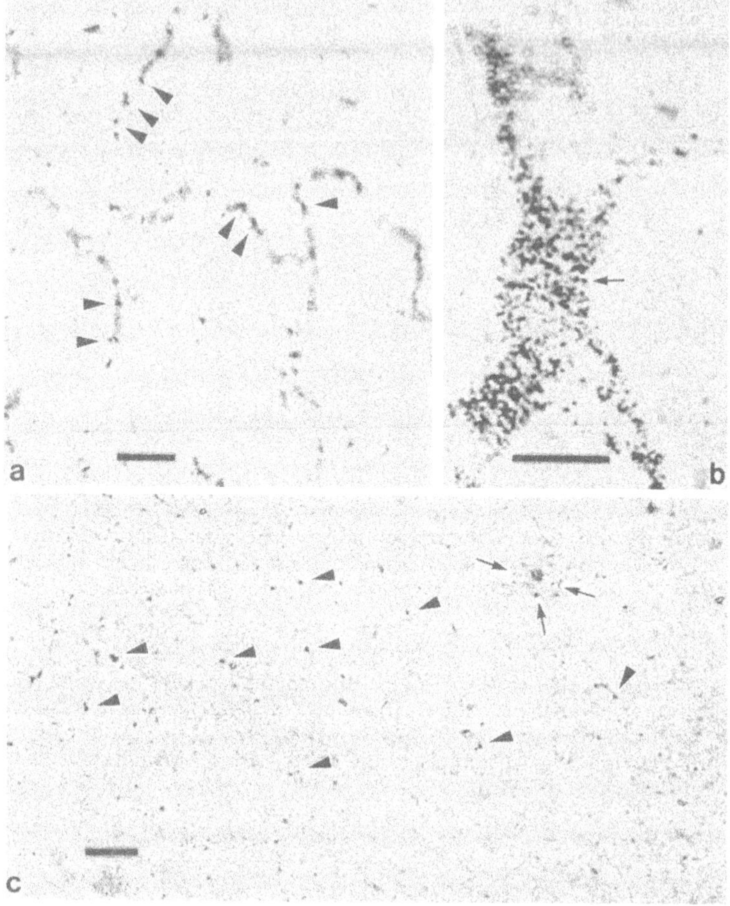

Fig. 6. Light micrographs of rat gastric mucosa infused with ³H-pyrilamine.
a, b, c: In upper portion of the gastric mucosa, the silver grains are recognized
on the true capillaries (arrowheads) and collecting venules (arrows). Few grains
are recognized on the epithelial cells (**a, b,** vertical section; **c,** horizontal section;
bars = 20 μm).

posed by Renkin[13] than with the opening of the intercellular junction postulated by Majno.[14]

In our previous paper,[15] the binding sites of muscarinic antagonist, quinuclidinyl benzilate (QNB), was found more richly on the endothelial cells than on the epithelial cells, showing the significance of muscarinic cholinergic mechanism in the regulation of the endothelial and vascular smooth muscle cell function by endothelium-derived relaxing facotr (EDRF). The localization of H_2 receptors on the luminal surface of the endothelium shown by the present study is similar with the data shown by QNB binding and may imply the importance of histamine in the function of the vascular smooth muscle cells by the EDRF-like mechanism in the arteriole and the muscular venule.

In the in vivo study, using cultured endothelial cells, some of these cells have been reported to form the capillary-like shape in certain conditions and show the reversed electrical polarity as compared to the capillary endothelium in vivo. In the present study, some epithelial cells forms the capillary-like structure. On these cells, the binding sites of pyrilamine were recognized on the luminal side of the cell membrane, supporting the reversed polarity of these endothelia.

156

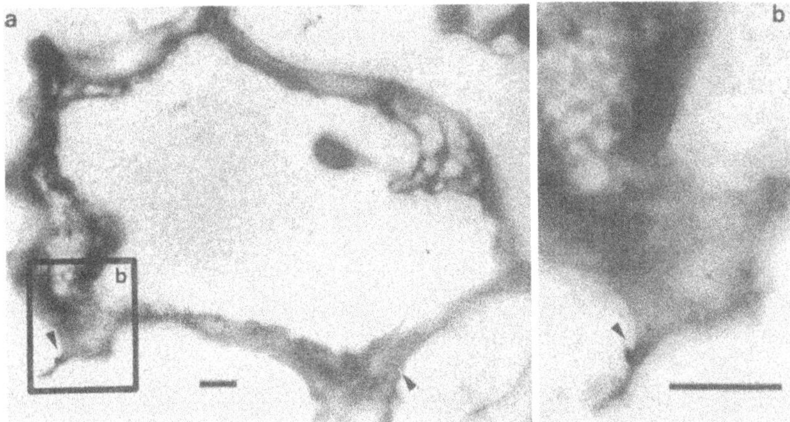

Fig. 7. Electron micrographs of rat gastric mucosa infused with ³H-pyrilamine. Electron microscopically, the silver graiins are recognized on the luminal surface of the endothelium of the collecting venule (bars = 2 μm; **b** is a magnification of the boxed area of **a**).

Table 2. Number of ³H-pyrilamine grains/cell

	³H-Pyrilamine alone	³H-Pyrilamine + cold Pyrilamine	³H-Pyrilamine + cold Histamine	³H-Pyrilamine + cold Cimetidine
Surface Mucous Cell	0.40 ± 0.20	0.20 ± 0.24	0 ± 0	0.40 ± 0.20
Mucous Neck Cell	0.40 ± 0.20	0 ± 0	0.40 ± 0.20	0.20 ± 0.24
Parietal Cell	1.0 ± 0.80	0.84 ± 0.42	0.40 ± 0.20	0.32 ± 0.20
Chief Cell	0.80 ± 0.40	0.40 ± 0.20	0.46 ± 0.24	0.40 ± 0.20
Collecting Venule	10 ± 4.8	2.4 ± 0.88	3.2 ± 0.80	12 ± 3.5
True Capillary (Upper Portion)	4.2 ± 1.4	1.2 ± 0.80	2.0 ± 0.68	4.0 ± 1.2
True Capillary (Lower Portion)	0 ± 0	0 ± 0	0.40 ± 0.20	0.40 ± 0.20

Values are means ± SD (n = 5).
*$0.001 < P < 0.01$ **$P < 0.001$

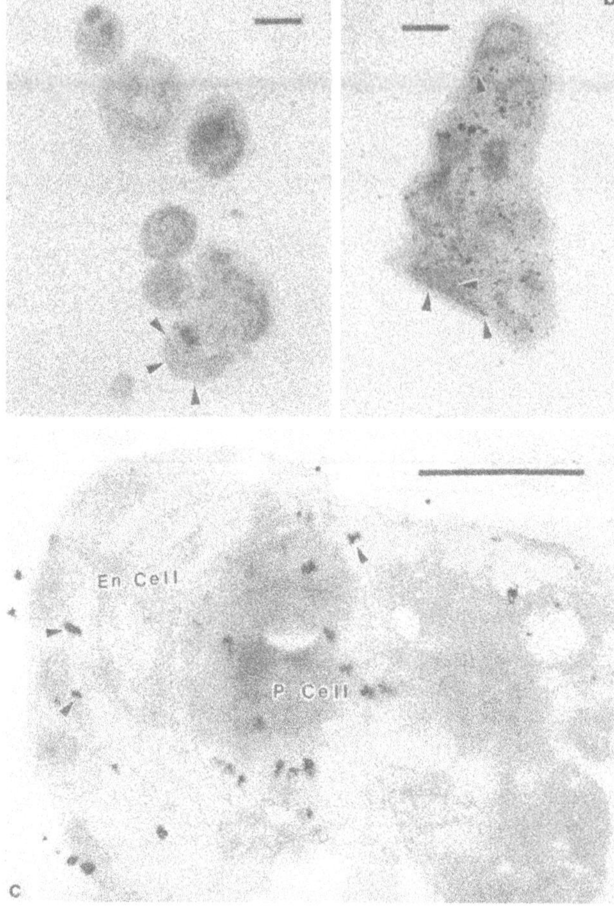

Fig. 8. Light and electron microscopic radioautographs of isolated fundic epithelial and endothelial cells incubated with ³H-cimetidine. The grains on the endothelial cells (arrowheads) are found near the plasma membrane, while those on the epithelial cells are seen in the cytoplasm (bars = 5 μm). En Cell: endothelial cell, P Cell: parietal cell.

CONCLUSION

The binding sites of H_1 and H_2 receptor-antogonist on the rat gastric mucosa and isolated gastric endothelial cells were studied by the radioautography of the soluble compounds. H_1-receptor antagonist-binding sites were found on the endothelia of the collecting venules and the true capillaries in the tip portion of the gastric mucosa both in the in vivo and in vitro studies. H_2-receptor antagonist-binding sites were seen on the parietal cells and the endothelia of the collecting venules.

ACKNOWLEDGMENTS

The authors wish to express their thanks to Koji Kami and Tatsushi Fujiwara for their constant encouragement and valuable suggestions. This study was supported by a Grant-in-Aid for Scientific Research from the Ministry of Education, Science and Culture of Japan (#56107005).

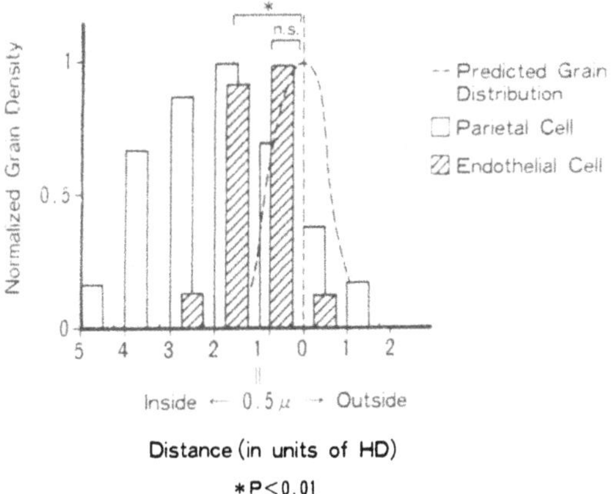

Fig. 9. Light microscopic radioautographic distribution of silver grains on ^{3}H-cimetidine-treated parietal and endothelial cell.

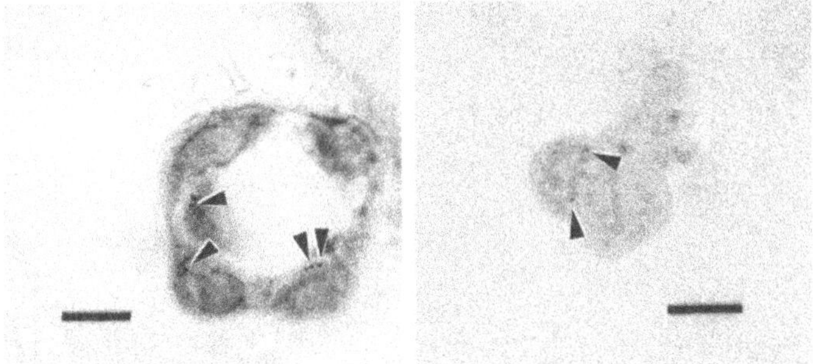

Fig. 10. Light microscopic radioautographs of the isolated epithelial cells incubated with ^{3}H-pyrilamine. The silver grains are exclusively found on the spindle-shaped endothelial cells. Most of the grains are localized on the luminal side of the endothelium (bar = 5 μm).

REFERENCES

1. A.S.F. Ash and H.O. Shild, Receptors mediating some action of histamine, *Br. J. Pharmacol.* **27**:427 (1966).
2. J.W. Black, W.A.M. Duncan, C.J. Durant, C.R. Ganellin and E.M. Parsons, Definition and antagonism of histamine H_2 receptors, *Nature* **236**:385 (1972).
3. G.A. Charbon, H.A.A. Brouwers and A. Sala, Histamine H_1- and H_2-receptors in the gastrointestinal circulation, *Naunyn-Schmiedeberg,s Arch Pharmacol* **312**:123 (1980).
4. J.G. Wood and H.W. Davenport, Measurement of canine gastric vascular permeability to plasma proteins in the normal and protein-losing states, *Gastroenterology* **82**:725 (1982).
5. B.P. Curwain and N.C. Turner, The involvement of histamine receptor subtypes in gastric acid secretion and mucosal blood flow in the anesthetized rabbit, *J. Physiol.* (London) **311**:431 (1981).
6. M. Nakamura, M. Oda, Y. Yonei, N. Tsukada, N. Watanabe, H. Komatsu and M. Tsuchiya, Demonstration of the localization of muscarinic acetylcholine receptors in the gastric mucosa — light and electron microscopic autoradiographic studies using ^{3}H-quinuclidinyl benzilate, *Acta Histochem. Cytochem.* **17**:297 (1984).
7. M. Nakamura, M. Oda, K. Kaneko, K. H. Komatsu, T. Fujiwara, I. Okazaki and M. Tsuchiya, Radioautographic demonstration of ^{3}H-QNB, ^{3}H-cimetidine, ^{3}H-TZU and ^{125}I-gastrin binding sites on the parietal cell: internalization of receptor-bound ligand, *J. Electron Microsc.* **35 (Suppl.)**:3553 (1986).
8. T. Nagata, T. Nawa and S. Yokota, A new technique for electron microscopic dry-mounting radio-

autography of soluble-compounds, *Histochemie* **18**:241 (1969).

9. M.M. Salpeter, L. Bachmann and E.E. Salpeter, Resolution in electron microscope radioautography, *J. Cell Biol.* **41**:1 (1969).

10. M. Nakamura, M. Oda, Y. Yonei, N. Tsukada, H. Komatsu, K. Kaneko and M. Tsuchiya, Muscarinic acetylcholine receptors in rat gastric mucosa a radioautographic study using a potent muscarinic antagonist, ^{3}H-pirenzepine, *Histochemistry* **83**:479 (1985).

11. D.J. Meiners, Y.G. Deshpande and D.L. Kaminski, The role of histamine in control of gastric mucosal blood flow in dogs, *J. Surg. Res.* **32**:608 (1982).

12. C. Heltianu, M. Simionescu and N. Simionescu, Histamine receptors of the microvascular endothelium revealed in situ with a histamine-ferritin conjugate: characteristic high-affinity binding sites in venules, *J. Cell Biol.* **93**:357 (1982).

13. E.M. Renkin, R.D. Carter and W.L. Joyner, Mechanism of the sustained action of histamine and bradykinin on transport of large molecules across the capillary walls in the dog paw, *Microvasc. Res.* **7**:49 (1974).

14. G. Majno and G.E. Palade. Studies on inflammation: I. the effect of histamine and serotonin on vascular permeability: an electron microscopic study, *J. Biophys. Biochem. Cytol.* **11**:571 (1961).

15. M. Nakamura, M. Oda, K. Kaneko, K. Honda, H. Komatsu and M. Tsuchiya, Radioautographic study of the binding sites of QNB on the isolated gastric glandular cell, *Histochemistry* (submitted).

16. M. Nakamura, M. Oda, Y. Yonei, K. Kaneko, H. Komatsu, N. Tsukada, M. Tsuchiya and Y. Fujishiro, Radioautographic demonstration of localization of histamine H_1 and H_2 receptors in the gastric mucosa, *in*: "Microcirculation Annual 1985. Japanese society for microcirculation," M. Tsuchiya, M. Asano, M. Oda and I. Okazaki, ed., Excerpta Medica, pp. 217 (1985).

ALTERATIONS IN GASTRIC MUCOSAL MICROVASCULAR ENDOTHELIUM IN A STRESSED CONDITION—RELEVANCE TO GASTRIC ULCEROGENESIS

Masaya Oda, Masahiko Nakamura, Koya Honda, Hirokazu Komatsu, Kotaro Kaneko, Toshifumi Azuma, Makoto Suematsu, Yoshikazu Yonei, Norihito Watanabe and Masaharu Tsuchiya

Department of Internal Medicine
School of Medicine
Keio University
Tokyo 160, Japan

INTRODUCTION

Since the pioneering reports of Bergmann[1] and Cushing,[2] it has been well known that stress greatly influences gastric functions such as acid secretion, blood flow and peristalsis, and is an important factor in the initiation and recurrence of gastric ulcer. A variety of stresses loaded on human and animal body are transmitted to the stomach via the autonomic nervous system,[3] which regulates the secretion, microcirculation and motility of the stomach.

It has been proposed that the formation of stress ulcers is primarily due to the hypersecretion of gastric acid, possibly triggered by stress-induced overactivity of the cholinergic nerves.[3] This ulcerogenic mechanism, however, has also been explained on the basis of the Reilly phenomenon, i.e. the autonomic nervous irritation syndrome (d'irritation neurovégétative), that an excessive irritation of the autonomic nerves results in hemorrhagic lesions in various visceral organs, concomitant with microcirculatory disturbances.[4] In fact, alterations of the gastric mucosal microcirculation were clearly demonstrated in the process of stress-induced ulcer formation in rats.[5-7] In this respect, the authors demonstrated the changes in the gastric mucosal microvascular endothelium in a stressed condition.[8]

The aim of this article is to review our recent stuides on hemodynamics, architecture and autonomic innervation of the gastric mucosal microvascular system and on their pathophysiological alterations in relation to stress-induced ulcer formation.

STRESS AND HEMORRHAGIC ULCER FORMATION

A large number of studies have been performed on the relationship between psychogenic and physical stresses and gastric ulcer formation. The disease concept of stress-induced gastric ulcer is originally based on "Cushing ulcers"[2] that follows brain trauma, cerebral bleeding, infarction and brain surgery. The following is a typical case of Cushing ulcers the authors had recently experienced. The patient, a 68 year-old housewife, slipped after heavy drinking of alcohol and stroke her head on the wall on June 14, 1987. Eleven days later she suddenly developed bloody stool and was immediately admitted to the Keio University Hospital. On admission, physical examination revealed no abnormal findings except anemia and hypotension (B.P. 78/48 mmHg). Examination of the blood disclosed a hemoglobin of 9.6 gm per 100 ml. Liver function tests showed no abnormalities. Bleeding time and coagulation time were within normal limits. Computed tomography of the brain revealed massive subdural hematoma on the right side, compressing the right hemisphere of the cerebrum to the left side (Fig. 1-a). Emergency gastroendoscopy revealed fresh severe bleeding from acute gastric ulcers on the posterior wall of the corpus of the stomach (Fig. 1-b). Immediately after the surgical removal of the subdural hematoma (Fig. 1-c), the gastric bleeding stopped and the gastric ulcers rapidly regressed and led to the healing stage (Fig. 1-d), indicating an intimate relationship between the intracranial disturbances and the acute hemorrhagic gastric ulcer formation. This is supported by the previous elegant study that experimentally focal electrolytic lesions of the anterior and the posterior hypothalamus result in acute gastric hemorrhage and ulcer formation respectively.[9]

Psychogenic and physical stresses also cause gastric hemorrhagic ulcers similar to those in brain lesions. This type of stress-induced ulcers has been experimentally demonstrated in a restrained rat (Fig. 2)[8].

THE TRANSMISSION PATHWAYS OF STRESS TO THE STOMACH FROM THE CENTRAL NERVOUS SYSTEM

A variety of physical and psychogenic stresses induce impulses from the limbic system of the cerebrum, which are further transmitted to the hypothalamus. The hypothalamus is an integrating center for autonomic, somatic and endocrine functions, controlling all the essential homeostatic processes in the body and keeping the internal milieu constant.[10] Anatomically the efferent and afferent neuronal pathways are connected in the hypothalamus, where the centers for the sympathetic and the parasympathetic nerves exist, contributing to the superordinate control of various autonomic functions, including the gastrointestinal and cardiovascular

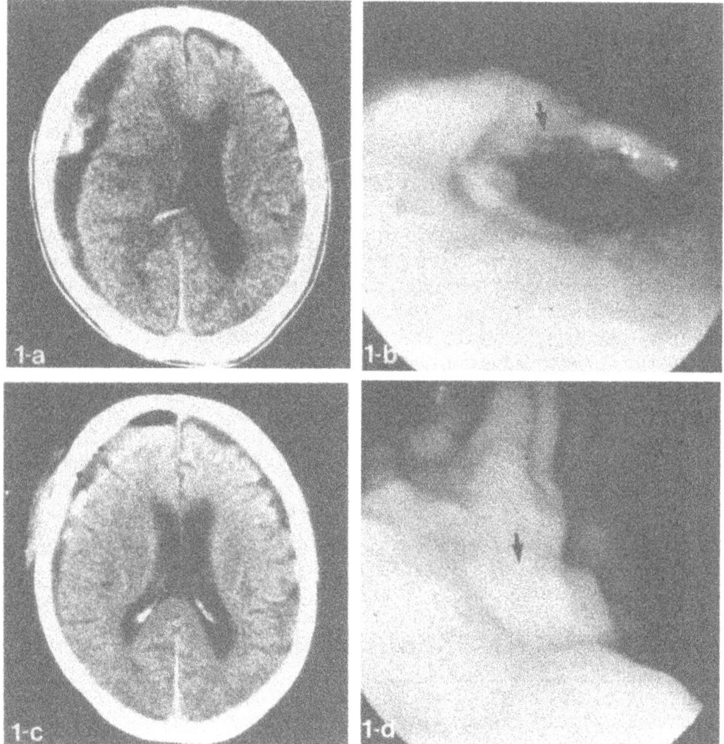

Fig. 1. Relationship between the intracranial lesion and the gastric hemorrhagic ulcer formation. 1-a: Computed tomography of the brain reveals subdural hemorrhage on the left side. The left cerebral hemisphere is remarkably shifted to the right side. 1-b: Gastroendoscopic view. Note a large hemorrhagic ulcer (arrow) formed in the corpus of the stomach. 1-c: Computed tomography after surgery reveals the removal of subdural hematoma concomitant with no shift of the left hemisphere. 1-d: No hemorrhage is noted in the ulcer (arrow) after the removal of subdural hematoma.

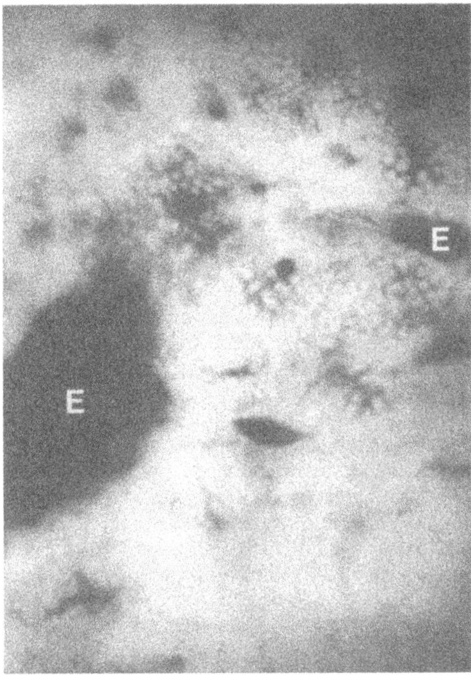

Fig. 2. An experimental model of stress-induced gastric hemorrhagic ulcer. Intravital microscopic view showing that hemorrhagic erosions (E) are formed in the gastric mucosa in the corpus. These hemorrhagic lesions are explained, at least in part, by autonomic nervous irritation syndrome, i.e. the Reilly phenomenon.

systems. From the hypothalamus, stress-induced impulses are conducted not only to the peripheral sympathetic and parasympathetic nervous systems via the medulla and the spinal cord, but also to the anterior pituitary — adrenal gland system via the medial hypothalamus. The former pathway concerns the Reilly phenomenon,[4] while the latter enhances the general adaptation syndrome proposed by Selye.[11]

Stresses are known to stimulate both sympathetic and parasympathetic nervous systems, the impulses from which are transmitted to the stomach throught the routes described below.

PERIPHERAL AUTOMONIC INNERVATION OF THE STOMACH

A. The autonomic nervous pathway to the stomach[10,12]

In general the peripheral autonomic nervous system is entirely efferent. Each autonomic visceral efferent pathway always consists of two nerves. One extends from the central nervous system to a ganglion, and the other extends directly from the ganglion to the effector. Thus preganglionic neurons convey efferent impulses from the central nervous system to autonomic ganglia. Postganglionic neurons relay the impulses from the autonomic ganglia to visceral effectors such as the stomach.

1. Sympathetic system

The cell bodies of the preganglionic sympathetic neurons coursing to the upper abdominal organs are located in the lateral horn of the spinal cord at the level of the fifth to the ninth thoracic

163

segments. The axons of these preganglionic neurons are thin and myelinated, leaving the spinal cord in the ventral roots and the white rami communicantes and terminating in the paired paravertebral ganglia or the unpaired prevertebral ganglia. The axons arising from preganglionic neurons of the sympathetic division at the level of the fifth to the ninth thoracic segments, pass through the sympathetic trunk, known as paravertebral (lateral) ganglia, without terminating in the trunk to form the greater splanchnic nerve that ends at the celiac ganglion, one of the prevertebral (collateral) ganglia, and synapses with the dendrites or cell body of the postganglionic sympathetic neuron. From the celiac ganglion, the postganglionic sympathetic fibers reach the upper abdominal organs, partly terminating in the stomach (Fig. 3). These postganglionic sympathetic fibers are relatively long and unmyelinated. Some postganglionic sympathetic fibers extending from the cervical paravertebral ganglion pass through the vagus nerve, reaching the stomach.

In the sympathetic system, acetylcholine is released as a neurotransmitter from the preganglionic sympathetic nerve endings, whereas noradrenaline is released from the postganglionic nerve endings, acting on the postganglionic effectors via α and β receptors.[12] Therefore the postganglionic sympathetic neurons are called adrenergic neurons.

2. Parasympathetic system

The cell bodies of the preganglionic parasympathetic neurons coursing to the upper abdominal viscera are located in the brainstem (medulla). The preganglionic parasympathetic neurons extending to abdominal organs such as the stomach run in the vagus nerve (cranial nerve X) (Fig. 3). These preganglionic neurons are very long as compared with those of the sympathetic system, passing to the terminal ganglia, which are situated near or within the walls of the gastrointestinal tract as intramural ganglia. Thus the unmyelinated, postganglionic parasympathetic fibers are very short.

In the parasympathetic system, acetylcholine is released as a neurotransmitter both from the

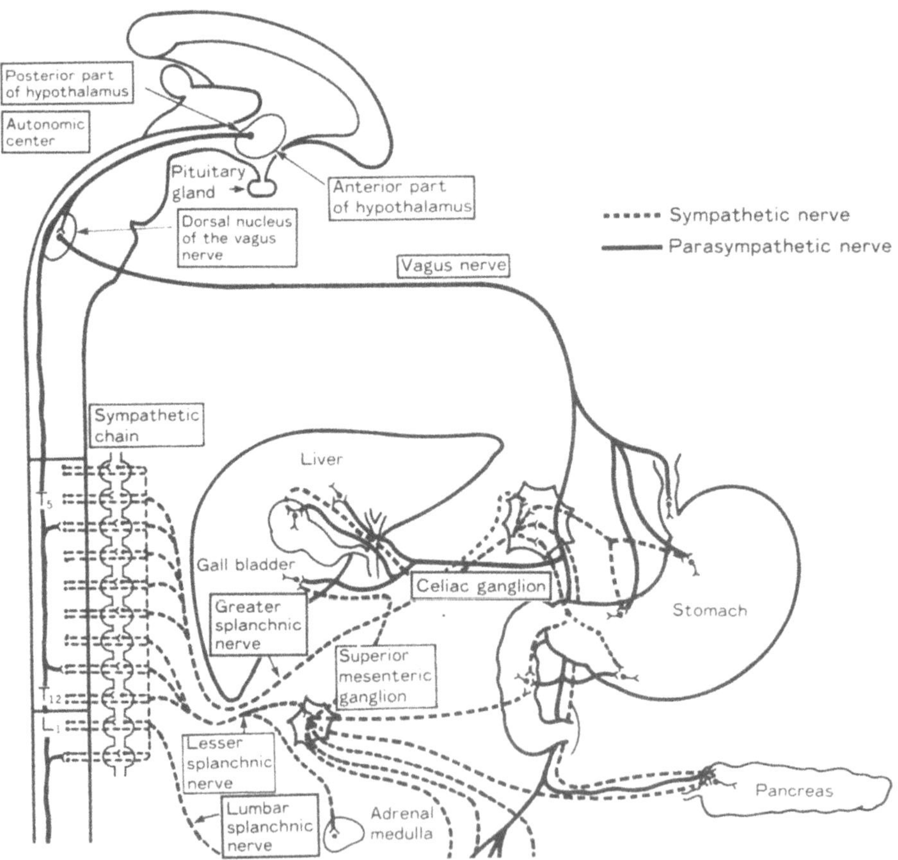

Fig. 3. A schematical illustration of the autonomic nervous system extending to the stomach.

preganglionic and from the postganglionic nerve endings. In the latter, acetylcholine is transmitted to the postsynaptic membranes via the muscarinic receptors (M_1 and M_2 receptors) or the nicotinic receptors. The muscarinic action of acetylcholine is selectively blocked by atropine, while the nicotinic action is blocked by quaternary ammonium bases. The postganglionic parasympathetic neurons are called cholinergic neurons.

B. Features of autonomic nervous distribution to the gastric mucosal microvasculature — Evidence for direct cholinergic innervation

1. Histochemical and fluorescence microscopy

Histochemical distribution of the cholinergic nerves in the rat gastric wall was examined by the method of Karnovsky & Roots,[13] in order to the localization of acetylcholinesterase (AChE), i.e. the enzyme which catabolizes acetylcholine released from the cholinergic nerve endings. The AChE activity, which is stained as reddish brown and indicates the localization of cholinergic nerve fibers, is distributed in linear form mainly along the microvessels throughout the gastric wall.[8,14-16] The AChE-positive nerve fibers are also located in the myenteric nerve plexuses (Auerbach plexuses) and in the submucosal nerve plexuses (Meissner plexuses). The distribution of choline acetyltransferase (ChA), i.e. the enzyme for synthesizing acetylcholine, was visualized by the indirect immunofluorescence antibody method using anti-ChA antibody obtained from the rabbit immunized with ChA.[17] The distribution of ChA is similar to that of AChE, indicating that the AChE-positive fibers correspond to the cholinergic nerve fibers. In the longitudinal sections, the cholinergic nerve fibers are found to reach the muscularis mucosae, via the myenteric and submucosal nerve plexuses supplying some branches. After piercing the muscularis mucosae along the blood vessels, they give rise to a large number of ramified fibers extending along the capillaries up to the mucosal surface. In the tangenital sections, the AChE-positive nerve fibers appear to be closely associated with the capillaries and venules, as well as the epithelial cells. This close relationship between the nerve fibers and the capillaries and postcapillary venules is clearly demonstrated in the Epon-embedded, methylene blue-stained 1 μm sections.[16]

The distribution of adrenergic nerve fibers was identified by a modification of the method of Falck and Hillarp,[18] with perfusion of glyoxylic acid followed by aluminum sulfate and formaldehyde.[19] The adrenergic varicose fibers showing the bluish green fluorescence under a fluorescence microscope are distributed mainly along the blood vessels, particularly along the arterioles in the submucosa and near the arterioles and arterial capillaries in the basal portion of the mucosa. They are also located near the muscular venules in the submucosa. The noradrenergic fluorescence is present in linear form within the myenteric and submucosal plexuses, but not in the nerve cells, indicating that the postganglionic adrenergic fibers do not change synapses in these intramural plexuses.

Morphometric analysis of the cholinergic and the adrenergic nervous distribution described above reveals that the cholinergic nerves are predominant throughout the gastric mucosal layer.[13] Neuroendocrine cells are found to be present in the myenteric and submucosal plexuses,[20] containing a variety of neuropeptides such as vasoactive intestinal polypeptide (VIP), substance P and somatostatin, cholecystokinin (CCK) and enkephalin and providing an autonomity in the regulation of gastric functions.[21,22] Thus, these intrinsic neuropeptidergic regulations are considered to be modified by adrenergic and cholinergic neurons entering the stomach wall as extrinsic nerves.

2. Electron microscopy

Scanning electron microscopic observation of hydrogen chloride and collagenase-digested preparations[23,24] reveals that the nerve fibers are terminated both on the outer surfaces of the capillary and venular walls and on those of the epithelial cells in the gastric mucosa.[8,15,16] By transmission electron microscopy, the unmyelinated nerve endings, including small clear vesicles, 20—50 nm in diameter, are found to be located in the close vicinity of the true capillary and postcapillary venular endothelium.[8,14,16] The adrenergic nerve endings, characterized by the presence of small cored vesicles, 40-50 nm in diameter, are located near the arteriolar and capillary wall in the basal portion of the mucosa. They sometimes coexist with the cholinergic nerve endings within a single Schwann cell,[14] possibly relating to the complexity of autonomic nervous control of gastric activities. By electron microscopic cytochemical observation of the AChE localization, the AChE reaction products are proved to be specifically deposited not only on the axonal membranes of the unmyelinated nerve endings but also on the basal site of the endothelial plasma membrane of the capillary and postcapillary venule, implying that acetylcholine is transmitted from the former to the latter. In the uranyl acetate en bloc stained preparations, the microfilaments, 5—7 nm in diameter, i.e. actin filaments, are evident within the capillary and postcapillary venular endothelium.[8] These intracytoplasmic microfilaments are closely associated with the endothelial plasma membrane and with the vesicles and vaculoes in the endothelium. These findings imply that the microfilaments may be involved in the contraction of endothelium and in the formation and movement of vesicles and vacuoles across the endothelium, regulating the permeability of the capillary and postcapillary venule. This hypothesis has recently been supported by the time-lapse cinematographic study[25,26] demonstrating that the primary monolayer-cultured capillary endothelium isolated from the gastric mucosa make contractions with Brownian movement of vesicles and that these dynamic motilities are completely suppressed by cytochalasin B, an actin filament-depolymerizing agent, whereas they are enhanced by acetylcholine and histamine.

3. Light and electron microscopic radioautography for the demonstration of muscarinic acetylcholine receptors in the gastric mucosa

In order to obtain direct evidence for cholinergic innervation of capillary and venular vessels, it is essential to demonstrate the presence of muscarinic acetylcholine receptors (m-AChR) on these vascular walls. Autoradiography for soluble compounds[27] is one of the useful methods for obtaining such evidence.

Under anesthesia with sodium pentobarbital, a tritium-labeled muscarinic acetylcholine receptor antagonist, ^{3}H-quinuclidinyl benzilate (^{3}H-QNB:250 μCi; 0.05 mg, Amersham) or a high dose of ^{3}H-pirenzepine (^{3}H-PZ:1 mCi; 1.5 mg, New England Nuclear) was infused for 30 min with a constant rate of 23 μl per min via an abdominal aortic catheter in the rat, followed by the procedures previously reported.[16,28] Tissue pieces of the corpus of the stomach obtained immediately after the infusion of ^{3}H-QNB or ^{3}H-PZ were quickly fixed by a freeze-drying method, followed by dry sectioning and mounting to prevent diffusion artifacts and translocation or loss of water-soluble ligands from the binding sites. Autoradiographic light microscopy revealed that the silver grains showing the binding sites of ^{3}H-QNB and the high dose of ^{3}H-PZ, i.e. the localization of m-AChR, are predominantly located in the middle and lower zones of the mucosa in the corpus of the rat stomach. At high magnifications, these grains are evident on the capillaries and venules, as well as near the basolateral plasma membranes of the epithelial cells corresponding to the parietal and chief cells.[16,29] By transmission electron microscopy the silver grains are proved to be present not only on the plasma membrane of the parietal cell, but also on the plasma membrane of the capillary and postcapillary venular endothelium.[16]

The histochemical, radioautographic and scanning and transmission electron microscopic findings described above lead to the tentative conclusion that the cholinergic nerves would directly innervate both the parietal cells and the capillaries and venules in the gastric mucosa, as schematically shown in Fig. 4.

Acetylcholine is considered to be transmitted from the nerve endings both to the mucosal microvascular endothelium and to the parietal cell via the m-AChR on each effector cell surface, acting on the microfilaments in both types of effector cells.[15] In the microvascular endothelium, the intracytoplasmic microfilaments[8,13,15,] would be involved in endothelial contraction and vesicular transport in the regulation of microvascular permeability. In the parietal cell, they may contribute to the membrane rearrangement and recycling in the mutual transformation between intracellular canaliculi and tubulovesicles in the control of gastric acid secretion.[31,32] This dual action of the cholinergic nerves in the gastric mucosa would explain, at least in part, the hypersensitivity of the stomach to stress which is transmitted via the parasympathetic pathway as well as the sympathetic from the central nervous system. The overactivity of the cholinergic nerves innervating the gastric mucosa would contribute to the pathogenesis of stress-induced gastric ulcer as described below.[15]

C. Features of gastric mucosal microvasculature

A major supplying artery entering the submucosa ramifies three or four times, giving rise to a number of arterioles approximately 100 to 50 μm in diameter, as its diameter decreases toward the base of the mucosa. These arterioles pierce through the muscularis mucosae, giving off the smaller arteriolar vessels corresponding to the metarterioles, approximately 15 to 10 μm in diameter, which are distributed just above the muscularis mucosae in the horizontal direction to the plane of the mucosa. From these terminal arterioles, a large number of capillaries arise at right angles to the plane of the mucosa, standing up toward the luminal surface of the mucosa. At the mucosal surface, most of these anastomosing capillaries drain into the collecting venules, approximately 30 to 50 μm in diameter, via the postcapillary venules, approximately 15 μm in diameter.[33] It is of importance for the understanding of the gastric mucosal microcirculatory mechanism to note that the drainage of the mucosal capillary blood flow into the collecting venules is restricted to the luminal surface of the mucosa.

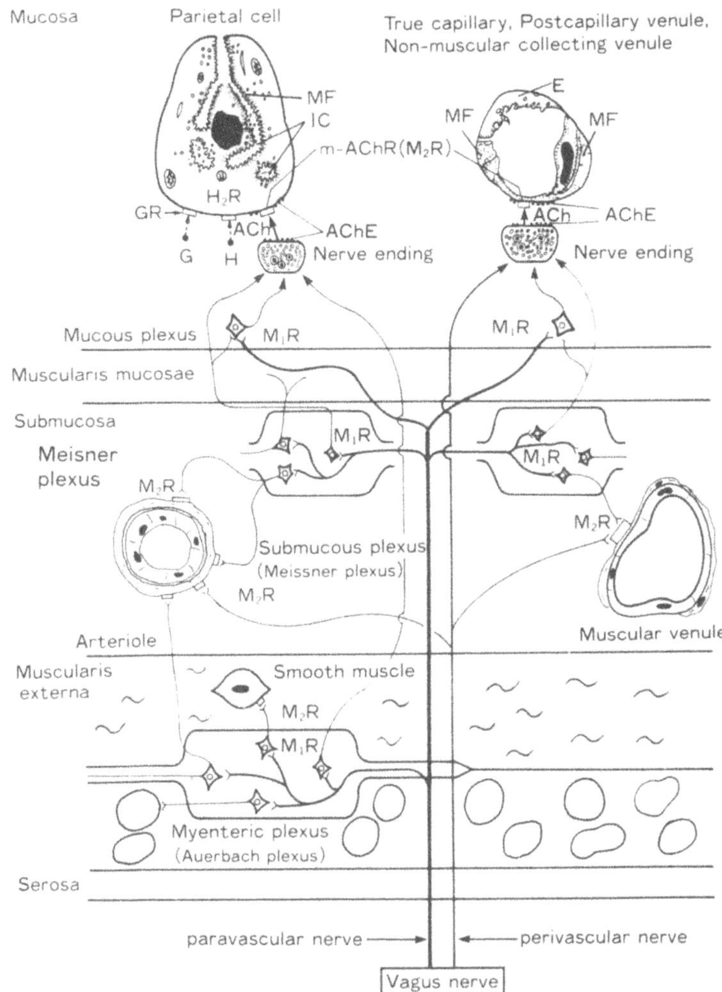

Fig. 4. Dual innervation of the intramural cholinergic nerves in the gastric mucosa. The cholinergic neurons directly innervate both parietal cells and mucosal capillaries and venules.

D. Intravital microscopic views of the hemodynamics in the gastric mucosal microvasculature

Intravital microscopic observation reveals the dynamic blood flow in the draining portion of the mucosal microvasculature (Fig.5-a).[8,33] Under an intravital microscope, the blood is seen flowing rapidly and uniformly in the anastomosing capillary network surrounding the gastric pits at the mucosal surface and ultimately draining into the collecting venules (Fig. 5-a,b).[8] Four percent pontamine sky blue administrated via an aortic catheter is evently distributed in the capillary network and immediately disappears into the collecting venules with no leakage from these microvessels.

ALTERATIONS IN THE GASTRIC MUCOSAL MICROVASCULAR SYSTEM IN A STRESSED CONDITION INDUCED BY IMMOBILIZATION OF A RAT WITH PLASTER BANDAGE

A. Intravital microscopic changes in the gastric mucosal microcirculation

Intravital microscopic observations of the gastric mucosal microcirculation of the restrain-

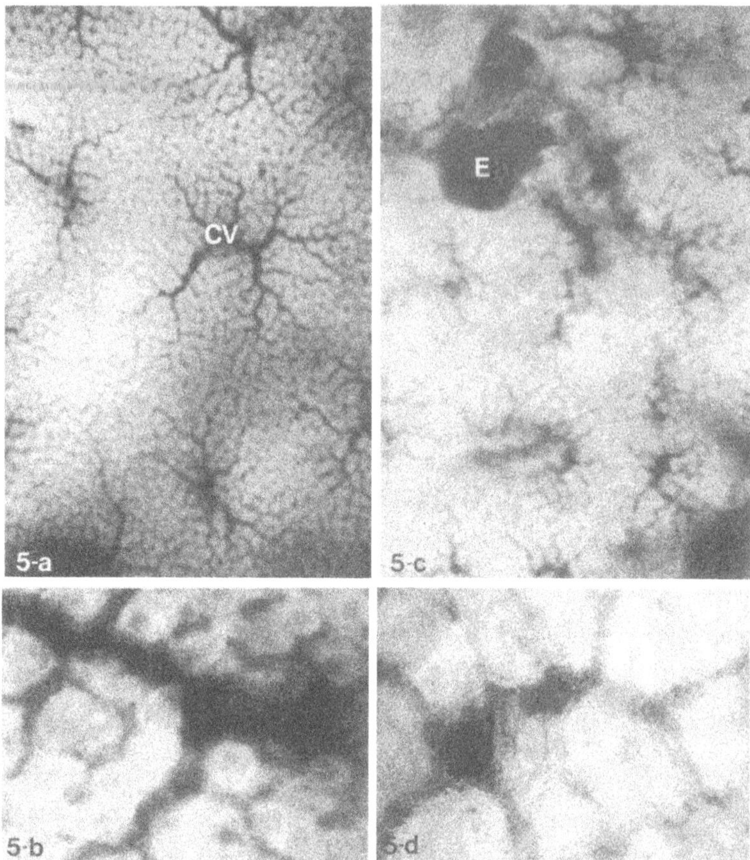

Fig. 5. Intravital microscopic view of the gastric mucosal microcirculatory system in control and restrained rats. 5-a: The capillary blood flow is rapid and uniform, draining into the collecting venules (CV) in the mucosa of control rat stomach. 5-b: At high magnification, the blood flow is clearly visualized. The flow is so fast that blood cells can not be recognized. 5-c: In the restrained rat stomach, focal hemorrhagic erosion (E) are noted in the mucosa. The capillary blood flow is irregularly interrupted. 5-d: At high magnification, the mucosal capillary hemodynamics is irregularly in a low flow state concomitant with sludging, regurgitation and flying thrombi.

ed rats reveal that focal bleedings occur in the capillary network and around the collecting venules (Fig. 5-c). At high magnifications, the blood flow is characterized by various forms of microcirculatory disturbances, even in areas distant from the hemorrhagic changes. Sludge phenomenon, stasis and regurgitation are observed in the capillary network, particularly around the collecting venules (Fig.5-d). In the low flow state, white blood cells are frequently seen sticking or rolling on the capillary and venular endothelium and flying thrombi are sometimes observed.

Pontamine sky blue infused via an abdominal aortic catheter permeates remarkably from the collecting venules and the surrounding capillaries, especially near the hemorrhagic erosion in the upper layer of the gastric mucosa (Fig. 6-a). Horseradish peroxidase (HRP) infused as above is also similarly extravasated from the collecting venules and capillaries surrounding the hemorrhagic erosion (Fig. 6-c). In the continuous tissue section, the acetylcholinesterase activity (AChE) is found to be greatly enhanced in the same portion as HRP is extensively permeated (Fig. 6-d).

B. Enhanced activity of the cholinergic nerves in the gastric mucosa under restraint stress

The AChE reaction products are also present in the increased pinocytotic vesicles of the capillary endothelium (Fig. 7-a), which correlates well with the cholinergic nervous activity,[15]

168

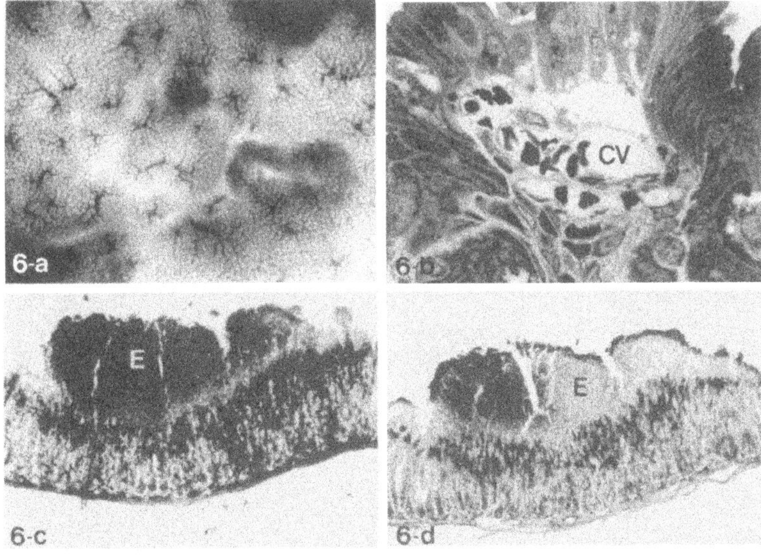

Fig. 6. Correlation between an increase in microvascular permeability and acetylcholinesterase activity in the gastric mucosa in the restrained rat. 6-a: Intravital microscopy reveals that pontamine sky blue infused via an abdominal aortic catheter markedly permeates from the collecting venules and surrounding capillaries. 6-b: The tip area of the lamina propriae mucosae appears to be edematous, particularly around the collecting venule (CV). A number of erythrocytes are extravasated. 6-c: Horseradish peroxidase (HRP) infused via an abdominal aortic catheter permeates markedly, particularly in the area surrounding the hemorrhagic erosion (E) in the longitudinal section of the restrained rat stomach. 6-d: In the continuous section of Fig. 6-c, acetylcholinesterase activity is markedly increased in the same area as HRP is excessively permeated.

indicating that the intramural cholinergic nerves are overstimulated in the gastric mucosa under the restraint-stressed condition. By transmission electron microscopy the AChE reaction products are remarkably increased both in the axonal membranes of the unmyelinated cholinergic nerve endings and in the basal site of the endothelial plasma membrane of the true capillary (Fig. 7-a) and postcapillary venule (Fig. 7-b), implying that the cholinergic neurotransmitter, acethylcholine, is excessively transmitted from the former to the latter.

C. Ultrastructural alterations of the gastric mucosal microvascular endothelium under the restraint-stressed condition

In the Epon-embedded, toluidine blue-stained 1 μm sections of the corpus of the restrained rat stomach, the lamina propria mucosae appears to be edematous with extravasation of red blood cells near the collecting venules and surrounding capillaries at the upper portion of the mucosa even in the area quite distant from the hemorrhagic erosion (Fig. 6-b). By transmission electron microscopy a number of erythrocytes are proved to be extravasated in the vicinity of the postcapillary venules and capillaries.

The true capillary endothelial cells tend to be swollen, especially in the area surrounding the collecting venule (Fig. 7-c). Horseradish peroxidase infused as a tracer via an abdominal aortic catheter permeates excessively from the capillary through the increased pinocytotic vesicles and the widened gaps between the adjacent capillary endothelial cells (Fig. 7-c).

HRP is also found to leak abnormally from the postcapillary and collecting venules in the gastric mucosa under the restraint-stressed condition. Thorium dioxide similarly infused as a tracer is found electron microscopically to be abnormally extravasated from the mucosal capillaries, mainly by the enhanced vesicular transport across the capillary endothelium (Fig. 7-d). The mechanism of these increased microvascular permeabilities could be explained as follows. Excessive acetylcholine released from the nerve endings of the cholinergic neurons, which have

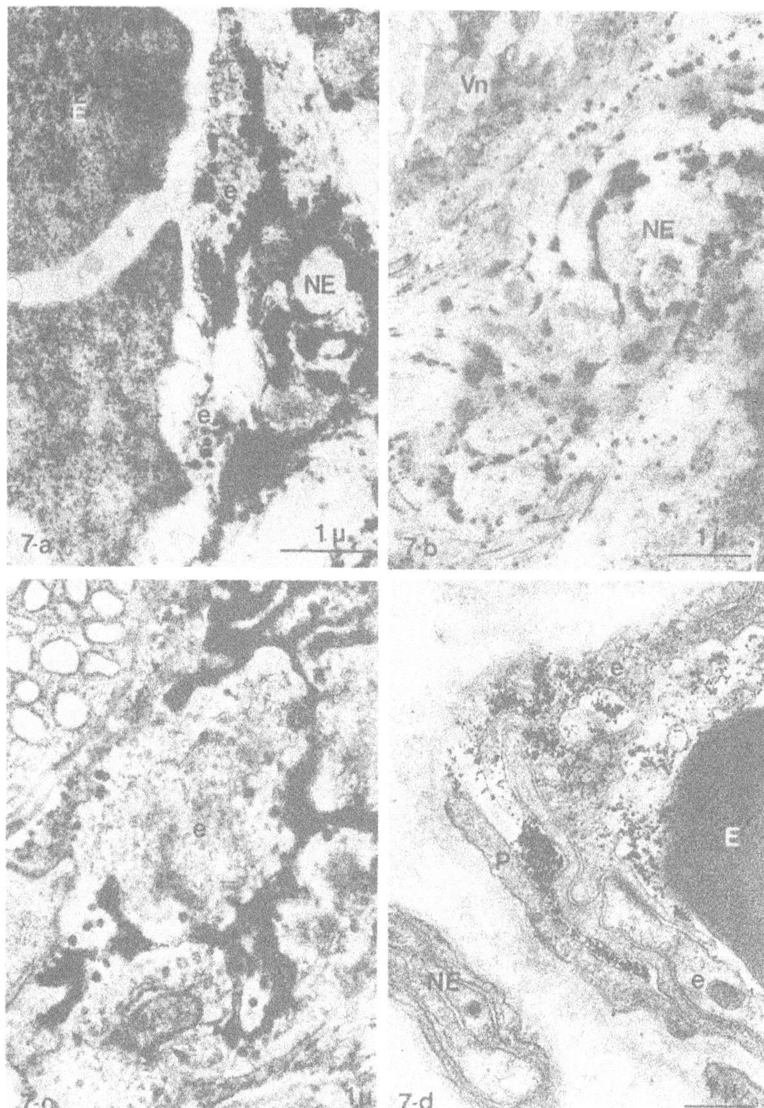

Fig. 7. Electron microscopic evidence for increase in acetylcholinesterase activity and in capillary permeability in the gastric mucosa under restraint stress. 7-a: The acetylcholinesterase (AChE) reaction products are markedly increased both on the axonal membranes of the unmyelinated nerve endings (NE) and on the basal site of the plasma membrane of capillary endothelium (e), implying that acetylcholine released from the cholinergic nerve endings is excessively transmitted to the capillary endothelium, possibly enhancing the vesicular transport. The erythrocyte (E) shows its own activity. AChE stain. 7-b: At the level of the postcapillary and collecting venule (Vn), the AChE activity is also proved to be increased not only on the axonal membranes of the nerve endings (NE) but also on the basal site of endothelial plasma membrane. AChE stain. 7-c: Horseradish peroxidase infused via an abdominal aortic catheter is seen to be excessively translocated across the capillary endothelium (e) from the luminal side to the abluminal side through vesicular transport. The endothelium appears to be swollen and the lumen is narrowed. E: erythrocyte, Graham-Karnovsky reaction. 7-d: Thorium dioxide (Thorotrast) infused via an abdominal aortic catheter is also abnormally extravasated via vesicles and vacuoles in the capillary endothelium (e). NE: nerve ending, E: erythrocyte, P: pericyte, Uranyl acetate and lead citrate stain.

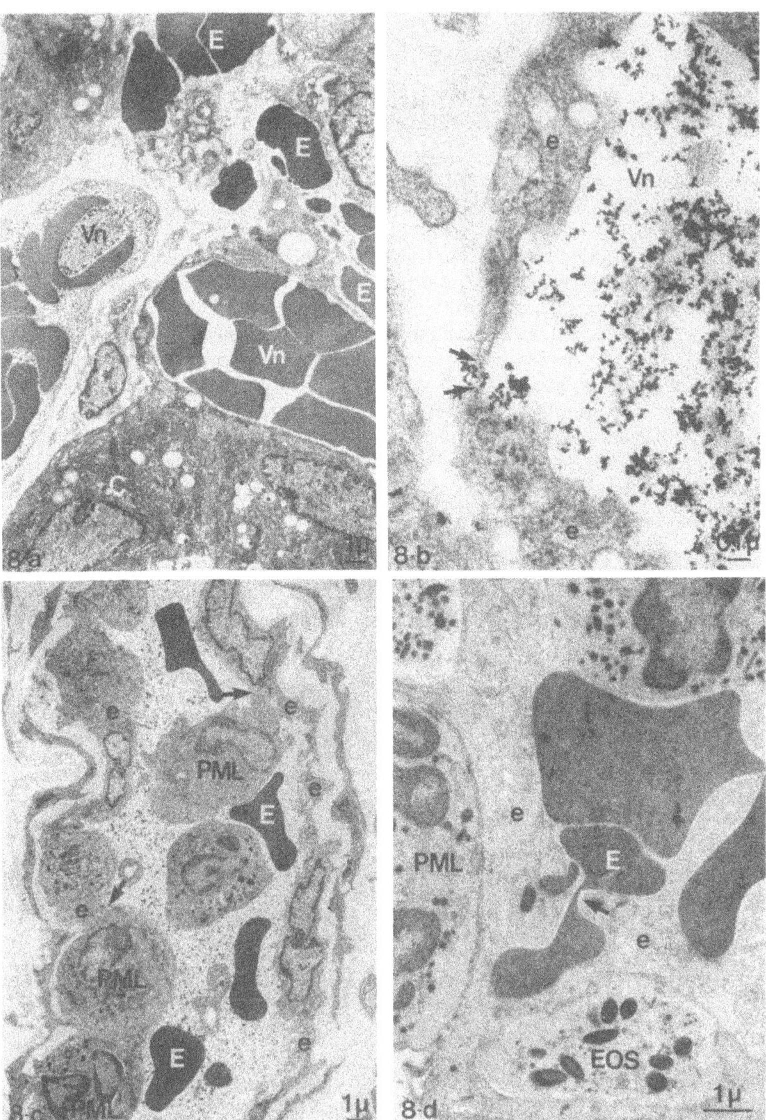

Fig. 8. Electron microscopic evidence for increased permeability and extravascular migration of blood cells at the level of the postcapillary venules under restraint stress. 8-a: A number of erythrocytes (E) are extravasated around the postcapillary venule (Vn) in the gastric mucosa. C: chief cell. Uranyl acetate and lead citrate stain. 8-b: Thorium dioxide infused via an abdominal aortic catheter leaks through a gap between the endothelial cells (e) of the postcapillary venule (Vn) (arrows). Uranyl acetate and lead citrate stain. 8-c: A couple of polymorphonuclear leukocytes (PML) are found to be closely associated with the postcapillary venular endothelial cells (e). This electron microscopic finding corresponds to the intravital microscopic view that white blood cells are rolling on or sticking to the venular endothelium. Note the close association of leukocytes with the endothelial cells (arrows), implying that the interaction between these two types of cells may play an important role in increasing vascular permeability. E: erythrocyte. Uranyl acetate and lead citrate stain. 8-d: The erythrocyte (E) is seen protruding to the extravascular space through a widened gap between the postcapillary venular endothelial cells (e) (arrow). A polymorphonuclear leukocyte (PML) and an eosinophile leukocyte (EOS) are extravasated. Uranyl acetate and lead citrate stain.

been overstimulated by restraint stress, would act chiefly on the capillary and non-muscular venular endothelium via the muscarinic acetylcholine receptors and activate the intracytoplasmic actin filament system,[8,26,30] enhancing not only the movement of vesicles and vacuoles across the endothelium but also the endothelial contraction.[26] The former concerns the enhancement of endothelial vesicular transport from the luminal side to the abluminal side, while the latter contributes to the widening of a gap between the endothelial cells through which blood constituents pass to the extravascular space. Intracytoplasmic calcium ions (Ca^{++}) and Ca^{++}-binding protein, calmodulin, are involved in the mechanism of actin filament contraction within the microvascular endothelium.[35]

The extravasation of erythrocytes possibly induced by overstimulation of the cholinergic neurons under restraint stress are most prominent at the postcapillary and collecting venules in the upper portion of the gastric mucosa (Fig. 8-a). Thorium dioxide or HRP infused via an abdominal aortic catheter is found electron microscopically to permeate from the widened endothelial gap (Fig. 8-b). Widening of the endothelial gap is also observed at the postcapillary venule, particularly when polymorphonuclear leukocytes are sticking on the luminal surface of the endothelial cells (Fig. 8-c), suggesting that the interaction between polymorphonuclear leukocytes and endothelial cells[36,37] is also related to the mechanism of endothelial contraction which allows leukocytes and erythrocytes to emigrate to the extravascular area. The erythrocyte is shown protruding into the extravascular space throgh the widened gap between the endothelial cells, possibly following the extravasation of leukocytes (Fig. 8-d).

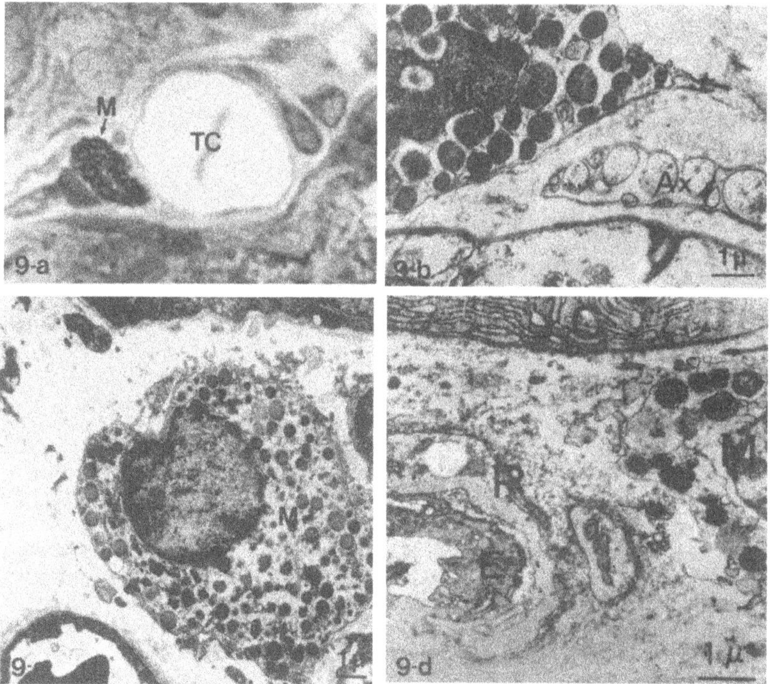

Fig. 9. Involvement of mast cell degranulation in the gastric mucosal microvascular alterations under restraint stress. 9-a: The mast cell (M) containing metachromatic granules are located in the vicinity of the true capillary (TC) in the gastric mucosa. Epon-embedded 1 μm section. Toluidine blue stain. 9-b: Electron microscopically the unmyelinated nerve axons (Ax) containing small clear vesicles (the cholinergic nerve endings) are located near the mast cell (M). Uranyl acetate and lead citrate stain. 9-c: Electron micrograph showing the mucosal mast cell (M). Uranyl acetate and lead citrate stain. 9-d: Electron micrograph demonstrating the degranulation of mucosal mast cell (M) under restraint stress. The granules containing histamine and serotonin (arrows) are scattered around the true capillary. E: capillary endothelium, P: pericyte. Uranyl acetate and lead citrate stain.

D. Involvement of mast cell degranulation in the gastric mucosal microvascular changes under restraint stress

Two types of mast cells containing metachromatic granules, i.e. the mucosal mast cells and the connective tissue mast cells, exist in the gastric wall. The former are located mainly near the capillaries and venules in the mucosa (Fig. 9-a), while the latter are located mainly near the arterioles and venules in the submucosa. Mucosal mast cells are smaller in cell size and more varied in size of granules in comparison with connective tissue mast cells (Fig. 9-c). It is of interest to note that the unmyelinated cholinergic nerve endings are found to be frequently situated in the close vicinity of mast cells (Fig. 9-b), implying that acetylcholine released from the nerve endings would directly affect mast cells to cause degranulation.[38]

Mucosal mast cells are frequently degranulated under restraint stress, and the granules are found to be scattered around the capillaries and venules (Fig. 9-d). Vasoactive substances such as histamine and serotonin released from mast cell granules would influence microvascular permeability, disturbing the hemodynamics of the microcirculatory system.[39]

SUMMARY AND CONCLUSIONS

The present paper describes the morphological and functional alterations of the gastric mucosal microvascular endothelium under restraint-stressed condition. On the basis of the direct cholinergic innervation of capillaries and non-muscular venules in the gastric mucosa, these endothelial changes would be caused by the stress-induced overstimulation of the cholinergic nerves and modified by the degranulation of mast cells, contributing to the stress-induced ulcer formation as schematically illustrated in Fig. 10.

ACKNOWLEDGMENT

This study was supported by the Grant-in-Aid for Scientific Research of the Ministry of Education, Science and Culture (#59370025, 61770504).

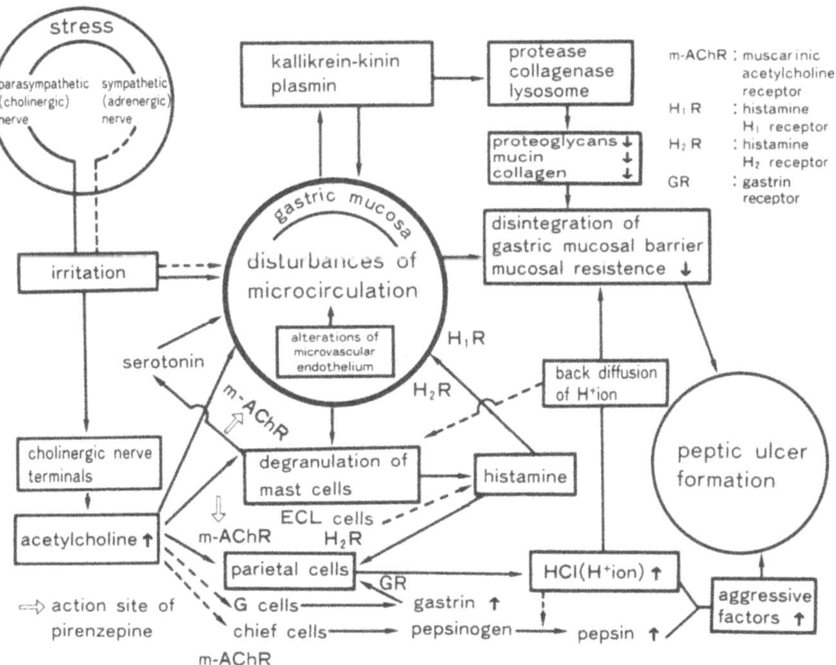

Fig. 10. Involvement of mucosal microvascular endothelial alterations in the mechanism of stress-induced ulcer formation.

REFERENCES

1. G. Bergmann, Das Spasmogene Ulcus Pepticum, *Münch. Med. Wöchenschr.*, **60**:169-174 (1913).
2. H. Cushing, Peptic ulcers and the interbrain, *Surg. Gynecol. Obstet.*, **55**:1-34 (1932).
3. H. Shay, Stress and gastric acid secretion, *Gastroenterology*, **26**:316-319 (1954).
4. Y. Yamaguchi, M. Tsuchiya, T. Akiba, K. Kobayashi, K. Shiraishi and H. Nozaki, Experimental studies on the pathological changes in the several organs due to irritation of the autonomic nervous system, *Keio J. Med.*, **9**:91-99 (1960).
5. M. Tsuchiya, T. Shishido, Y. Kamisaka, M. Oda and Y. Fujishiro, The alteration of gastric microcirculation in the restraint-induced gastric lesion, *in*: "Microcirculatory Approach to Current Therapeutic Problems," Proceedings of the 6th European Conference for Microcirculation, Aalborg, Demmark, 138-141 (1970).
6. T. Hase and B.J. Moss, Microvascular changes of gastric mucosa in the development of stress ulcer in rats, *Gastroenterology*, **65**:224-234 (1973).
7. M. Kitajima, R.R. Wolfe, R.L. Trelftadt, J.R. Allsop and J.F. Burk, Gastric mucosal lesion after burn injury: Relationship to H^+-back diffusion and the microcirculation, *J. Trauma*, **18**:644-650 (1978).
8. M. Oda, M. Nakamura, N. Watanabe, N. Tsukada, Y. Ohya, E. Sekizuka and M. Tsuchiya, Autonomic nervous regulation of gastric mucosal microcirculation — with special reference to the pathogenesis of stress-induced gastric ulcer, *in*: "Basic Aspects of Microcirculation," Proceedings of Tokyo International Symposium on Microcirculation, July 26, 1981, Tokyo, Japan, M. Tsuchiya, M. Oda, M. Asano, ed, Excerpta Medica, Amsterdam, 209-229 (1982).
9. J.D. French, R.W. Porter, F.K.von Amwrongen and R.B. Raney, Gastrointestinal hemorrhage and ulceration associated with intracranial lesions, *Surgery*, **32**:395-407 (1952).
10. G.J. Tortora, N.P. Anagnostakos, The autonomic nervous system, *in*: "Principles of Anatomy and Physiology," G.J. Tortora, N.P. Anagnostakos, ed, Harper & Row Publishers, New York, 356-369 (1978).
11. H. Selye, The physiology and pathology of exposure to stress, A treatise based on the concepts of the general adaptation syndrome and the disease of adaptation, Acta Inc. Medical Publishers, Montreal (1950).
12. W. Jänig, The autonomic nervous system, *in*: "Human Physiology," R.F. Schmidt, G. Thews, ed, Springer-Verlag, Berlin, Heiderberg, New York, 111-144 (1983).
13. M.J. Karnovsky and L. Roots, A direct coloring thiocholine method for cholinesterase, J. Histochem. *Cytochem.*, **12**:219-221 (1964).
14. M. Nakamura, N. Watanabe, N. Tsukada, M. Oda and M. Tsuchiya, Demonstration of the adrenergic nerves in the rat gastric mucosa — a histofluorescence and electron microscopic study in comparison with the distribution of the cholinergic nerves —, *Okajimas Folia Anat. Jpn.*, **59**:65-86 (1982).
15. M. Oda, M. Nakamura, N. Tsukada, Y. Yonei, H. Komatsu, Y. Ohya, E. Sekizuka and M. Tsuchiya, Dual action of the parasympathetic nerve in the gastric mucosa; significance of its overactivity in the pathogenesis of gastric ulcer, *in*: "Gastronintestinal Function, Regulation and Disturbances," Proceedings of the 1st Symposium of the Regulation and Disturbances of Gastrointestinal Function, September 18, 1982, Tokyo, Japan, Y. Kasuya, M. Tsuchiya, F. Nagao, Y. Matsuo, ed, Excerpta Medica, Amsterdam, 145-173 (1983).
16. M. Oda, M. Nakamura, Y. Yonei, K. Kaneko, H. Komatsu, N. Tsukada, K. Honda, Y. Akaiwa and M. Tsuchiya, Features of autonomic innervation of the gastric microvasculature evidence for cholinergic innervation of the mucosal capillaries in the rat stomach —, *in*: "Microcirculation Annual 1985. Japanese Society for Miscrocirculation," M. Tsuchiya, M. Asano, M. Oda, I. Okazaki, ed, Excerpta Medica, Amsterdam, 205-216 (1985).
17. M. Nakamura, M. Oda, N. Watanabe, N. Tsukada, Y. Yonei, H. Komatsu, Y. Akaiwa and M. Tsuchiya, Significance of the cholinergic innervation in the gastric mucosa, *in*: "Experimental Ulcer Research Trends in Japan," Proceedings of the 11th Annual Meeting for Experimental Ulcer Research, November 25, 1983, Tokyo, Japan, M. Tsuchiya, M. Oda, I. Okazaki, ed, Yurinsha Ltd., Tokyo, 127-136 (1984).
18. B. Falck and N. Hillarp, Fluorescence of cathecolamine and related compounds condensed with folmaldehyde, *J. Histochem. Cytochem.*, **10**:348-354 (1973).
19. V. Ajelis, A. Björklund, B. Falck, O. Lindvall, J. Loren and B. Walles, Application of the aluminium formaldehyde (ALFA) histofluorescence method for demonstration of peripheral stores of cathecolamines and indolamines in freeze-dried parafine-embedded tissue, cryostat sections and whole mounts, *Histochemistry*, **65**:1-15 (1979).
20. Y. Matsuo and A. Seki, The coordination of gastrointestinal hormones and the autonomic nerves, *Am. J. Gastroenterol.*, **69**:21-50 (1978).
21. G. Gabella, Innervation of the gastrointestinal tract, *Int. Rev. Cytol.*, **59**:129-193 (1979).
22. I.J. Llewellyn-Smith, J.B. Furness, A.J. Wilson and M. Costa, Organization and fine structure of

enteric ganglia, *in:* "Autonomic Ganglia," L.-G. Elfvin, ed, John Wiley & Sons, Chinchester, 145-182 (1983).

23. A.P. Evan, W.G. Dail, D. Dammrose and C. Palmer, Scanning electron microscopy of cell surface following removal of extracellular material, *Anat. Rec.,* 185:433-445 (1976).

24. T. Fujiwara and Y. Uehara, The cytoarchitecture of the wall and the innervation pattern of the microvessels in the rat mammary grand: a scanning electron microscopic observation, *Am. J. Anat.,* 170:39-54 (1984).

25. K. Honda, M. Oda, M. Nakamura, N. Tsukada, H. Komatsu, K. Kaneko, T. Azuma and M. Tsuchiya, Involvement of actin filaments in the motility of the primary cultured capillary endothelium, *in:* "Microcirculation Annual 1987. Japanese society for Microcirculation," M. Tsuchiya, M. Asano, Y. Mishima, ed, Nihon-Igakukan, Tokyo, 117-118 (1987).

26. M. Oda and K. Honda, Cytoskeletal regulation of endothelial permeability, IVth World Congress for Microcirculation, Symposium, The cell biology of endothelium: permeability, July 27, 1987, Tokyo, Japan.

27. T. Nagata, T. Nawa and S. Yokota, A new technique for electron microscopic dry-mounting radioautography of soluble compounds, *Histochemie,* 18:241-249 (1969).

28. M. Nakamura, M. Oda, Y. Yonei, N. Tsukada, N. Watanabe, H. Komatsu and M. Tsuchiya, Demonstration of the localization of muscarinic acetylcholine receptors in the gastric mucosa-light and electron microscopic autoradiographic studies using ^{3}H-quinuclidinyl benzilate, *Acta Histochem. Cytochem.,* 17:297-309 (1984).

29. M. Oda, M. Nakamura, Y. Yonei, N. Tsukada, H. Komatsu, K. Kaneko, Y. Akaiwa, E. Ichikawa, I. Okazaki and M. Tsuchiya, Effect of the muscarinic receptor antagonist pirenzepine on the gastric mucosal microcirculation — its possible action sites in the stomach, Proceedings of the Symposium on Pirenzepine: New Aspects in Research and Theraphy, September 18, 1984, Lisbon, Portugal, A. Bettarello, ed, Excerpta Medica, Amsterdam, 19-40 (1985).

30. K. Honda, M. Oda, M. Nakamura, N. Tsukada, Y. Yonei, H. Komatsu, K. Kaneko, Y. Akaiwa, T. Fujiwara and M. Tsuchiya, Ultrastructural and cytochemical characterization of the monolayer-cultured capillary endothelium, *J. Electron Microscopy,* 35 (supple):2761-2762 (1986).

31. H. Komatsu, M. Oda, M. Nakamura, Y. Akaiwa, N. Tsukada, K. Honda, Y. Yonei, K. Kaneko, T. Fujiwara and M. Tsuchiya, Electron microscopic and cytochemical studies on the mechanism of hydrochloric acid secretion — with special reference to actin filaments —, *J. Clin. Electron Microscopy,* 18:542-543 (1985).

32. H. Komatsu, M. Oda, K. Honda, K. Kaneko, Y. Yonei, N. Tsukada, M. Nakamura, T. Fujiwara and M. Tsuchiya, Possible involvement of actin filaments in the mechanism of gastric acid secretion — an ultrastructural and immunocytochemical study —, *J. Electron Microscopy* **(supple),** 35:2879-2880 (1986).

33. M. Oda, M. Nakamura, N. Watanabe, N. Tsukada, Y. Yonei, H. Komatsu, K. Kaneko, Y. Akaiwa, I. Okazaki and M. Tsuchiya: Ultrastructural characterization of the microvasculatory system in the stomach-from a terminological point of view-, *in:* "Microcirculation Annual 1985: Japanese Society for Microcirculation," M. Tsuchiya, M. Asano, M. Oda, I. Okazaki, ed, Excerpta Medica, Amsterdam, 191-204 (1985).

34. M. Nakamura, M. Oda, N. Watanabe, N. Tsukada, Y. Yonei and M. Tsuchiya, Evidence for direct parasympathetic innervation of parietal cells in the rat glandular stomach-Histochemical and electron microscopic cytochemical study. *Folia Okajimas Anat. Jpn.,* 59:167-179 (1982).

35. M. Oda, N. Tsukada, H. Komatsu, Y. Yonei, K. Honda and M. Tsuchiya, Mechanism of contraction and dilatation of sinusoidal endothelial fenestrae in the liver, *Hepatology,* 6:771 (1986).

36. G.W. Schmid-Schönbein, S. Usami, R. Skalak and S. Chien, The interaction of leukocytes and erythrocytes in capillary and postcapillary vessels, *Microvasc. Res.,* 19:45-70 (1980).

37. M. Suematsu, S. Miura, M. Suzuki, H. Nagata, T. Morishita, C. Oshio and M. Tsuchiya, 5-lipoxygenase inhibitor (AA-861) attenuates neutrophil-mediated oxidative stress on the venular endothelium in endotoxemia, *J. Clin. Lab. Immunol.,* 25:41-45 (1988).

38. Y. Yonei, M. Oda, M. Nakamura, N. Watanabe, N. Tsukada, H. Komatsu, Y. Akaiwa, E. Ichikawa, K. Kaneko, H. Asakura, T. Fujiwara and M. Tsuchiya, Evidence for direct innervation between the cholinergic nerve and mast cells in the rat colonic mucosa. An electron microscopic cytochemical and autoradiographic study, *J. Clin. Electron Microscopy,* 18:560-561 (1985).

39. M. Tsuchiya, M. Oda, Y. Kamisaka and C. Oshio, Influence of mast cell degranulation on venular permeability, *in:* "Atherogenesis vol II," Proceedings of the 2nd international symposium on atherogenesis, thrombogenesis and pyridinolcarbamate treatment, May 18-20, 1972, Tokyo, Japan, T. Shimamoto, F. Numao, G.M. Addison, ed, Excerpta Medica, Amsterdam, 152-158 (1973).

CELL BIOLOGY OF ENDOTHELIUM

CARBOHYDRATE REGULATED TRANSENDOTHELIAL TRANSPORT OF PROTEINS

Stuart K. Williams and Deborah G. Rose

Department of Surgery
Jefferson Medical College
Philadelphia, PA 19107, USA

INTRODUCTION

The study of vascular permeability has been focused in part on the structure of endothelial cells which line the vascular system. The importance of endothelial cell junctions, fenestra and vesicles in the regulation of vascular permeability is now well established. Newer ultrastructural techniques such as immuno-gold labelling[1] and rapid freezing[2] have confirmed numerous earlier studies which established that endothelial cell structure regulates the transendothelial transport of solutes.

A parallel, nearly unrelated, research path has been followed by many investigators to evaluate the effect of molecular structure on transendothelial transport. Our laboratory has examined several aspects of molecular structure on solute exchange, in particular:

- molecular size
- molecular charge
- carbohydrate content
- molecular shape

While all of these components appear to play a role in regulating vascular permeability, we will focus on the importance of carbohydrate structure during this chapter. When appropriate, we will include a description of the importance of molecular size, charge and shape on solute permeability.

MATERIALS AND METHODS

Microvessel Endothelial Cell Isolation

Microvascular endothelial cells were isolated from rat epididymal fat pads according to the procedures of Williams et al,[3] a modification of the procedures of Wagner and Matthews.[4] Briefly, epididymal fat was treated with crude collagenase for 30 minutes at 37°C. The cell digest was centrifuged in phosphate buffered saline, to remove adipoytes, and Percoll (Pharmacia Co., NJ) to purify endothelium. The microvascular EC were resuspended in phosphate buffered saline prior to studies of endocytosis.

Endocytosis studies of albumin, ferritin and glucosylated albumin were performed according to the procedures of Williams.[5] Albumin and glucosylated albumin were prepared according to the procedures of Williams.[3]

Urine Protein Analysis

Male, Speague Dawley rats (100-200 gm) were made diabetic by I.P. injection of streptozotocin (65 mg/kg, in 0.01 M citrate (pW 4.5) following a 48 hour fast. Diabetes was confirmed by the presence of hyperglycemia, glycosuria and failure to gain weight. Serum and urine proteins were studied after one month of untreated hyperglycemia.

Rats were anesthetized with Nembutal (I.P. injection 30 mg/kg body weight). Blood was collected by cardiac puncture and formed elements were removed by centrifugation. The serum was exhaustively dialyzed against distilled water (4°C). The dialyzed serum was cleared of pre-cipitated protein by centrifugation and then lyophilized. Urine samples were collected into flasks, bathed in an ice/water mixture. After each of 3 consecutive 8 hour intervals, urine volumes were measured, the samples were centrifuged and exhaustively dialyzed against distilled water (4°C). Precipitated proteins which appeared during dialysis were cleared by centrifugation and the urine proteins were filtered through 0.2 micron 'Acrodisc' (Gelman Co.) filters and then lyophilized.

The extent of glucosylation of albumin was evaluated by exposing 200 μg of urine or serum protein to a 200 molar excess of Na boro tritide (^{3}H – sodium borohydride). This reagent selec-tively labels reducing sugars which have covalently attached to protein. Both serum and urine proteins were separated by $NaDoSo_4$ polyacrylamide gel electrophoresis and the extent of albumin labelling was subsequently quantified.

RESULTS AND DISCUSSION

Our original investigations of carbohydrate selective transendothelial solute transport were initiated following studies of a non glycoprotein, serum albumin. This 69 K-dalton serum pro-tein is synthesized by hepatocytes and is not enzymatically glycosylated prior to its secretion into the blood. Using a system of isolated microvessel endothelial cells, we evaluated the endocytosis and transcytosis of glycoproteins and the non glycoprotein serum albumin. Our original reason to use albumin as a probe of endocytosis was its abundance and ease of isolation. However, as shown in Figure 1, we observed the exclusion of native serum albumin from endocytosis by isolated microvessel endothelium (Wagner et al[6]).

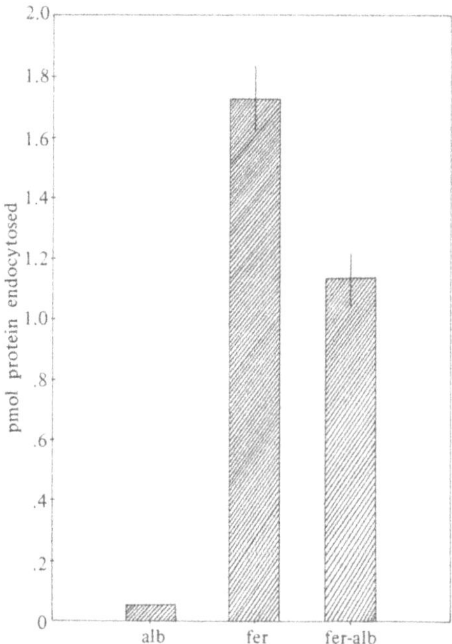

Fig. 1. Endothelial cells exhibit the ability to exclude albumin from endocytosis while ferritin is ingested. When albumin and ferritin were incubated with endothelium together, a reduction in ferritin ingestion was observed. (Reprinted with permission from Annals New York Acad. Sciences 416:457).

In addition to the exclusion of albumin from endocytosis, we also observed reduced ferritin ingestion in the presence of albumin. To explain the exclusion of albumin from vesicular ingestion we reviewed its structure and found albumin is similar to many other serum proteins with respect to size, and charge, but differed since it contains no carbohydrates. The lack of enzymatic attachment of carbohydrates during albumin synthesis was of greater interest when the process of nonenzymatic glycosylation was considered. This process is a chemical reaction which takes place between glucose and almost all proteins.

HC = 0		HC = N – R		CH₂NH – R		HCN – R
HCOH		HCOH		C = 0		HCOH
	+ H₂N – R →		AMADORI →		H⁺ →	
HOCH		HOCH *in vivo*		HOCH		HOCH
HCOH		HCOH		HCOH		HCOH
HCOH		HCOH		HCOH		HCOH
CH₂OH		CH₂OH		CH₂OH		CH₂OH
GLUCOSE		ALDIMINE		KETOAMINE		GLUCOSYL – R

The major driving force in this reaction is the concentration of glucose; thus in the diabetic, this reaction results in a higher level of glucosylated proteins. Our work focused on glucosylated albumin since the attachment of glucose would change this protein into a glycoprotein.

As seen in Figure 2, the glucosylation of albumin results in the reversal albumin exclusion

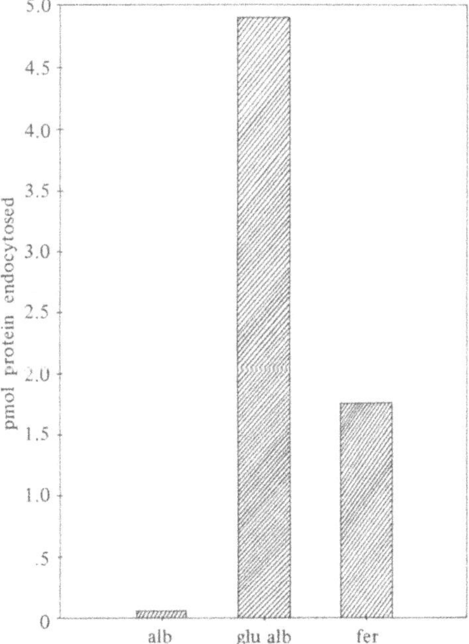

Fig. 2. Endothelial cells exhibit differential endocytic capacity for solutes depending in part on their carbohydrate content. While native, non glucosylated serum albumin is excluded from endocytosis, glucosylated albumin and ferritin are endocytosed (Reprinted with permission from Annals New York Acad. Sciences 416:457).

and its avid endocytosis by microvessel endothelium. The exact mechanism of this change in albumin handling by endothelial vesicles following glycosylation is, as yet, not known. We do know that the level of glucosylation is two moles glucose per mole albumin which results in minimal change in molecular weight and charge. Thus some other property of albumin must be changed following glucosylation.

To evaluate the effects of albumin glucosylation on its *in vivo* permeability, we evaluated the level of albumin glucosylation in serum and urine albumin isolated from normal and diabetic rats. As shown in Figure 3, the level of glucosylated albumin in the urine was significantly higher than in the serum. As expected, diabetic serum also contained a higher level of glucosylated albumin as compared to the level of glucosylated albumin the serum from non diabetic rats. The highest level of glucosylated albumin appeared in the urine of normal rats. We conclude that nonenzymatic glucosylation takes place under both normal and diabetic conditions. Furthermore, glucosylated albumin is transported across the glomerular filtration apparatus preferentially to unmodified albumin.

The increased permeability of glucosylated albumin provides clear evidence for a molecular selection which favors the appearance of glucosylated albumin in the urine. Since the glomecular endothelium has open ferestrations, the enhanced escape of glucosylated albumin may reflect selective permeability of the basement membrane, or alterations in the permeability of the tubules to albumin. Moreover, we suggest that glucosylated albumin may enhance the escape of normal albumin from the nephron.

In addition to molecular weight and molecular charge, we must now consider the carbohydrate content of proteins as an additional determinant of vascular permeability. We cannot rule out the possibility that all these molecular properties collectively affect transendothelial solute exchange. Future studies will focus on the molecular specificity of vascular permeability.

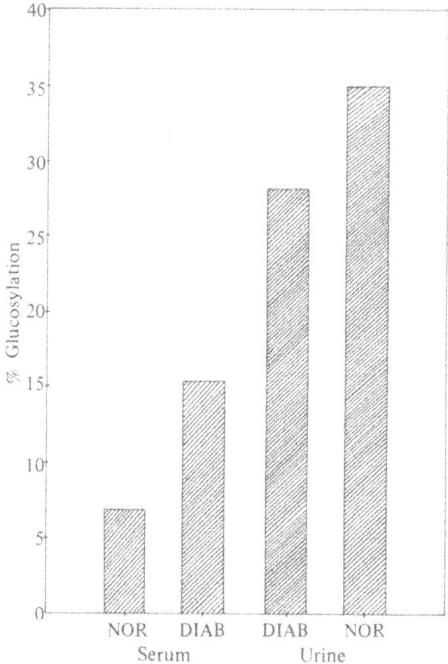

Fig. 3. Extent of glucosylation of albumin in normal and diabetic rat serum and urine. Albumin concentrations were calculated by integration of densitometric scans of polyacylamide gels. After scanning to determine albumin concentrations, the albumin band was cut out and counted for tritium. The % glucosylation is based on the observed 7% glucosylation of albumin found in normal rat serum.

REFERENCES

1. A.J. Milici, N.E. Watrous and G.E. Palade, Immunogold Localization of Exogenous Albumin in Murine Myocardial Capillaries, *J. Cell. Biol.* **103**: p. 718 (1986).
2. R.C. Wagner and S.B. Andrews, Ultrastructure of the Vesicular System in Rapidly Frozen Capillary Endothelium of the Rete Mirabile, *J. Ultrastruct. Res.* **90**:172-182 (1985).
3. S. Williams, J. Devenny and M. Bitensky, Micropinocytic ingestion of glucosylated albumin by microvessels: Possible role in the pathogenesis of diabetic microangiopathy, *Proc. Natl. Acad. Sci. U.S.A.* **78**:2393-2397 (1981).
4. R. Wagner and M. Matthews, The isolation and culture of capillary endothelium from epididymal fat, *Microvascular Res.* **10**:286-297 (1975).
5. S. Williams, D. Greener and N. Solenski, Endocytosis and exocytosis of proteins by capillary endothelium, *J. Cell Physiol.* **120**:157-162 (1984).
6. R. Wagner, S. Williams, M. Matthews and S. Andrews, Exclusion of albumin from vescicular ingestion by isolated microvessels, *Microvascular Res.* **19**:127-130 (1980).

COMPUTER TRACKING OF ENDOTHELIAL ACTIVATION RESPONSES

Una S. Ryan and Linda J. Mayfield

Department of Medicine (R58)
University of Miami School of Medicine
P.O. Box 016960
Miami, FL 33101, USA

INTRODUCTION

Endothelial cell responses to stimuli may involve structural, functional or behavioral alterations or a combination of all these.[1] Understanding of the role of endothelial cells depends on the ability of investigators to measure these responses. Considerable progress has been made in measuring some, but not all, endothelial responses. Functional responses can usually be quantified by bioassay or by biochemical analysis of endothelial products, enzymes or receptors. Structural responses can be recorded by light and electron microscopy and, to a certain extent, quantification of structural alterations can be achieved by morphometric means. However, analysis of endothelial behavior in terms of migration and division activity has been hampered by existing methods for quantitative assay. Thus, in this paper we have focused on these less well-documented areas. We describe studies that consider methods for measuring endothelial cell behavior.

BEHAVIORAL RESPONSES

Wounded monolayer assay

Previously, the most widely used methods for measurement of directed endothelial growth have involved the rabbit eye assay,[2] the chorioallantoic membrane (CAM) assay[3] and estimation of migration through filters in a Boyden chamber.[4] Each of these has disadvantages, either of requiring the use of live animals, or by being tedious, cumbersome and difficult to perform. Previously[5] we have shown by time-lapse cinematography that if a confluent endothelial monolayer is wounded by scraping away part of it, a proportion of the endothelial cells remaining, will migrate out unidirectionally from the wound edge, and subsequently divide such that the daughters also migrate in the same direction.

We now employ the same monolayer wounding assay described earlier[5] but involving video time-lapse recording of the unidirectional growth (migration and division) of endothelial cells repopulating the denuded area (Fig. 1, a and b), followed by automated data analysis and graphical display using an IBM PC XT. The cells are tracked individually and the data are analyzed using a new computer program, QuikTrak, a software package developed in our laboratory, that provides graphical and statistical reports.[6] It has the particular advantage of allowing assessment not only of the average rate of migration or division but also the precise kinetics of rate changes. QuikTrak allows tracking of individual cells and clones as well as analysis of the population dynamics. The method is suitable for studies of angiogenesis, chemotaxis and endothelial activation phenomena in response to a wide variety of chemical and mechanical stimuli.

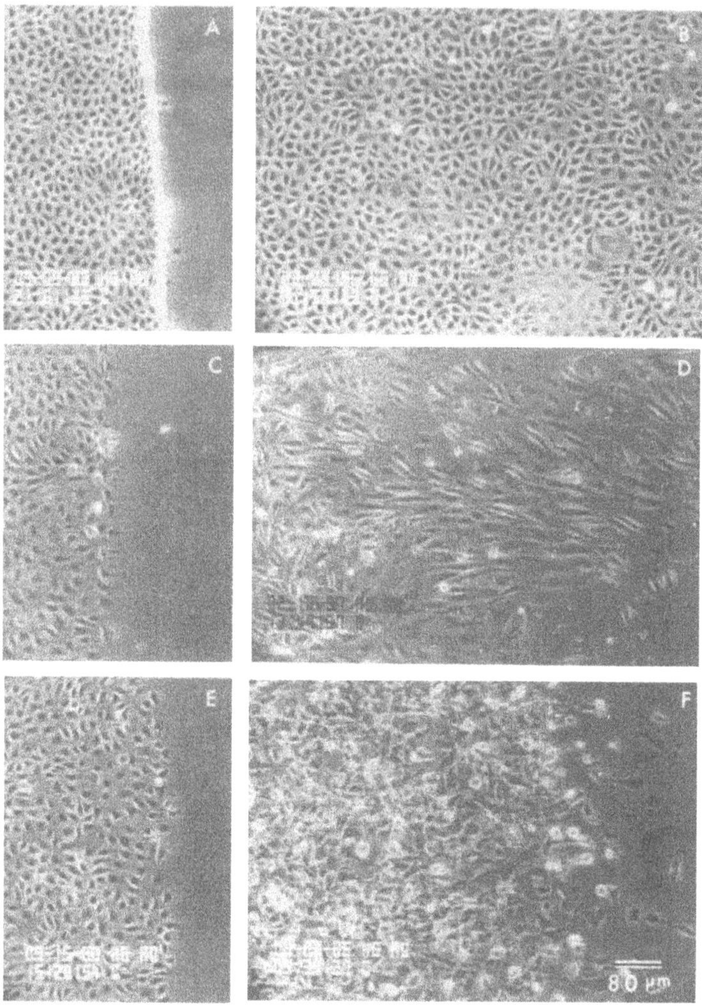

Fig.1 . Cultures of bovine pulmonary endothelial cells at time of wounding and after cells were allowed to grow to confluence. a) Untreated culture at time of wounding. b) Untreated culture 4 days after wounding. c) Culture treated with 50 nM α-thrombin at time of wounding. d) 5 days after wounding. e) Culture treated with 5 μl/ml TGF-ß at time of wounding. f) 7 days after wounding.

Data Acquisition

QuikTrak and the Micro-comp data acquisition system (Southern Micro Instruments SMU-051, version 6.1) tracks and analyzes the chemotactic and mitotic behavior of endothelial cell growth. The Micro-comp system as described[6] is the software and hardware that interfaces the time-lapse recording of the experiment under analysis with a digitizing tablet and an IBM PC XT. All data are obtained via this system and entered into Micro-comp data files which are essentially standard ASCII files. The only data that are entered into the computer manually are related to time, e.g. time of division or time a cell begins and ends a migratory path. In addition, if there is to be a study on cell migration and division patterns as they relate to cell genealogy, each cell must be identified with an appropriate ID number and entered into a separate data file manually.

QuikTrak takes these data files, reads them and compiles them into a master data base. QuikTrak then sorts through these data and produces four varieties of report summaries.[6] Each report type concentrates on different aspects of analysis. The first is a general organization of the data by cell identification number. This report provides the data on cell interdivision times. The second report organizes data related to cell migration (e.g. distance travelled and migration rates). The third report is an organization of data on population density of selected regions of the culture at a given time interval throughout the experiment. Each of the three above-mentioned report summaries includes standard statistics on the data listed. In addition, a final report summary can be selected that will provide statistics (standard deviation, standard error, variance, median, and mean) on a particular data point, e.g. distance travelled, interdivision time, or region of division, according to a specified time period or region in the culture. Finally QuikTrak will plot clone genealogy for each cell.

Time-lapse video cinematography is a powerful technique for studying cell migration and division behavior. Fig. 1(a-f) shows three different cultures, each at the time of wounding, and after 4-7 days growth to confluence. The morphologic differences between these three cultures are striking. Time-lapse analysis provides a permanent record of the events leading to repopulation and a means of determining the method by which the cells fill the wounded area. Anyone who has watched cell movement on a time-lapse video is soon overwhelmed by the amount of information contained in such recordings. Consequently, investigators have been deterred from this approach to the analysis of cell movement and division behavior. The deterrent is two fold. First, one must determine the nature of the cellular response to a stimulus (chemotactic, mitogenic, or morphologic). This requires the ability to transcribe what is seen into a data set that quantifies the response. Second, after the data has been collected, it must be compiled, sorted and statistically analyzed so as to reveal the observed phenomenon. This task was not realizable without the application of the computer technology available today.

A good strategy for determining the response elicited in cells of a wounded monolayer, is to track the speed of the advancing wound edge and density of the culture at 4 hour intervals. If the advancement of the wound edge is the same for both the treated and untreated cultures but there is an increase in the cell density of the treated culture, the response is exclusively mitogenic. A more detailed data set is obtained and sorted by QuikTrak according to time of division. A report summary of the data will reveal the number of cells that divided during a selected 8 hour time interval. This will show whether the mitogenic response was one of in-creased number of dividing cells and/or decrease in interdivision time (IDT). If the advance-ment of the wound edge is accelerated, regardless of any change in population density, the response could be any one of the three responses mentioned above. A more detailed data set must be obtained to determine the response. The following are a few examples that illustrate the complexities and problems that may arise in data analysis.

In phase contrast video time-lapse microscopy, division is noted by cells in the monolayer becoming birefringent or bright. The cell then splits and the two daughters reattach approxi-mately 1 hour later and return to a grey color. Fig. 2 shows a culture wounded and exposed to thrombin (30 nM). Cells rapidly began lifting off 1 hour after wounding as if dividing, but as shown, these cells remained detached 9 hours later. After exposure to thrombin the number of dividing cells was found to be 4 times fewer than that of the untreated culture while the migration rate was found to be twice that of the untreated culture (21 μ/hr versus 10 μ/hr). The cells that lifted off but did not divide, clumped together and then reattached, undivided, 72 hours after lift off.

Fig. 1(e and f) illustrates a culture exposed to 5 μl/ml TGF-ß. The cells showed an enor-mous increase in the number of dividing cells as well as a decrease in the IDT. The cells were transformed such that they no longer grew as a monolayer but divided piling one on another, without ever repopulating the denuded area of the flask. The cells could not be analyzed by computer and alternative methods such as reducing the concentration of the stimulant or analysis using a fluorescence activated cell sorter would be preferable ways to obtain data on mitogenic responses.

Fig. 3(a-c) shows a culture that had been wounded and then exposed to 50 nM prothrom-bin. The cells became oriented in three distinct regions. Fig. 3a shows the culture at time of wounding. The area of preserved confluence (1/3 cell population) remaining after wounding is defined as region 1. These cells showed no migration for the duration of the experiment with the exception of those cells just at the wound edge. These cells migrated into the denuded area in a trajectory perpendicular to the wound edge for 19 hours without dividing, forming region 2 (Fig. 3b). The migration pattern of region 2 was highly directed. 24 hours after wounding, the cells in region 2 stopped migrating and the cells at the edge of this region began to divide rapidly. This was the first significant sign of division in the culture. Finally, the cells at the edge of region 2 migrated in a random manner forming a third region (Fig. 3c).

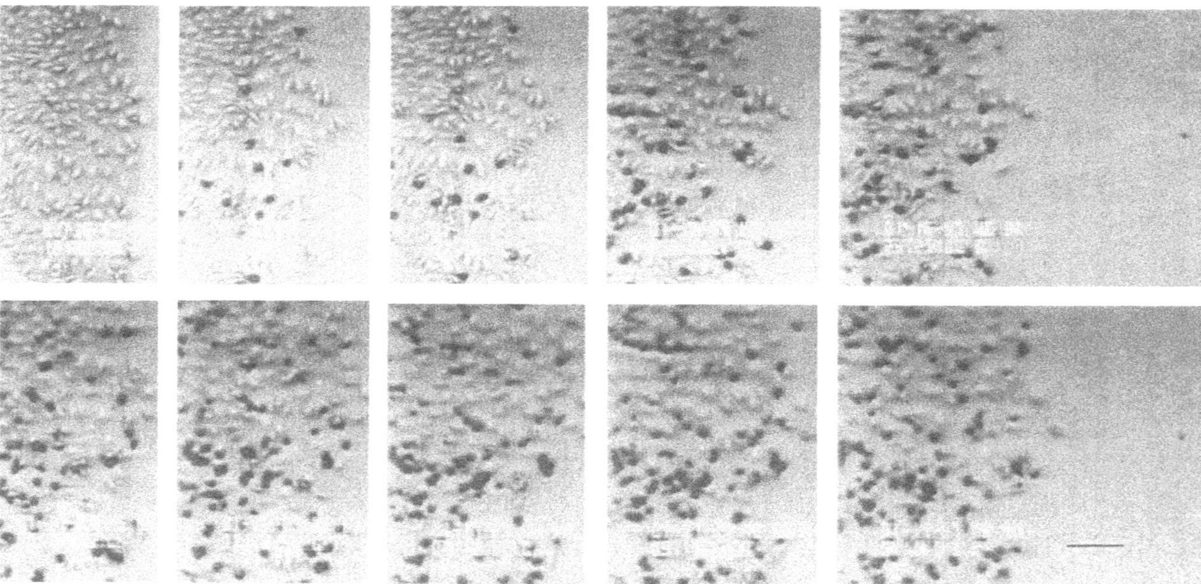

Fig. 2. Culture of bovine pulmonary endothelial cells exposed to 50 nM thrombin at time of wounding and 1 hour intervals after wounding for 10 hours. Cells have lifted off as if entering division but remain detached without dividing, (printed negative so dividing cells are depicted as dark spots on field and become more visible).

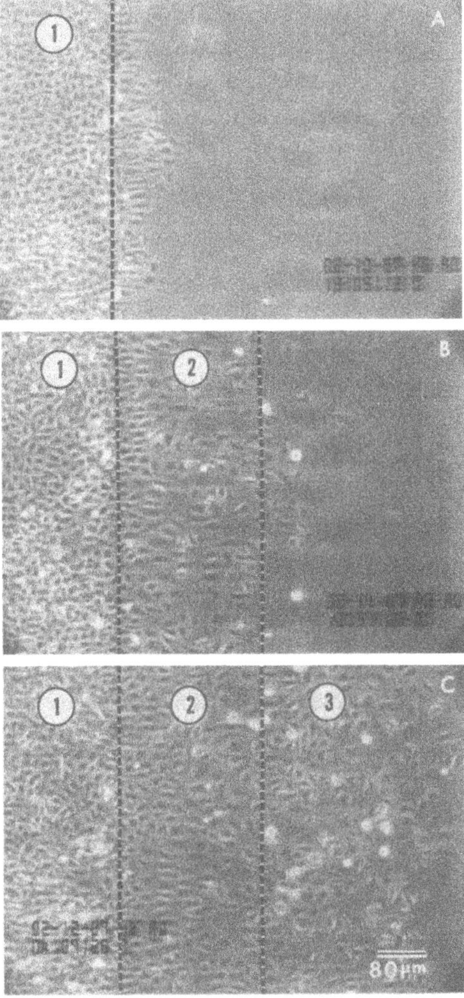

Fig. 3. Culture of bovine pulmonary endothelial cells exposed to 50 nM prothrombin at time of wounding forming 3 regions a) 5 hours after wounding. Cells at edge of region 1 migrate in direction perpendicular to wound edge. b) 24 hours after wounding. No division or migration in region 1 or 2. Cells at edge of region 2 begin rapid division and random movement. c) 64 hours after wounding. Three distinct regions are seen.

This type of "regional" migratory behavior, directed or random, lends itself to describing cell motility in terms of classical models (see Fig. 4). Once data is obtained and sorted with QuikTrak it can be described in terms of one of these models and if a model is found applicable, the cells' speed and orientation of migration can be predicted and quantified.

THEORIES FOR ANALYSIS OF MOVEMENT

Random Walk Theory

Two dimensional random walk theory has been applied to the study of cell chemotaxis, however several difficulties arise when this theory is used to analyze cell migratory behavior. Ran-

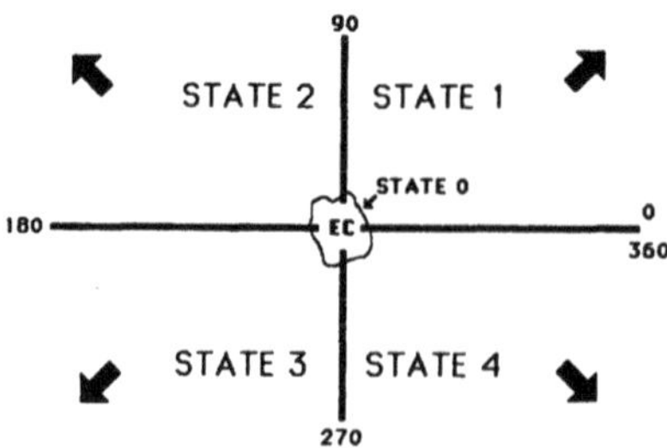

Fig. 4. State diagram of five states of endothelial cell (EC) migration. Cell migration between 0° and 90° with respect to the x-axis is defined as state 1; 90° and 180°, state 2; 180° and 270° state 3; and 270° and 360° state 4. State 0 is defined as no migration in any direction for a minimum time (30 minutes).

dom migration is a type of locomotion that is not necessarily oriented in an axis related to a stimulus. The probability that a cell will change direction along its migratory path is the same for any direction. The initial steps of any migrating object are highly directed, It is only after these initial steps, when conditions allowing independent free movement become manifest, that Random Walk theory can be applied. As shown in Fig. 3a the cells at the wound edge migrate in a nonrandon manner. In actual fact, the random walk theory is not applicable at time of wounding because initially the cells are only able to move through a 180° angle due to the population behind the wound edge. Eventually the cells migrate into the wounded area and reach a level of confluence such that the neighboring cells are in close contact. Cell-cell interactions and collisions are frequent and begin to play an important role. The duration of this intermediate time interval beginning shortly after wounding and ending prior to confluence is not only determined by cell type, but can be dramatically altered by the presence of varying stimulatory factors. Thus, as described above, the migration may only be truly random in defined regions within the culture for limited periods of time.

Markov Theory

The continuous time Markov theory[8] is a probability oriented theory to predict the probable step-length, speed and chemotactic direction of a cell in response to a hormone, cytokine, angiogenesis or growth factor. It can only be applied to endothelial cell migration if the Markov property is verified. This is achieved by tracking each cell's migratory path, and determining the amount of time, T_j, spent by a cell in each of the states (1, 2, 3, 4, and 0) and the number of times a cell spent that amount of time in a given state, X_j. A histogram of these two parameters can then be plotted ($T(j)$ as abscissa and X_j and ordinate). If the histogram can be fitted to the probability density function:

$$f(t) = (1/\Theta)e - (t/\Theta)$$

where $\Theta = T(j)$, a continuous-time Markov chain theory can be used to quantify cell locomotory trajectories.[9]

The Markov property assumes that the present and future states (of cell migration in this case) are independent of previous states. The location of a cell in future states can depend only on its location at present not on how it got there. The trajectories of the migrating cells are defined by five directional states with respect to the x-axis of a two-dimensional Cartesian plane. (Fig. 4a) shows the five states bounded by the four quadrants of a Cartesian plane.

Each cell's migratory path is characterized by these five states (Fig. 5a) and is traced via a digitizing tablet and an IBM PC XT (Fig. 5b); the path length and direction of subtrajectories is computed by Micro-comp and integrated with the master database by QuikTrak. Consider the cell movement shown in Fig. 5a. Employing the continuous-time Markov chain for this single path one can estimate the probability, $\hat{p}(j/l)$, of the cell migrating from state 1 to state

190

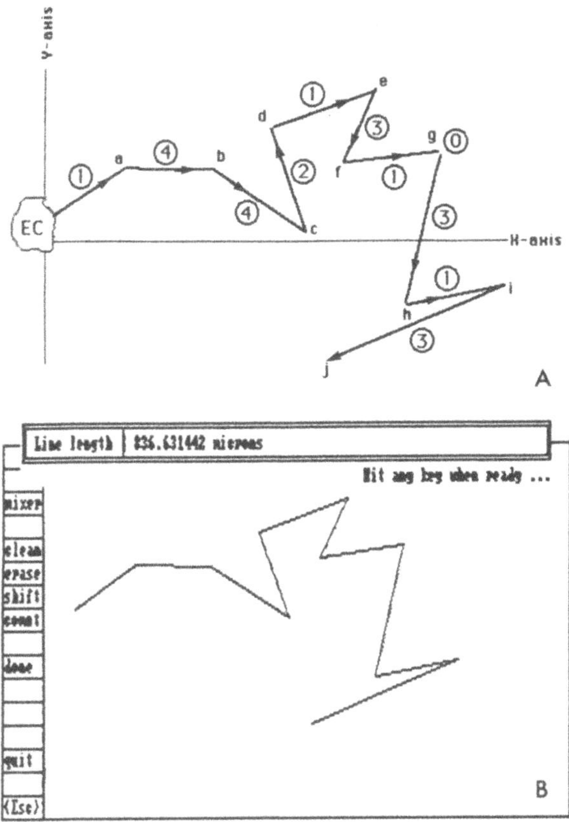

Fig. 5. a) Migratory path of an endothelial cell divided into subtrajectories each identified by its directional state. b) The path is then tracked with Micro comp image analysis system on an IBM PC XT and its length is calculated.

j, l ≠ j and, Q(j), where $1/Q(j)$ = the expected value of T(j).

$$\hat{p}(j/l) = \frac{\text{number of transitions from l to j}}{\text{number of transition from l to any state}}$$

and

$$Q(j) = \frac{\text{number of subtrajectories in state j}}{\text{cumulative time spent in state j}}$$

The two state probabilities, $\hat{p}(j/l)$ and $Q(j)$, can be estimated from the data. These data can relate to a single cell path, but can also be collected from any number of cell paths. The time spent in state j is determined by summation of time spent, not for the single cell, but all cells in the population combined (see ref. 8 for worked example).

In chemotactic movement we are interested in knowing the most probable direction(s) in which a culture is heading. In quantifying these probabilities one can determine the degree of intensity of the migratory response. Mathematically, this means we wish to know the limiting distribution of the continuous-time Markov chain such that for any starting state, i, as $t \to \partial$, $p_t(j/i) \to p(j)$.

Then to determine the state(s) for which a culture has most affinity, $p(j)$, $j = 0,...,4$, one must find the unique solution to the set of linear equations:

$$Q(j)p(j) = \sum_{l=0}^{4} p(j/l)Q(l)p(l)$$

where $l \neq j$ and $j = 0,...,4$.

These 5 equations can be solved for $\{p(j); j = 0,...,4\}$ by Gaussian elimination on computer (see ref. 10 for derivation of this set of equations). If $p(0),...,p(4) = 0.20$ the migration is purely random.

CONCLUDING COMMENTS

Endothelial cells normally exist as a stationary monolayer of cells linked by intercellular junctions. This monolayer provides a selective permeability barrier, a surface for processing circulating vasoactive substances and a clot resistant, non-thrombogenic, immunologically unreactive surface.[11] However, in response to a variety of agonists, inflammatory mediators, viruses, bacteria or their products, endothelial cells can become activated.[1,12] Activated endothelial cells may express procoagulant activities, unmask latent Fc and C3b receptors, and can present antibody.[11,12] We sought to investigate the mechanisms of signal transduction and stimulus-response coupling by studying the receptor-mediated responses of endothelial cells to agonists such as bradykinin, histamine, thrombin, ATP and platelet activating factor.[13,14] Activation responses have been measured in terms of the release of endothelium derived relaxing factor, prostacyclin, thromboxane, and in terms of alterations in cell shape, migration, division and phagocytic activities.[15] We have measured the cytosolic free calcium levels using the intracellular calcium indicators FURA-2 and INDO-1 and have measured calcium fluxes using ^{45}Ca-loaded endothelial cells.[16,13] In addition we have measured adenylate cyclase, activation of protein kinase C and the phosphoinositide turnover levels in challenged endothelial cells.[14] We have also demonstrated agonist-induced endothelial cell ion channels using the patch clamp technique.[13,17] However, full understanding of endothelial cell behavior has lacked methods for tracking endothelial cell activation responses in terms of migration, division and phagocytosis.

In this paper, we have discussed just a few of the complexities in the analysis of endothelial cell migration in the wounded monolayer assay. Although a large number of endothelial responses are known to occur to a diverse variety of stimuli, the mechanisms underlying endothelial responses are not well understood. Our aim is to provide useful tools and techniques to challenge the researcher to investigate morphologic, mitotic and chemotactic properties of endothelial cells, and thus to explore the fundamental basis for the responses of the microcirculation to acute and chronic signals.

ACKNOWLEDGMENT

We wish to thank Dr. David Stern for providing the thrombin, pro-thrombin and α-thrombin and Dr. Vincent Falanger for providing the TGF-ß. We also thank Jeffrey Goodwin for his patience in filming the cultures provided here as examples. Supported by grants HL21568, HL33064 from the National Heart Lung and Blood Institute and Council for Tobacco Research, 814.

REFERENCES

1. U.S. Ryan, Endothelial cell activation responses, *in*: "Pulmonary Endothelium in Health and Disease," U.S. Ryan, ed., Marcel Dekker, Inc., New York (1987).

2. M.A. Gimbrone Jr., R.S. Cotran, S.B. Leapman and J. Folkman, Tumor growth and neovascularization an experimental model using the rabbit cornea, *J. Natl. Cancer Inst.* **52**:413 (1974).

3. J. Folkman, Angiogenesis and its inhibitors, *in*: "Important Advances in Oncology Part 1," V.T. Devita Jr., S. Hellman, S.A. Rosenberg eds., J.B. Lippincott, Philadelphia (1985).

4. S.B. Boyden, The chemotactic effect of mixtures of antibody and antigen on polymorpho—nuclear leucocytes, *J. Exp. Med.* **115**:453 (1962).

5. U.S. Ryan, M. Absher, B.M. Olazabal, L.M. Brown and J. W. Ryan, Proliferation of pulmonary

endothelial cells: Time-lapse cinematography of growth to confluence and restitution of monolayer after wounding, *Tissue & Cell* 14:637 (1982).

6. U.S. Ryan and L.J. Mayfield, Video analysis of endothelial cell genealogy, migration and division, *J. Tissue Cult. Methods* 10:55 (1986).

7. M.H. Gail and C.W. Boone, The locomotion of mouse fibroblasts in tissue culture, *Biophys. J.* 10:980 (1970).

8. A. Boyarsky, A markov chain model for human granulocyte movement, *J. Math. Biol.* 2:69 (1975).

9. A. Boyarsky and P.B. Noble, A markov chain characterization of human neutrophil locomotion under neutral and chemotactic condition, *Can. J. Physiol. Pharmacol.* 55:1 (1977).

10. L. Breiman "Probability and Stochastic Processes," Addison-Wesley, Massachusetts (1967).

11. U.S. Ryan, Metabolic activity of pulmonary endothelium: Modulation of structure and function, *Ann. Rev. Physiol.* 48:263 (1986).

12. U.S. Ryan, Endothelial cell activation responses, *in*: "Pulmonary Endothelium in Health and Disease," U.S. Ryan, ed., Marcel Dekker, Inc., New York (1987).

13. A. Johns, T.W. Lategan, U.S. Ryan, C. van Breemen and D.J. Adams, Calcium and excitation - secretion coupling in cultured pulmonary endothelial cells, *Tissue & Cell* 19:1-13 (1987).

14. G.Y. Grigorian and U.S. Ryan, Platelet-activating factor effects on bovine pulmonary artery endothelial cells, *Circulation Research* 61:389-395 (1987).

15. U.S. Ryan, Phagocytic properties of endothelial cells, *in*: "Endothelial Cells," U.S. Ryan, ed., CRC Press, Boca Raton (1988).

16. U.S. Ryan, P.V. Avdonin, E.Ya. Pozin, E.G. Popov, S.M. Danilov and V.A. Tkachuck, Influence of vasoactive agents on cytoplasmic free calcium concentration in INDO-1 loaded vascular endothelial cells, *J. Applied Physiology,* in press (1988).

17. P. Bregestovski, A. Bakhramov and U. S. Ryan, Effect of platelet activating factor on the membrane of endothelial cells, *Circulation Research,* submitted (1988).

EFFECTS OF CYTOCHALASIN B ON THE PRIMARY
CULTURED CAPILLARY ENDOTHELIUM

Koya Honda, Masaya Oda, Masahiko Nakamura, Hirokazu Komatsu, Kotaro Kaneko, Toshifumi Azuma, Yasuhiro Nishizaki, Norihito Watanabe and Masaharu Tsuchiya

Department of Internal Medicine
School of Medicine, Keio University
Tokyo 160, Japan

INTRODUCTION

Actin filaments, one of the cytoskeletal components in non-muscle cells, are known to be involved in cell contractility, implying that they are one of the mediators regulating the microcirculation system. Recently we have reported that endothelial actin filaments are present in the cytoplasm of capillary endothelium both in the gastric mucosa and in primary monolayer culture. The present study is designed to characterize the functional significance of the actin filaments using an in vitro experimental model.

MATERIALS AND METHODS

Wistar strain male rats were used. The stomach was perfused with $Ca^{++}Mg^{++}$free-Hanks balanced salte solution (BSS) containing 0.01% collagenase (Sigma, type I). The mucosal layer was stripped off and shaked in Hanks BSS containing 1000 PU/ml of dispase (Godo Shusei, Tokyo). The cell suspension obtained was passed through 250 μm stainless mesh and was left for 10 min to permit cells to sediment by gravity. The endothelium-rich supernatant was centrifuged and the pellet was resuspended in Dalbecco minimal essential medium with 15% fetal calf serum and incubated in a petri dish using a CO_2 incubator. The monolayer cultured cells were characterized by the indirect immunofluorescence methods using the monoclonal OKM5, anti-human Factor VIII antibody and anti-actin antibody. The cultured cells were fixed with 1.2% glutaraldehyde and processed for scanning (SEM) and transmission electron microscopy (TEM). For observation of intracytoplasmic microfilaments, some cultured cells were subjected to uranyl acetate en bloc stain before dehydration. Cytochalasin B (CB; Aldrich, USA) was added to the culture medium at 1 and 10 μg/ml. The time-lapse cinematographic analyses were made before and after the addition of CB to the culture medium. Film was taken at a speed of 1 frame per 4 sec.

RESULTS

By phase contrast microscopy, oval-shaped cell aggregates composed of 5-50 cells were observed 24 hr after the beginning of culture (Fig. 1-a). The endothelial cells forming these cell colonies showed the specific immunofluorescence for OKM5 and Factor VIII related antigen by the indirect immunofluorecsence antibody method (Fig. 1-b). The filamentous immunofluorescence for actin filaments was demonstrated in the cytoplasm of the cultured capillary endothelium (Fig. 1-c). By SEM, the microvilli were found to be sparsely scattered on the surface of the cultured cells loosely connected (Fig. 1-d). In the uranyl acetate en bloc stained

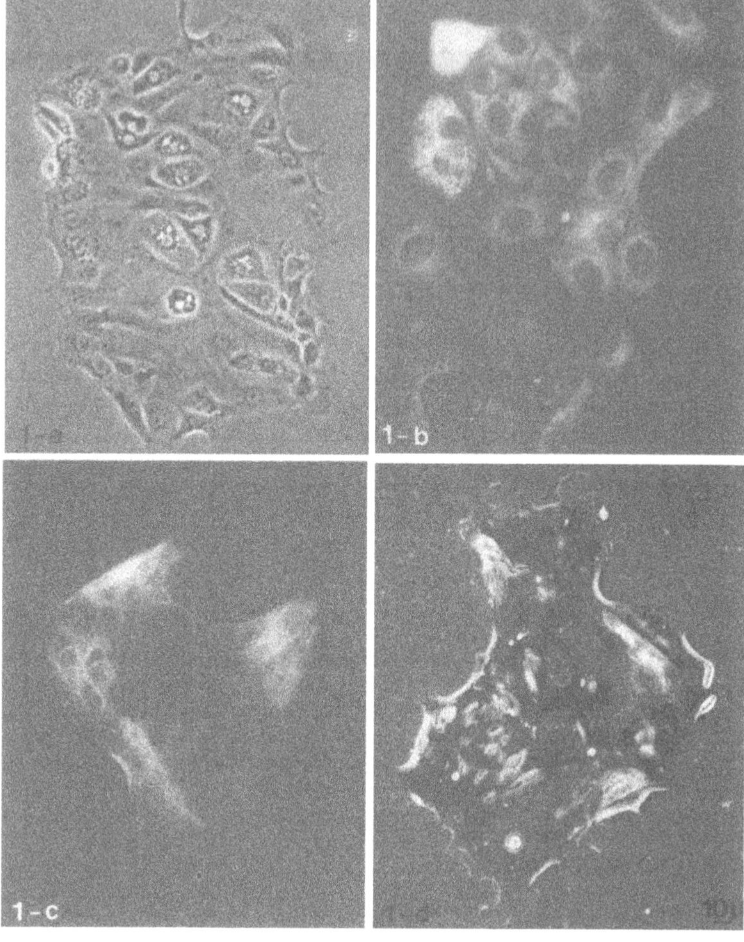

Fig. 1-a: Phase contrast micrograph of the primary monolayer-cultured cells isolated from the gastric mucosa 24 hr after the beginning of culture. Fig. 1-b: Most of the cultured cells show the specific immunofluorescence for OKM5, indicating that these cells largely correspond to the capillary endothelium. Fig. 1-c: The filamentous immunofluorescence for actin filaments is clearly demonstrated in the cytoplasm of cultured capillary endothelium. Fig. 1-d: Scanning electron micrograph of the primary cultured capillary endothelium.

preparations, the microfilaments, 5-7 nm in diameter, were evident within the cytoplasm of cultured capillary endothelium. A bundle of microfilaments, i.e. stress fibers, were present in the cell periphery in parallel with the long axis of the cell (Fig. 2-a). These intracytoplasmic microfilaments were closely associated with not only the plasma membrane, but also the vesicles and vacuoles formed in the endothelium (Fig. 2-b). By time-lapse cinematographic analysis, dynamic membrane ruffling and rhythmic contraction of the cultured capillary endothelium and a Brownian movement of the vesicles in the cytoplasm were clearly demonstrated. The addition of 1 μg/ml of CB resulted in cessation of membrane ruffling. By the addition of 10 μg/ml of CB, bleb formation and microarborization were prominent in the cell periphery. Dynamic contraction of cultured cells and vesicular movement ceased completely. Just after the removal of CB from the culture medium, endothelial cell motility became restored and returned to previous state (Fig. 3-a-d). The specific immunofluorescence for actin was irregularly distributed with focal aggregation after the addition of CB (Fig. 4-a). By SEM, the microspikes were found to protrude from the cell body, with a decrease of the microvilli (Fig. 4-b). By TEM,

196

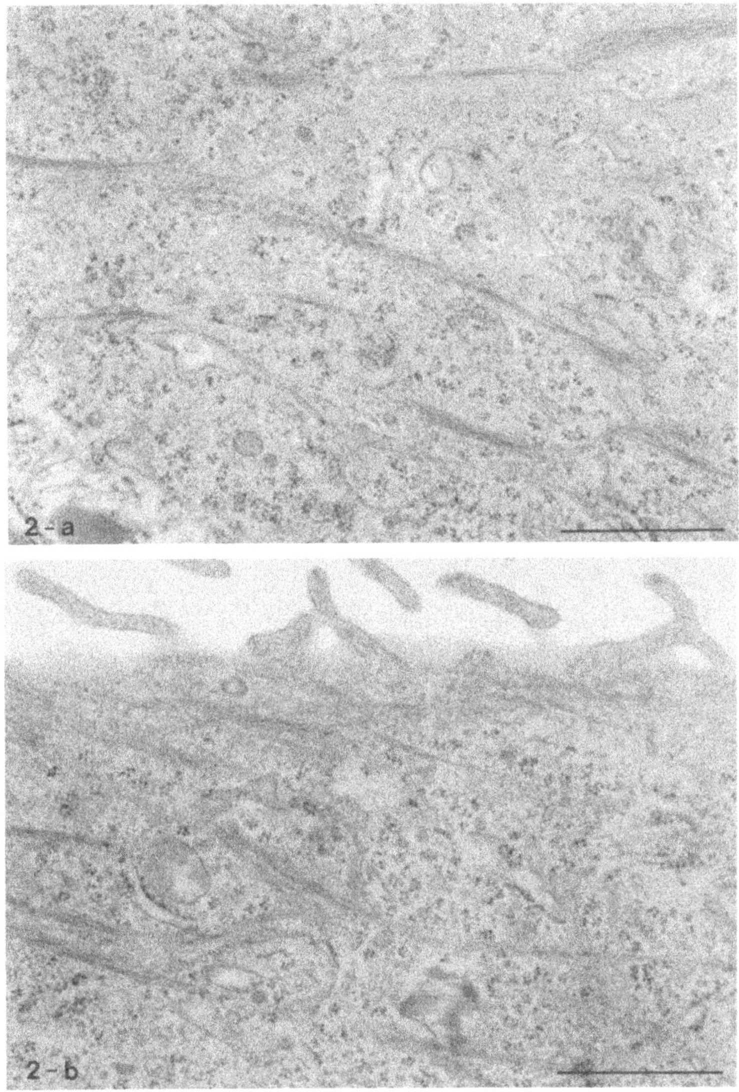

Fig. 2-a: Transmission electron micrograph of the cultured capillary endothelium, showing the stress fibers (bundle of actin filaments) in the cytoplasm. Uranyl acetate en bloc stain. Fig. 2-b: The microfilaments, 5-7 nm in diameter, are evident within the cytoplasm of cultured capillary endothelium and are closely associated not only with the plasma membrane, but also with the vesicles or vacuoles. Uranyl acetate en bloc stain.

the microfilaments in the cytoplasm appeared to be granular and the filamentous structure were hardly seen (Fig. 4-c).

DISCUSSION

The cytoskeletal system in non-muscle cells are involved in a wide variety of cell functions.[1-3] According to a current concept, the actin filaments associated with the plasma membrane in non-muscle cells are considered to be involved in plasma membrane motility.[4,5] There have been several reports concerning whether endothelial contractility exists or not. It has been postulated that endothelial filaments may serve as a design to originate tensile strength and

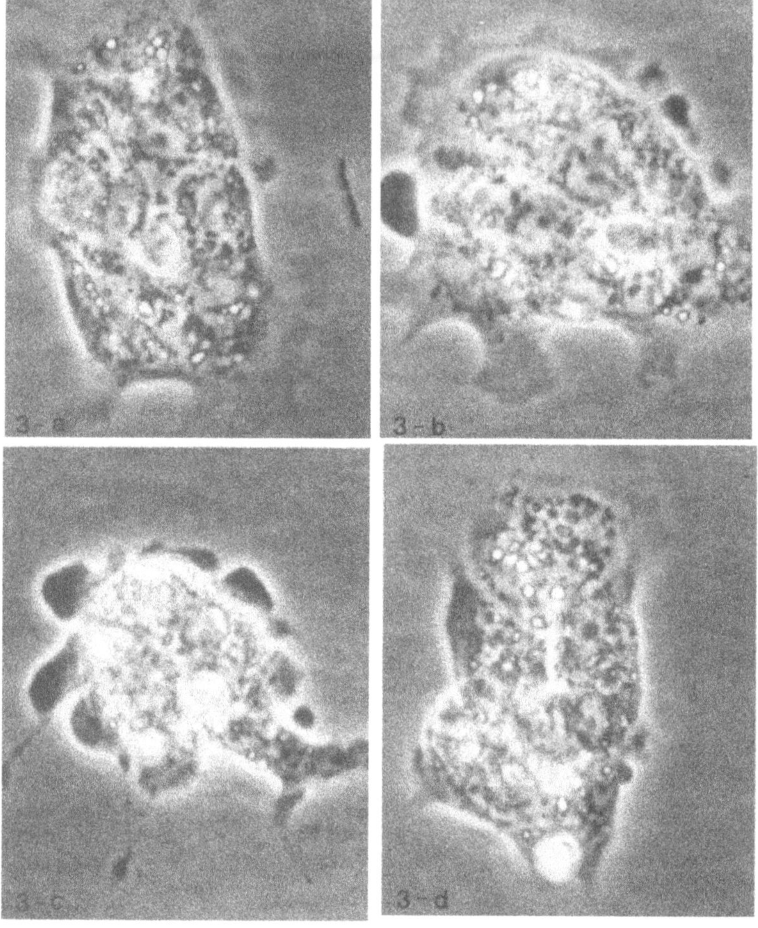

Fig. 3. One frame of the time-lapse cinematography of primary cultured capillary endothelium. a: Before the addition of cytochalasin B (CB). b: 5 min after the addition of CB (10 μg/ml) to the culture medium. c: 30 min after the addition of CB to the culture medium. d: 30 min after the removal of CB from the culture medium.

to provide for a firm attachment to the substratum.[6] On the other hand, it has been reported that the endothelium of small vessels can contract, although its mechanism remains obscure.[7] Our light and electron microscopic study revealed that the rat gastric mucosal microvasculature comprises a large number of true capillaries and a small number of non-muscular collecting venules and terminal arterioles[8] and that actin filaments are evident in the true capillary in the gastric mucosa by uranyl acetate en bloc stain and indirect immunofluorescence antibody method using anti-actin antibody.[9-12] Recently isolation and monolayer culture of vascular endothelium from various organs have been established.[13-16] In an attempt to elucidate morphological and functional properties of capillary endothelium, we developed a new method for primary monolayer culture of capillary endothelium isolated from the rat gastric mucosa.[17-20] In the present study, evidence for the specific immunofluorescence of actin in the cytoplasm of the primary cultured capillary endothelium represents the existence of actin contractile protein. The microfilaments, 5-7 nm in diameter, demonstrated in the cultured capillary endothelium by electron micros-copy, are considered to be actin filaments similar to those of smooth muscle. Time-lapse cinematographic analysis proved dynamic contraction and vesicular movement of the primary cultured capillary endothelium. These endothelial motilities were completely inhibited by CB, the actin-depolymerizing agent, indicating that actin filaments associated with plasma membrane

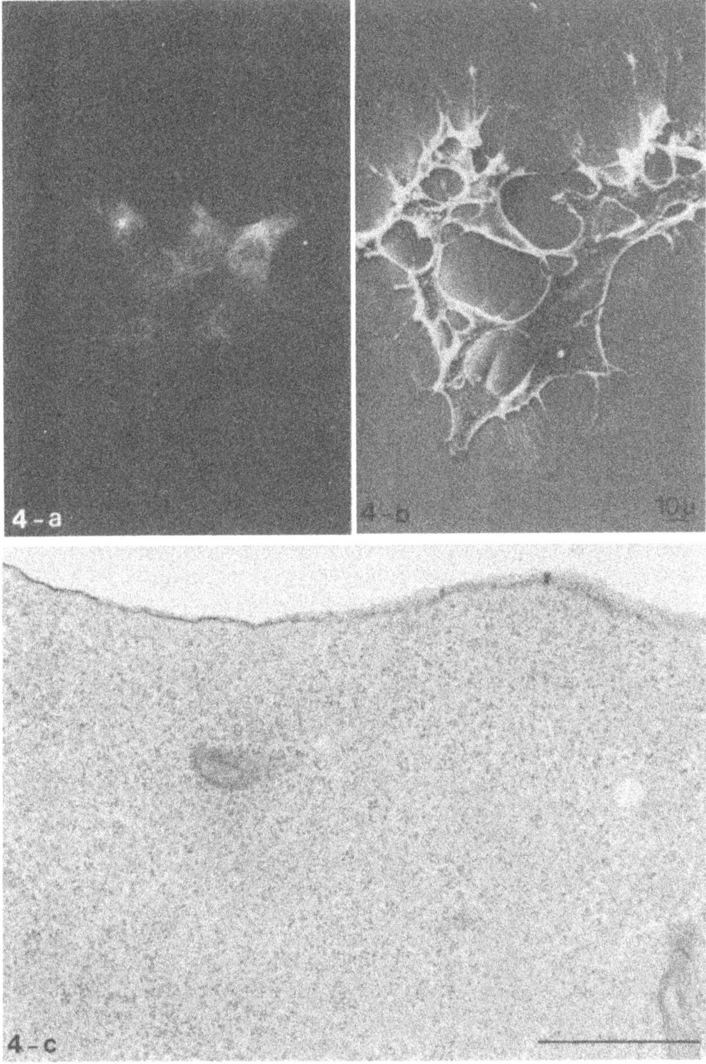

Fig. 4-a: 30 min after the addition of CB to the culture medium, the specific immunofluorescence for actin is irregulary distributed with focal aggregation. Fig. 4-b and c: Ultrastructural alterations of the primary cultured capillary endothelium 30 min after the addition of CB (10 μg/ml) to the culture medium. b: Scanning electron micrographs. The microspikes protrude from the cell body with a decrease of microvili. c: Transmission electron micrographs. The actin filaments in the cytoplasm appear to be granular and the micro-filamentous structures are hardly seen. Uranyl acetate en bloc stain.

or vesicles are involved in the contraction of capillary endothelium and vesicular movement within the cell.

CONCLUSIONS

By using a technique of time-lapse cinematography, the contractility of primary monolayer-cultured capillary endothelium was demonstrated. The addition of CB resulted in complete cessation of endothelial contraction. Thus, the actin filaments within the capillary endothelium are considered to play an important role in the endothelial contraction and vesicular transport, possibly regulating the capillary permeability and blood flow in the gastric mucosa.

ACKNOWLEDGMENT

This study was supported by the Grant-in-Aid for Science Research of the Ministry of Education, Science and Culture (#61770504)

REFERENCES

1. M. Oda, V.M. Price, M.M. Fisher and M.J. Phillips, Ultrstaructure of bile canaliculi, with special reference to the surface coat and the pericanalicular web, *Lab. Invest.*, **31**:314-323 (1974).
2. C. Oshio and M.J. Phillips, Contractility of bile canaliculi: implication for liver function, *Science*, **212**:1041-1042 (1981).
3. T.C.S. Keller and M.S. Mooseker, Ca^{++}-calmodulin-dependent phosphorylation of myosin, and its role in brush border contraction in vitro, *J. Cell Biol.*, **95**:943-959 (1982).
4. S.E. Hichcock, Regulation of motility in nonmuscle cells, *J. Cell Biol.*, **74**:1-15 (1977).
5. T.D. Pollard, Cytoplasmic contractile proteins, *J. Cell Biol.* **91**:156-165 (1981).
6. F. Hammersen, Endothelial contraction- Does it exist?, *in*: "Vascular Endothelium and Basement Membranes. Advance in Microcirculation, Vol 9," B.M. Altura and N.Y. Blooklyn, ed, S. Karger, Basel, München, Paris, London, New York, Sydney, 95-134 (1980).
7. G. Majino, S.M. Shea and M. Leventhal, Endothelial contraction induced by histamine-type mediators. An electron microscopic study, *J. Cell Biol.*, **42**:647-672 (1969).
8. M. Oda, M. Nakamura, N. Watanabe, N. Tsukada, Y. Yonei, H. Komatsu, K. Kaneko, Y. Akaiwa, I. Okazaki and M. Tsuchiya, Ultrastructural characterizations of the microcircuratory system in the stomach — from a terminological point of view, *in*: "Microcirculation Annual 1985, Japanese Society for Microcirculation," M. Tsuchiya, M. Asano, M. Oda and I. Okazaki, ed, Excerpta Medica, Amsterdam, 191-204 (1985).
9. N. Watanabe, M. Oda, M. Nakamura and M. Tsuchiya, Electron microscopic studies on a relation between the autonomic nerves and true capillaries in the gastric mucosa — with special reference to the endothelial microfilaments, *Bibl. Anat.*, **20**:120-125 (1981).
10. M. Oda, M. Nakamura, N. Watanabe, N. Tsukada, Y. Ohya, E. Sekizuka and M. Tsuchiya, Autonomic nervous regulation of gastric mucosal microcirculation — with special reference to the pathogenesis of stress-induced gastric ulcer, *in*: "Basic Aspects of Microcirculation, Proceedings of Tokyo International Syposium on Microcirculation, July 26, 1981, Tokyo, Japan," M. Tsuchiya, M. Asano, M. Oda, ed, Excerpta Medica, Amsterdam, 209-229 (1982).
11. M. Oda, M. Nakamura, N. Watanabe, N. Tsukada, Y. Yonei, H. Komatsu, Y. Ohya, E. Sekizuka and M. Tsuchiya, Dual action of the parasympathetic nerve in the gastric mucosa — significance of its overactivity in the pathogenesis of gastric ulcer, *in*: "Gastrointestinal Function, Regulation and Disturbances," Y. Kasuya, M. Tsuchiya, F. Nagao, Y. Matsuo, ed, Excerpta Medica, Amsterdam, 145-173 (1982).
12. N. Watanabe, M. Oda, M. Nakamura, E. Sekizuka, N. Tsukada, Y. Yonei, H. Komatsu and M. Tsuchiya, Mechanism of increased permeability of the capillary induced by histamine — possible involvement of the endothelial microfilaments, *in*: "Progress in Microcirculation Research II, F.C. Courtice," D.G. Garlic and M.A. Perry, ed, Postgraduate Medical Education, University of NSW, 479-485 (1984).
13. Y. Murayama, The human endothelial cell in tissue culture, *Z. Zellforsch. Mikrosk. Anat.*, **60**:69-79 (1963).
14. R.C. Wagner and M.A. Mathews, The isolation and culture of capillary endothelium from epididymal fat, *Microvasc. Res.*, **10**:286-297(1975).
15. D. Shepro, M. Rosenthal, J. Batbouta, L.S. Roflee and F.A. Belamarich, The cultivation of aortic endothelium. *Anat. Rec.*, **178**:523 (1974).
16. J.D. Gitlin and P.A. D'Amore, Retinal capillary endothelial cells: long-term culture using selective growth media, *Microvasc. Res.*, **26**:74-80 (1983).
17. M. Oda, K. Honda, H. Komatsu, Y. Yonei, K. Kaneko, N. Tsukada and M. Tsuchiya, Primary monolayer culture of capillary endothelium from the rat gastric mucosa. -immunocytochemical and ultrastructural characterizations-. The 33th American Microcirculatory Society Meeting. St. Louis, April (1986).
18. K. Honda, M. Oda, M. Nakamura, N. Tsukada, Y. Yonei, H. Komatsu, K. Kaneko, Y. Akaiwa, T. Fujiwara and M. Tsuchiya, Ultrastructural and cytochemical characterization of the monolayer-

cultured capillary endothelium, *J. Electron Microscopy 35,* (supple):2761-2762 (1986).

19. K. Honda, M. Oda, M. Nakamura, N. Tsukada, Y. Yonei, H. Komatsu, K. Kaneko, Y. Akaiwa and M. Tsuchiya, Primary monolayer culture of capillary endothelium from the rat gastric mucosa — a morphological and immunocytochemical study-, *in*: "Microcirculation Annual 1986. Japanese Society for Microcirculation," M. Tsuchiya, M. Asano, H. Hayashi and T. Kambara, ed, Nihonigakukan, Tokyo, Japan, 129-130 (1986).

20. K. Honda, M. Oda, M. Nakamura, N. Tsukada, Y. Yonei, H. Komatsu, K. Kaneko, T. Azuma, Y. Akaiwa, T. Fujiwara and M. Tsuchiya, Electron microscopic localization of actin filaments in the primary cultured capillary endothelium, *J. Clin. Electron Microscopy,* 19:470-471 (1986).

TUMOR MICROCIRCULATION

CAPILLARY ULTRASTRUCTURE AND
MICROCIRCULATORY FUNCTION OF MALIGNANT TUMORS

Bernhard Endrich, Frithjof Hammersen and Konrad Messmer

Department of Experimental Surgery
University of Heidelberg and Institute of Anatomy
Technical University of Munich, F.R.G.

INTRODUCTION

Organisation and recruitment of the vascular system comprises one of the fundamental aspects of tumor biology. In most neoplasms, there is a peculiar arrangement of living cells around some vascular arborizations on which they depend for nutrition, growth and metastasis. For studies of the vascular system in tumors, cellular implants have been employed primarily. Such techniques provided the opportunity to demonstrate distinct morphologic changes induced first in neighboring vessels of the host, with new capillaries sprouting from existing capillaries and venules.[1,2,3,4,5]

However, any consideration of the microcirculatory blood supply to tumors should not only cover the process of neovascularization itself but ought to distinguish three major topics:

1. The earliest development of tumor blood vessels,
2. The vascular morphology of the established tumor, and
3. The microvascular function of these channels.

Although the second topic encompasses the first (because as the tumor expands it recruits further blood supply by inducing capillary sprouts from the adjacent microcirculatory networks), we will review the development of the blood supply in tumors as listed above. Particular attention will be given to a possible clinical relevance.

THE EARLIEST DEVELOPMENT OF NEW TUMOR CAPILLARIES — TUMOR ANGIOGENESIS

Tumor angiogenesis is defined as the formation of capillary sprouts induced by a group of tumor cells associated with the subsequent development of a microcirculatory network within the mass.[6] Angiogenesis itself constitutes one of the main elements of any reaction upon tissue trauma because the restitution of tissue takes place after the invasion of the injured region by capillaries.[7,8] This new growth of blood vessels can be induced by a variety of factors such as blood cells, fibrin, histamine or the endothelial cell itself.[8] So called "tumor angiogenesis factors" have been isolated[9,10,11] but it appears that the net effect of angiogenesis will not only depend on factors released by a growing tumor (for a review see Reference 12).

Therefore, to define the angiogenesis in tumors as a specific feature occurring only during malignant growth, the analysis of the capillary ultrastructure should differentiate between neovascularization as a result of tissue trauma and truly new blood channels sprouting into a tumor. To the best of our knowledge, such distinction is possible only when experimental techniques like transparent chambers, quantitative intravital microscopy and a subsequent analysis of capillaries by electron microscopy are utilized (for a review see Reference 13) (Figures 1 and 2).

Although the tumor can be observed only during a limited period of time and may become necrotic as a result of external compression (by the tissue chamber),[14,15] such experimental set up provided very useful information. We have summarized the different characteristics of new vessel growth for both the tumor (amelanotic melanoma A-Mel-3 of the hamster) and the traumatized tissue in Table 1. In addition, a typical example of neovascularization induced by a tumor or by microsurgical tissue trauma is shown in Figure 3. It should be noted that there is a certain time lapse in our experimental set up because tumor cells were implanted 48 hrs after the implantation of the dorsal skin fold chamber. The analysis of ultrastructure was carried out three days after implantation of the chamber (tissue trauma = control) or three to ten days after tumor implantation into the chamber. 72 hrs after tumor cell implantation, the first sprouts were observed to be oriented toward the center of the amelanotic melanoma A-Mel-3. The most remarkable observation was that of *tumor cells incorporated into capillary sprouts,* thereby enhancing the growth rate of minute channels independently from endothelial proliferation.

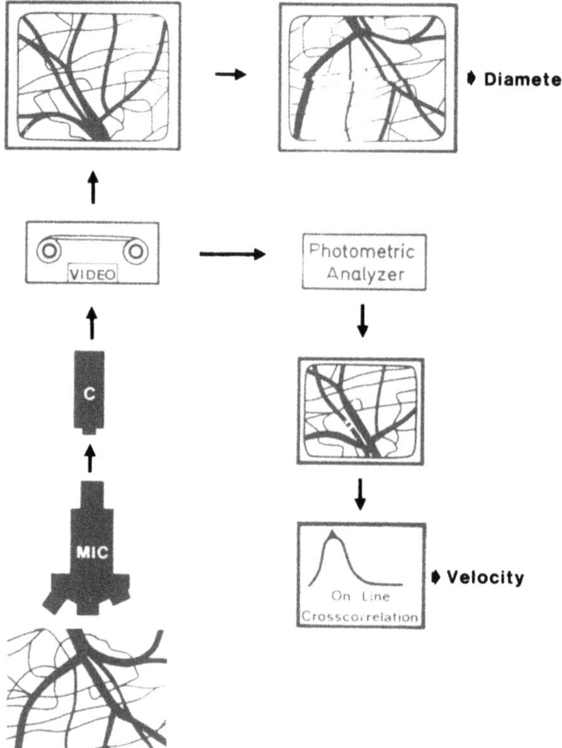

Fig. 1: Diagram of the experimental set up. A selected region within the skin fold preparation was observed through a microscope (MIC); the picture obtained at the eyepiece was recorded by a video camera (C) and stored on a video tape recorder (VIDEO) for subsequent analysis. Vessel diameters were measured using an electronic image shearing technique (upper part of the graph); measurements of blood cell velocity were performed by combining photometric analysis and crosscorrelation to determine the time for movement of red cells over a measured distance through the vessel lumen. The electronic equipment for microcirculatory measurements was obtained from IPM Inc., San Diego, California, USA.

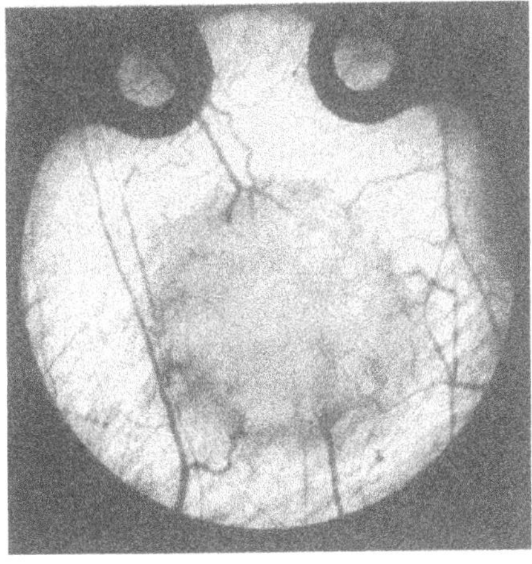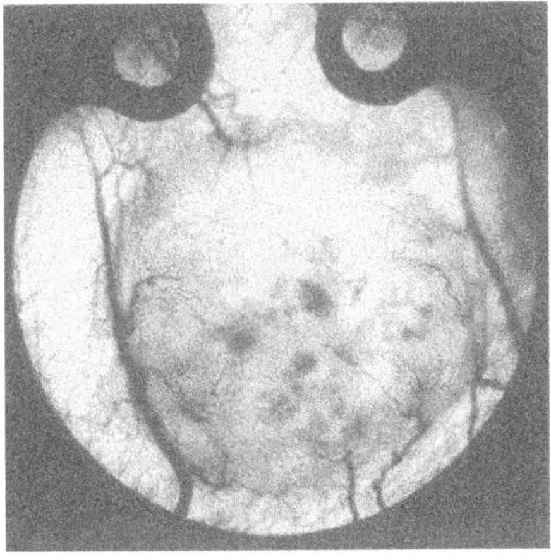

Fig. 2: Overview photographs from the amelanotic melanoma A-Mel-3 of the hamster implanted into a dorsal skin fold chamber. These pictures were obtained five (left) and ten days after tumor implantation. Note the tortuosity of draining blood vessels and the obstruction of some of the feeding vessels (11°°) particularly at the tumor's edge. Magnification app. 8×

Table 1. Characteristics of Neovascularization in Malignant Tumors and after Tissue Trauma

	Trauma	Tumor
Number of intraendothelial organelles	+	+ + +
Flattening of endothelium	−	+
Basal lamina	+	(−)
Tumor cells as part of the endothelial lining	−	+
Differentiation in arterioles and venules	+	−
Arteriolar vasomotion	+	−
Terminal lymphatics	+	−
Increased permeability	+	−

VASCULAR MORPHOLOGY OF THE ESTABLISHED TUMOR

The continuous observation of the tumor vasculature through a small window also provides the opportunity to study what has been described as "established microcirculation in tumors". These tumor capillaries were irregularly constricted or dilated and distorted with twisting, kinking and sharp bending (Figure 4). A chaotic capillary network, as seen in all malignant tumors studied so far, could impose a greater resistance to blood flow through the terminal vascular bed.[15,16] As the mass continuously enlarges, capillaries are elongated and more capillaries are formed in excess of the capacity of host arterioles and venules.[14]

Microvessels from the amelanotic melanoma A-Mel-3, the melanotic melanoma MOHR, and the BA 1112 sarcoma revealed common structural features:

1. The wall texture was that of a capillary irrespective of sometimes large diameters.
2. The endothelium was extremely flat in the non-nucleated part without becoming fenestrated.
3. The endothelium was frequently interrupted. Numerous gaps were bridged by a well-preserved basal lamina. These discontinuities provided the avenue for erythrocyte

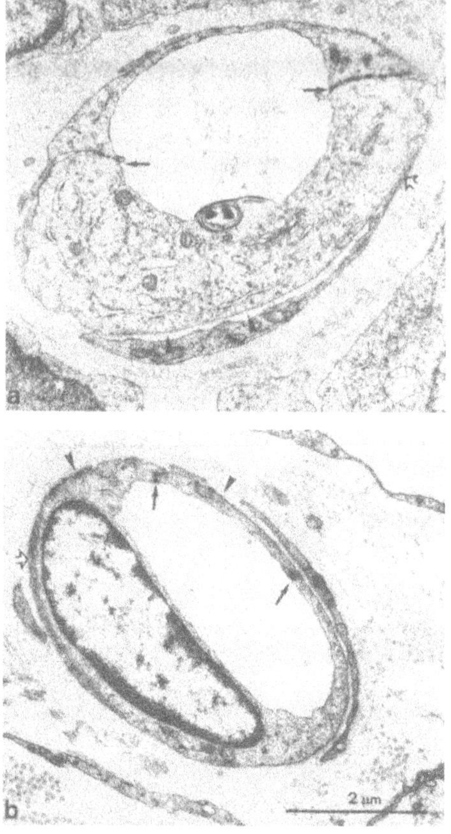

Fig. 3: A typical capillary sprout in the amelanotic melanoma A-Mel-3 (a) and in the tissue covered by the transparent chamber (b), both at the same magnification. (a) Angiogenesis induced by a tumor yields a thicker endothelium with plumpish endothelial cells which are well equipped with organelles. Intercellular attachment devices (◄—) and the basal lamina (◄) are poorly developed. ⇐ indicates the cellular expansion closely attached to the endothelium without an intervening basal lamina. (b) Angiogenesis as a result of microsurgical trauma is frequently observed within the first 72 hrs after implantation of the skin fold chamber. The new capillaries are more mature than new tumor capillaries. The interendothelial junctions (◄—) are tightened, the basal lamina (◄) rather well developed. ⇐ indicates subendothelial cells closely attached to the endothelium. For further details see Reference 17.

diapedesis. On occasion, platelets adhered to these sites, but leukocytes were never seen to penetrate these defects of mostly more than 1.5 μm.

4. Periendothelial cells and their elongated protrusions were closely attached to vascular endothelium in the melanoma; an intervening basal lamina was lacking. Therefore, these elements were very difficult to distinguish from the true endothelium, which are structurally similar. It has been suggested that these cell elements represent extensions of either undifferentiated mesenchymal or even tumor cells.[17]

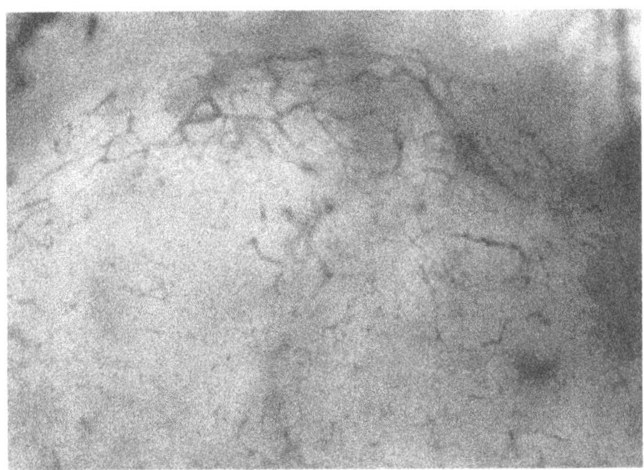

Fig. 4. Capillaries at the edge of the amelanotic melanoma
A-Mel-3 of the hamster. These minute channels are irregularly
aligned, their diameter changes frequently and there is kinking and
sharp bending. At the tumor margin (top), their is tissue edema.
In these regions, capillaries are non-existing or invisible because
they could not be visualized by FITC (fluorescent) — Dextran.
Magnification app. 60×

5. Evidence has been provided recently that tumor cells not only penetrated sinusoidal
   vessels, but they were also integrated into the lining endothelium over longer distances;
   thus, they contribute actively to the rapid growth of tumor capillaries[17] (Figure 5, Table
   2).

Further support for the above observations can be added by most recent studies of our group
in another melanotic cell line: numerous electron dense and membrane bound granules were found
in this tumor; they also occurred in lower numbers within the cells forming a capillary sprout
as well as in those rather mature and differentiated blood perfused tumor vessels.[18]

In our opinion, these findings are corroborated by earlier studies carried out with entirely different techniques. TANNOCK[19] analyzed population kinetics of cancer and endothelial
cells as well as that of fibroblasts in a transplantable mouse mammary tumor. He found a
significantly higher turnover rate for endothelial cells as compared to fibroblasts. The labeling
index with ^{3}H-thymidine reached a maximum close to a blood channel and decreased continuously with increasing distance from a capillary. These data are basically confirmed by HIRST[20]
who noted the highest turnover rate of endothelial cells in most rapidly proliferating tumors. Similar
conclusions can be derived from the work of DENEKAMP.[21] These data justify already the
assumption that an integration of tumor cells into the vascular lining occurs in newly formed
vessels. It should further be noted that the techniques employed by these authors do not permit
a precise differentiation between malignant and true endothelial cells; thus, all cells encircling
a vascular lumen were classified as "endothelial" in the studies cited above.

If an unknown number of these cells are derived from a malignant tumor, the turnover time
of the total number of endothelial cells must be above that of fibroblasts. Furthermore, it
becomes evident why the highest values are found near a capillary and within the most rapidly
proliferating tumors. Therefore, it is likely that the total number of true endothelial cells is
much lower in tumors than previously assumed.

From our own observations in implanted tissue chambers, several conclusions can be
derived:

1. In contrast to earlier reports (for a review see References 6, 8 and 22), our data strongly suggest that tumor angiogenesis is a specific and spezialized reaction of the microvasculature to generate as quickly as possible an adequate network of minute channels
   to meet the metabolic demands. This is further substantiated by the fact that initial values
   of capillary density are remarkably elevated at least in melanomas.[14,15]
2. Tumor cells are integrated in varying numbers into the linings of capillary sprouts as

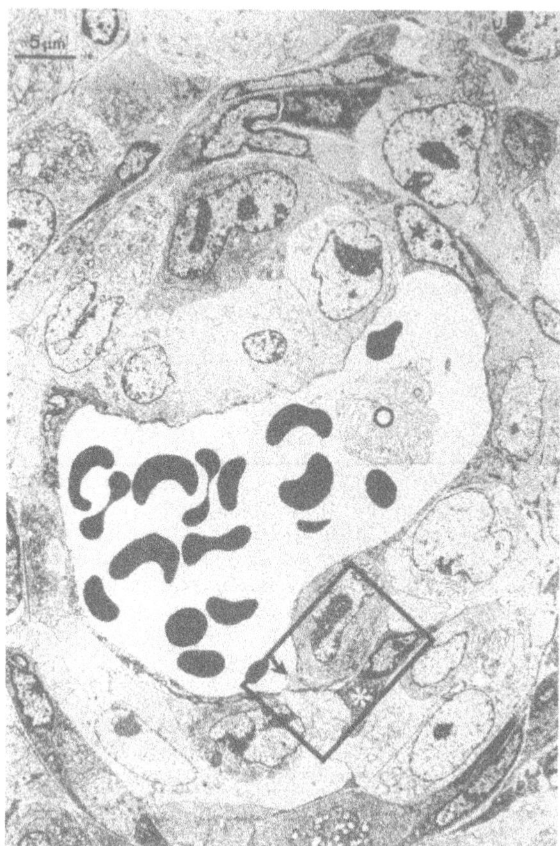

Fig. 5. Capillary from the amelanotic melanoma A-Mel-3 with an extremely attenuated endothelium and a few erythrocytes as well as a tumor cell ($\bigcirc$) within the vascular lumen. Parts of the endothelial nucleus have lost their contact with the vessel lumen and are far away as plumpish elements between tumor cells ($\bigstar$). These melanoma cells form cytoplasmic processes that protrude into the vessel lumen ($\longleftarrow$). Thus, the encircled box could be a region of tumor cell invasion. Magnification 2400×. For further details see Reference 17.

well as rather large, blood perfused vessels thereby facilitating their establishment, remodeling and adaptation, particularly at the tumor's edge.
3. Proliferating tumor cells will generate external pressure on fragile capillaries; thus, the tumor itself might determine growth and alignment of vessels.
4. Tumor capillaries are mostly young, premature vessels; their reactivity is likely to be much different when therapeutic measures such as hyperthermia are applied.

Any response of a tumor and its vasculature will not only depend on a peculiar morphology of the capillaries but on their function within a network of nutritive channels. Therefore, the present knowledge of the hemodynamic function of the tumor microcirculation should be reviewed before the medical impact of both pathomorphology and hemodynamic changes is being discussed.

MICROCIRCULATORY FUNCTION IN MALIGNANT TUMORS

The ultrastructural appearance of the microvessels varies in different tumor types, as it

Table 2. Comparison of Ultrastructural Observations in Different Malignant Tumors Implanted in a Dorsal Skin Fold Chamber of the Hamster (for more information see References 17 and 18)

	TUMOR CAPILLARIES	
	Capillary sprouts	*Mature Capillaries*
Intraluminal diameter (μm)	4 - 12	5 - 33
Feature of the endothelial wall texture	two cells with close membrane appositions	extremely attenuated
Adjacent cells within the endothelium	+	−
Pseudoendothelium formed by tumor cells	+	−
Great number of intra-endothelial organelles (cisternae, Golgi complexes, mitochondria)	+ +	(+)
Endothelial discontinuities	−	+
Increased permeability	−	+

dose the arrangement of tumor capillaries. The latter is different in different tumors and even in individual animals. Based on daily *in vivo* observation and direct *in situ* measurements of the microcirculation, remarkable differences were found between tumor-free and melanoma-bearing animals:

1. There are short, tortuous capillaries around the tumor edge (see Figure 4).
2. The capillary density per unit tissue tends to decrease with tumor growth after reaching high values initially, while in tumor free preparations capillary density and surface area was greatly enhanced.[14] The latter was very pronounced if a tissue chamber was left in situ for several weeks. Furthermore, if pieces of non malignant tissue were implanted,[23] angiogenesis was seen mostly at the edge with pinpoint hemorrhages, dilation of vessels and sluggish flow. In general, the capillary density in these regions was lower than in tumor free preparations.
3. The blood cell velocity in precapillaries and capillaries of tumors studied by intravital microscopy is lower than in the normal microcirculation.
4. In tumors, spontaneous arteriolar vasomotion with concomitant diameter changes in arterioles and precapillaries is almost absent. It is a consistent phenomenon in chamber preparations of unanesthetized animals and also in tissue implants from the myocardium.[13,24,25]
5. In tumors, there is a progressive and pronounced tissue hypoxia.[14,15,26]

Tumor hypoxia is primarily related to the increase in intercapillary distances, the peripheral alignment of tumor capillaries and their temporary or even permanent embolization. Data obtained from a hamster melanoma are summarized in Table 3.

Undoubtfully, there are also similarities between the normal microcirculation (as reflected by s.c. tissue and skeletal muscle in the skin fold preparation[13,24]) and the melanoma microcirculation:

1. A majority of capillaries were consistently perfused, the flow rate showed little variation.
2. A minority of capillaries shifted between low flow and zero flow at irregular intervals varying from seconds to several minutes.
3. A fair number of capillaries were visible but the flow was arrested during a 60 min period of observation and video recording.
4. Contercurrent capillary flow and plasma perfused capillaries (visualized by FITC-Dextran 150) were seen in both preparations.

Table 3. Skin Fold Preparation of the Hamster — Comparison of Data Between the Normal and the Tumor (A-Mel-3) Microcirculation

Parameter		Normal	Melanoma A-Mel-3	
			Day 4	Day 12
Capillary diameter	(μm)	7 (3-14)	7 (3-20)	14 (3-34)
Capillary density	(cm^{-1})	170-230	240	150
Capillary length	(μm)	440	220	270
Blood flow in capillaries (ml/min $\times$ 10^{-4})		0.11-0.13	0.08-0.37	
Tissue perfusion (ml/min/100 gm)		10	7.6	5.4
Tissue/Tumor PO$_2$ (mm Hg)		20 - 25	10	8

It should be noted that the FITC-filling time of the tumor capillary network was delayed by a factor of 6; in addition, there was a very uneven distribution of this marker. Moreover, the prolonged recording of blood cell velocity in the amelanotic melanoma A-Mel-3 of the hamster demonstrated a sometimes sudden decrease of flow to the point of complete or temporary stagnation. As a result, the flow through tumor capillaries was at a stand still; vascular stasis eliminated the normal function of the microcirculation despite obviously intact vessels causing acute ischemia and subsequently local necrosis. It has been previously shown[27] that numerous intact blood vessels penetrate necrotic tumor regions. This will imply that cell death can occur not only after a gradual decrease of capillary density but quite frequently after the interruption of blood flow.

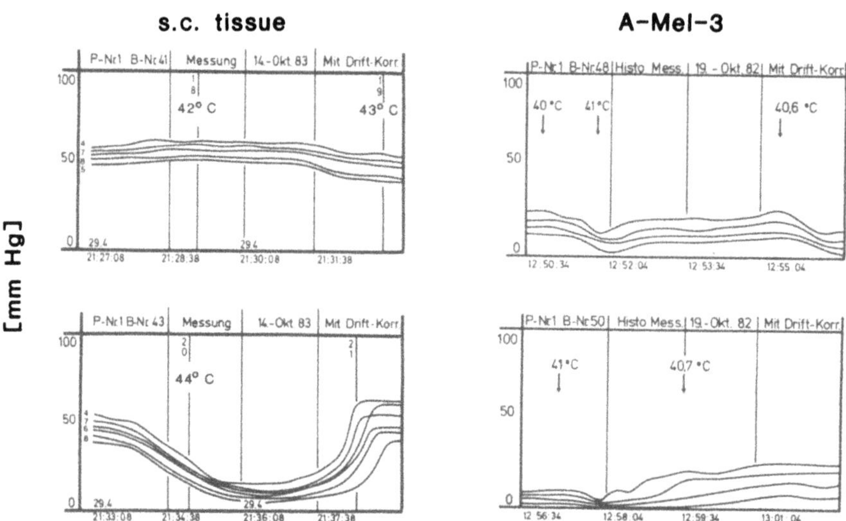

Fig. 6. Original recording of local tissue oxygenation using a platinum multiwire electrode to demonstrate a difference in thermal sensitivity between the normal (s.c. tissue) and the tumor microcirculation (A-Mel-3). It should be noted that there are much lower PO$_2$-values in the tumor. These values drop almost to zero as soon as a tumor temperature of app. 41°C is established. In the normal microcirculation, tissue oxygenation deteriorates at app. 44°C from initial values around 40-50 mm Hg, which were achieved by stepwise heating.

CONCLUSION

Variations in local perfusion of a tumor might indicate that any effective chemical or physical treatment of malignant lesions will strongly depend on extra- and intravascular transport properties of capillaries which are indeed different both in terms of their morphology and function. From quantitative intravital microscopy in malignant tumors, it appears that the transport of a cytotoxic agent will be limited to a great extent by the low tumor blood flow while the numerous and large discontinuities of the endothelium permit an easy penetration even of large size molecules. A consequence of these findings were recent attempts to improve tumor blood flow by means of isovolemic hemodilution.[28,29]

On the other hand, the tumor microcirculation seems to react more sensitive to physical measures. The effect of hyperthermia is particularly significant because, as show in Figure 6, a critical level of tumor temperature that would lead to a further deterioration of tumor oxygenation is already found around 41°C; any value above will aggravate tumor hypoxia and induce stasis in capillaries. In fact, many studies have shown that the microcirculation of malignant tumors cannot tolerate a longer lasting elevation of temperature (for a review see Reference 30). The difference in thermal sensitivity might provide the possibility to obstruct the tumor's microvasculature, thereby destroying preferentially neoplastic cells while leaving surrounding normal tissue unaffected.

REFERENCES

1. H.A. Eddy and W. Casarett, Development of the vascular system in the hamster malignant neurilemmoma, *Microvasc Res* 6:63-82 (1973).
2. E. Eriksson and H.A. Zarem, Growth and differentiation of blood vessels, *In*: "Microcirculation." Vol. I. G. Kaley, B.M. Altura, eds., University Park Press, Baltimore, London, Tokyo pp. 393-419 (1977).
3. M.A. Gimbrone, R.S. Cotran, S.B. Leapman and J. Folkman, Tumor growth and neovascularization: an experimental model using the rabbit cornea, *JNCI* 52:413-427 (1974).
4. C.M. Goodall, A.G. Sanders and P. Shubik, Studies of vascular patterns in living tumors with a transparent chamber inserted in the hamster cheek pouch, *JNCI* 35:497-521 (1965).
5. B.A. Warren, The vascular morphology of tumors, *In*: "Tumor blood circulation. Angiogenesis, vascular morpholoy and blood flow of experimental and human tumors." H.I. Petersen, ed., CRC Press, Boca Raton, Florida, USA, pp. 1-47 (1979).
6. B.A. Warren, Tumor angiogenesis, *In*: "Tumor blood circulation. Angiogenesis, vascular morphology and blood flow of experimental and human tumors." H.I. Petersen, ed., CRC Press, Boca Raton, Florida, USA, pp. 48-75 (1979).
7. T.E. Dudar and R.K. Jain, Microcirculatory flow changes during tissue growth, *Microvasc Res* 25:1-21 (1983).
8. J.G. Simpson and R.A. Fraser, Angiogenese in malignen Tumoren, *Prog Appl Microcirc* 2:1-14 (1983).
9. J. Folkman and C. Haudenschild, Angiogenesis in vitro, *Nature* 288:551-556 (1980).
10. J. Folkman, E. Merler, C. Abernathy and G. Williams, Isolation of a tumor factor responsible for angiogenesis, *J Exp Med* 133:275-288 (1971).
11. S. Kumar, A. Keegan, A. Erroi, D. West, P. Kumar and J. Gaffney, Responses of tissue cultured endothelial cells to angiogenesis factors — a review. TAF and endothelial cells, *Prog Appl Microcirc* 4:54-75 (1984).
12. O. Hudlicka and K.R. Tyler, "Angiogenesis. The growth of the vascular system." Academic Press, Harcourt Brace Jovanovich Publishers, London, Orlando, San Diego, New York, Austin, Montreal, Sydney, Tokyo, Toronto (1986).
13. B. Endrich and K. Messmer, Quantitative analysis of the Microcirculation in the awake animal, *In*: "Handbook of Microsurgery." Vol. I, W.L. Olszewski, ed., CRC Press, Boca Raton, Florida, USA, pp 79-105 (1984).
14. B. Endrich, A. Goetz and K. Messmer, Distribution of microflow and oxygen tension in hamster melanoma, *Int J Microcirc Clin Exp* 1:81-99 (1982).
15. B. Endrich, F. Hammersen, A. Goetz and K. Messmer, Microcirculatory blood flow, capillary morphology and local oxygen pressure of the hamster amelanotic melanoma A-Mel-3, *JNCI* 68:475-485 (1982).
16. B. Endrich and F. Hammersen, Morphologic and hemodynamic alterations in capillaries during hyperthermia, *In*: "Hyperthermia in Cancer Treatment." Vol. II. L.J. Anghileri, J. Robert, ed., CRC Press, Boca Raton, Florida, USA, pp 17-47 (1986).

17. F. Hammersen, U. Osterkamp-Baust and B. Endrich, Ein Beitrag zum Feinbau terminaler Strombahnen und ihrer Entstehung in bösartigen Tumoren, *Prog Appl Microcirc* **2**:15-51 (1983).
18. F. Hammersen, B. Endrich and K. Messmer, The fine structure of tumor blood vessels: I. Participation of non-endothelial cells in tumor angiogenesis, *Int J Microcirc Clin Exp* **4**:31-43 (1985).
19. I.F. Tannock, Population kinetics of carcinoma cells, capillary endothelial cells and fibroblasts in a transplanted mouse mammary tumor, *Cancer Res* **30**:2470-2476 (1970).
20. D.G. Hirst, J. Denekamp and B. Hobson, Proliferation kinetics of endothelial and tumor cells in three mouse mammary carcinomas, *Cell Tiss Kinet* **15**:251-262 (1982).
21. J. Denekamp, Vasculature as a target for tumor therapy, *Prog Appl Microcirc* **4**:28-38 (1984).
22. W.D. Thompson, K.J. Shiach, R.A. Fraser, L.C. Mc Intosh and J.G. Simpson, Tumours acquire their vasculature by vessel incorporation, not vessel ingrowth, *J Path* **151**:323-332 (1987).
23. W. Funk, B. Endrich and K. Messmer, A novel method for follow-up studies of the microcirculation in non malignant tissue implants, *Res Exp Med* **186**:259-270 (1986).
24. W. Funk, B. Endrich, K. Messmer and M. Intaglietta, Spontaneous arteriolar vasomotion as a determinant of peripheral vascular resistance, *Int J Microcirc Clin Exp* **2**:11-25 (1983).
25. M. Intaglietta and K. Messmer, Microangiodynamics, peripheral vascular resistance and the normal microcirculation, *Int J Microcirc Clin Exp* **2**:3-10 (1983).
26. P. Vaupel: Oxygen supply to malignant tumors, *In*: "Tumor blood circulation. Angiogenesis, vascular morphology and blood flow of experimental and human tumors." H.I. Petersen, ed., CRC Press, Boca Raton, Florida, USA, pp. 143-168 (1979).
27. P. Rubin and G. Casarett, Microcirculation of tumors. Part I: Anatomy, function and necrosis, *Clin Radiol* **17**:220-229 (1966).
28. T. Oda, A. Lehmann and B. Endrich, Capillary blood flow in the amelanotic melanoma of the hamster after isovolemic hemodilution, *Biorheology* **21**:509-520 (1984).
29. P. Vaupel and W. Mueller-Klieser, Hemodilution in isolated tumor perfusion, *Biorheology* **21**:521-528 (1984).
30. H.S. Reinhold and B. Endrich, Tumor microcirculation as a target for hyperthermia, *Int J Hyperthermia* **2**:111-137 (1986).

TRANSVASCULAR AND INTERSTITIAL
TRANSPORT IN TUMORS

Rakesh K. Jain

Department of Chemical Engineering
Carnegie Mellon University
Pittsburgh, PA 15213-3890, USA

INTRODUCTION

The advent of hybridoma technology and genetic engineering has led to a large scale production of monoclonal antibodies and other biologically useful molecules. Some of these molecules can bind to intra- or extracellular sites in tumors for detection and treatment, while others (e.g., lymphokines) have the ability to activate certain immune cells for killing cancer cells. Since these molecules or cells do not have the biological selectivity for tumors *in vivo* as previously envisioned, methods must be developed to deliver them selectively to the target *in vivo*. Since no molecule or cell can reach the tumor cells without passing through the vascular and interstitial compartments, it seems reasonable to find out more about the structure and function of these two compartments. In the past few years, we have focused our research on the experimental and mathematical characterization of transport through these spaces. I would like to share the results of some of these studies with you, and point out their implications for tumor growth, detection and treatment.

MATHEMATICAL CONSIDERATIONS

The transport of various solutes across vessel walls and through the interstitium occurs by both diffusion and convection. Concentration gradients of solute in the medium lead to diffusive transport. Movement of fluid molecules caused by pressure gradients leads to convective transport of solute molecules by "solvent-drag". For low molecular weight hydrophilic and lipophilic molecules, diffusion is the primary mechanism. For large molecules both convection and diffusion determine the transport. Mathematically, the transvascular transport is given by the Staverman-Kedem-Katchalsky equation:[1,2]

$$J_S = PA \, (C_v - C_i) + J_F \, (1 - \sigma_F) \, (C_v - C_i) \, / \, \ell n \, (C_v / C_i) \tag{1}$$

where, J_S (g/s) and J_F (cm³/s) are the net transvascular transport rates of solute and fluid, respectively; P is the diffusive permeability (cm/s); A is the exchange surface area (cm²); σ_F is the solvent-drag reflection coefficient while $(1 - \sigma_F)$ is a measure of coupling between fluid and solute transport; and C_v and C_i are, respectively, the plasma and interstitial concentrations of solute (g/cm³).

Similarily the transinterstitial transport of solute in x direction (I_S; g/s) is given by:[3]

$$I_S = - DA \frac{dC_i}{dx} + uA \, r_F \, C_i \tag{2}$$

where, D is the diffusion coefficient of the solute in the interstitium (cm²/s); C_i is the interitial concentration (g/s); u is the interstitial fluid velocity resulting from pressure gradients (cm/s); A is the area across which transport occurs (cm²); r_F is the retardation factor similar to $(1 - \sigma_F)$; and dC_i/dx is the solute concentration gradient.

It is sometimes convenient to "lump" the convection term into the diffusive term, and describe transvascular and interstitial transport in terms of an effective vascular permeability, P_{eff} and an effective interstitial diffusion coefficient, D_{eff}:

$$J_S = P_{eff} A (C_v - C_i) \tag{3}$$

$$I_S = - D_{eff} A \frac{dC_i}{dx} \tag{4}$$

In what follows I will describe our results on D_{eff} and P_{eff} in tumors obtained using intravital fluorescence microscopy, and then discuss our attempts to discriminate between convection and diffusion using fluorescence recovery after photobleaching (FRAP).

EFFECTIVE DIFFUSION AND PERMEABILITY COEFFICIENTS

The effective transport coefficients of various molecules (sodium fluorescein, MW = 376; bovine serum albumin, MW = 67,000; dextrans, MW = 19,400 − 150,000) in normal and neoplastic tissues grown in the rabbit ear chamber were measured using intravital quantitative fluorescence microscopy.[4] In this method a fluorescent tracer was injected into the auricular vein of the contralateral ear, and the movement of molecules in the microvascular bed of the tissue grown in the rabbit ear chamber was video-recorded using a SIT camera.[5] The optical set-up was calibrated so that the light intensity at a point in the video field after background subtraction was proportional to the tracer concentration.[6] The spatial and temporal distributions of intensity in the vascular and extravascular spaces were analyzed using a one-dimensional interstitial diffusion-vascular permeability model to yield D_{eff} and P_{eff}. The validity and details of the model are discussed in Nugent and Jain[6] and Gerlowski and Jain.[7]

Our studies on interestitial transport have shown that D_{eff} of various solutes is significantly higher in VX2 carcinoma than in mature granulation tissue, and this difference in transport rates increases with increasing molecular weight (Figure 1). For example, the D_{eff} of 150,000 MW dextran (D150) was about 33 times greater in the tumor than in the non-malignant tissue.[7,8] Further, D_{eff} of BSA was found to be about an order of magnitude less than that of dextran of the equivalent Stokes-Einstein radius. The low resistance to the interstitial transport in tumors could be attributed, at least in part, to the large interstitial volume, low glycosaminoglycans (GAG) content resulting from proteolytic enzymes released by cancer cells, and large interstitial convection in tumors compared to those in the homologous normal tissue.[3,9,10] The difference in the BSA versus dextran data could be attributed to the negative charge and globular nature of BSA.[9]

Our studies on microvascular permeability have shown that P_{eff} of D150 was about 8 times higher in the tumor than in the non-malignant tissue[7] (Figure 2). Glucose or galactose (0.2 and 2 g/kg, i.v.) or moderate hyperthermia (43°C × 1 h) had no significant effect on the permeability of D150 in either tissue type. Severe hyperthermia (50°C × 1 h) increased granulation tissue permeability about six-fold and the tumor permeability about two-fold.[4,11] The high permeability of tumor vessels is consistent with the ultrastructure studies of tumor vessels which show wide interendothelial junctions, fenestrae, transendothelial channels formed by vesicles, and discontinuous or absent basement membrane. The inability to increase P_{eff} of tumors at low thermal dose also supports the hypothesis that the transport pathways in tumors are maximally open to begin with, and that only physical destruction resulting from severe thermal stress may lead to a further increase in tumor vascular permeability.[2]

HETEROGENEITY IN TUMORS: ROLE OF INTERSTITIAL FLUID PRESSURE AND FLOW

These two key kindings — high D_{eff} and high P_{eff} — support the use of large molecules in cancer detection and treatment. These molecules can be monclonal antibodies or other macromolecules conjugated with drugs or toxins.[12,13] The conventional anti-cancer agents (MW < 2,000) do not have this transport selectivity, and hence their delivery is limited by poor

216

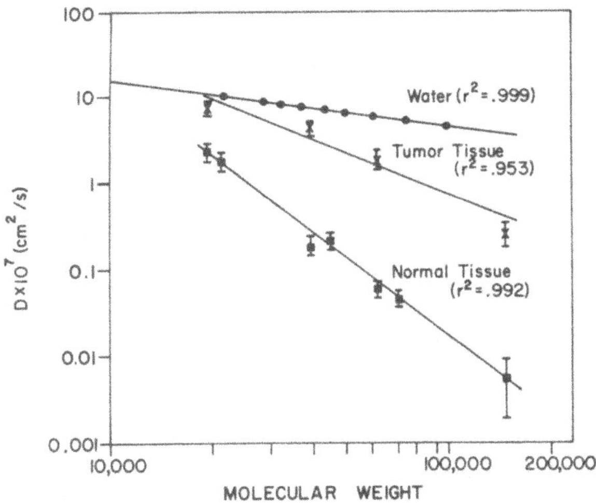

Fig. 1. Dependence of effective diffusion coefficients of dextrans on molecular weight in water, VX2 carcinoma and mature granulation tissue. [From Gerlowski and Jain,[7] with permission.]

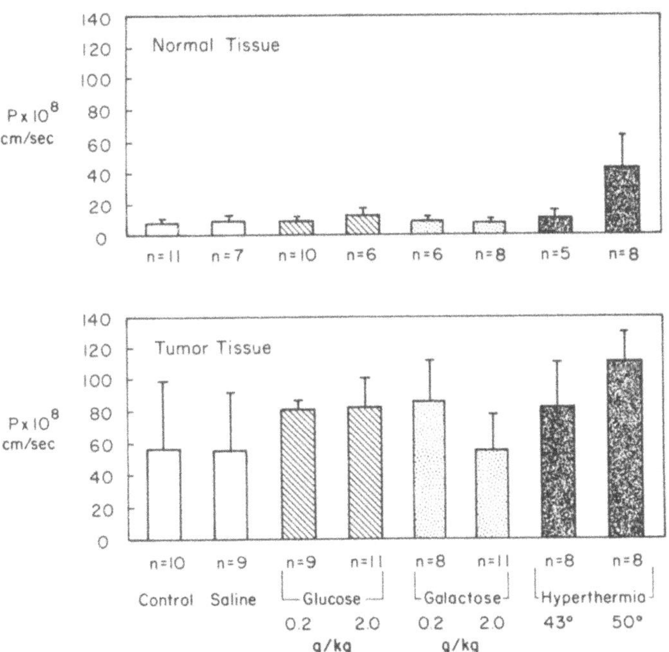

Fig. 2. Effective permeability coefficients of 150,000 molecular weight dextran in mature granulation tissue and VX2 carcinoma under various conditions: (a) control, (b) following saline injection, (c) following glucose injections, (d) following galactose injections, and (e) following hyperthermia. [From Jain,[4] with permission.]

perfusion rates of solid tumors and cell membrane transport.[14,15] The question is how well macromolecules accumulate in tumors.

Let us look at the data. Several investigators have measured uptake of various macromolecules (e.g. albumin, horseradish peroxidase, α-fetoprotein, IgG, IgM) in transplanted tumors. These investigators found the tissue uptake indices in tumors to be higher than in most normal tissues examined.[2,12] However, a closer examination of the data shows that while the *average* uptake of macromolecules in relatively high in tumors, there are regions in tumors with relatively poor concentration of these molecules. What are the causes of this heterogeneity?

It is well known that tumor blood supply is highly heterogeneous. (For a review, see, e.g. Jain and Ward-Hartley[16]). In a peripherally vascular tumor, one would expect the blood-borne macromolecules to accumulate primarily at the tumor periphery and relatively less in the center. However, diffusion should reduce these concentration gradients with time. As a matter of fact, this is what we found for small molecules.[17] However, large molecules remain at the periphery longer than several diffusion time constants. Why does this happen? One possibility is that the binding of these molecules to the cellular or extracellular sites would reduce the amount of "free" molecules available for diffusion. That may be true, especially in the case of monoclonal antibodies. We propose an alternate hypothesis for the peripheral localization of macromolecules in tumors: Net outward convection of interstitial fluid occurs from the tumor's periphery.

The question that follows is: Why is there net outward flow of fluid from tumors? Since the work of Young *et al* in 1950, several investigators have shown that the average interstitial pressure (IP) in tumors is significantly higher than that in normal tissues and that it increases with tumor growth. In addition, Wiig and our group have shown that the IP is highest in the center of tumors and it decreases to normal values at the tumor periphery (Figure 3). This increase in IP results presumably from the lack of anatomically well-defined, functioning lymphatics in tumors, growth of neoplastic cells in a relatively rigid space, increased vascular permeability to macromolecules, and from ischemic cell swelling.[3,18]

Existence of pressure gradients from the tumor center to the periphery suggests significant outward interstitial convection in tumors. Butler *et al*[19] calculated the net fluid loss from the tumor periphery (Q_{IF}) from the arteriovenous difference in blood hematocrit of isolated tumors. In four different mammary carcinomas, 2-5g, average Q_{IF} was found to be $\sim 0.14 - 0.22$ ml/h/g tissue which is significantly more than the lymph drainage in most normal tissues ($\sim 0.002 - 0.07$ ml/h/g). We can calculate the radial component of convective velocity at the tumor periphery, u_R, by dividing the fluid flow by tumor surface area (A)

$$u_R = \frac{\rho V Q_{IF}}{A} = \frac{\rho R Q_{IF}}{3} \tag{5}$$

where, ρ is the tumor density (g/ml); and R, A, and V are, respectively, the tumor radius, surface area and volume (cm, cm^2, cm^3).

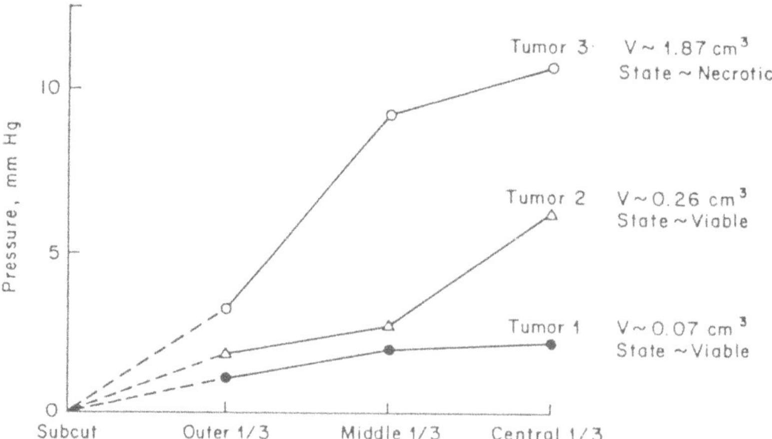

Fig. 3. Interstitial pressure gradients in VX2 carcinoma. [From Misiewicz and Jain, in preparation.]

Equation (5) implies that if Q_{IF} were constant u_R would increase with increasing tumor radius. However, Butler *et al* showed that Q_{IF} is proportional to the tumor blood perfusion rate, B [B (ml/h/g) = 1.90 + 12.66 Q_{IF}]. It is well established that B decreases with increasing tumor size (B = $\alpha e^{-\beta V}$ or B = $\alpha V^{-\beta}$; Jain and Ward-Hartley[16]). Therefore, one would expect Q_{IF} to decrease with increasing tumor size. Whether u_R would decrease with increasing tumor size depends upon how rapidly Q_{IF} decreases with R; this would vary from one tumor to another, and for the same tumor at different stages of growth.

Per equation (5), the value of fluid velocity at the periphery, u_R, for a tumor of 1 cm radius ($\sim$4g) is $\sim$0.1 − 0.2 μm/s! The value of convective velocity, u, inside the tumor is not known. A macromolecule has to have an inward diffusional velocity greater than the outward convective velocity to penetrate a tumor. Despite the overwhelming evidence of interstitial convection in tumors and the importance of this phenomenon, there are no *direct* measurements of the magnitude and direction of convective velocity of solute or solvent in the interstitium. This leads to the next question: Can we measure convection and diffusion in the tumor interstitium directly?

DIRECT MEASUREMENT OF INTERSTITIAL CONVECTION AND DIFFUSION

Fluorescence recovery after photobleaching (FRAP) has been utilized by biologists to measure movement of molecules on the cell surface and in the cytoplasm.[20] We have recently adapted this method to measure convection versus diffusion in the interstitium. In this technique, a well-defined concentration gradient of a fluorescent tracer is artificially imposed in the extravascular region of a tissue using a laser beam. The relaxation of the concentration profile is monitored using intravital fluorescence microscopy and quantified using computer-assisted image analysis to yield the diffusion coefficient and the convective velocity.[21]

To date we have tested the feasibility of this approach in the rabbit ear chamber and have found the convection to be space- and time-dependent. For 70,000 molecular weight dextran the *preliminary* estimates of the Peclet number (= convective velocity/diffusive velocity) range from one to four. Our current efforts include *in vitro* and *in vivo* calibrations as well as extensive data collection to map temporal and spatial distributions of convective velocity in the normal and tumor interstititum.

CONCLUSIONS

Effective microvascular permeability and interstitial diffusion coefficients of macromolecules are higher in tumors than in most normal tissues. Possible causes of these differences include "leaky" structure of the vessel wall, large interstitial space, low GAG contents and relatively high interstitial convection in tumors. While these factors favor the use of large molecules in the detection and treatment of solid tumors, increased interstitial pressure in the center coupled with lower intravascular pressure retards the extravasation and penetration of large molecules In the internal melieu of a tumor. Reduction in the number of tumor cells by proper doses of radiation or heat may modulate these pressures to increase extravasation and penetration of macromolecules in a tumor.

Despite overwhelming evidence of increased interstitial convection in tumors, there are no direct measurements of convective versus diffusive transport in tumors. Recent developments in fluorescence microscopy and image analysis should permit these measurements. Availability of such information would help in determining the optimal size of macromolecules to be used in cancer detection and treatment.

ACKNOWLEDGMENTS

The author wishes to express his sincere gratitude to Dr. P.M. Gullino for his pioneering work in the pathophysiology of tumors, and to his former and current students: Dr. L.J. Nugent, Dr. L.E. Gerlowski, M. Misiewicz, M.A. Young, S. Chary, and L. Baxter, for contributing in many ways to the research on transport in tumors. This article is based on research supported by grants from the National Cancer Institute, the National Science Foundation, and the Richard K. Mellon Foundation; by an NIH Research Career Development Award (1980-85); and by a Guggenheim Fellowship (1983-84).

REFERENCES

1. F.E. Curry, Mechanics and thermodynamics of transcapillary exchange, *In*: "Handbook of Physiology — The Cardiovascular System — Microcirculation," E.M. Renkin and C.C. Michel, eds, American Physiological Society, Bethesda, pp 309-374 (1984).
2. R.K. Jain, Transport of molecules across tumor vessels, *Cancer and Metastasis Reviews.* 6:559-594 (1987).
3. R.K. Jain, Transport of molecules in the tumor interstitium: A review, *Cancer Research,* 47:3038-3050 (1987).
4. R.K. Jain, Transport of macromolecules in tumor microcirculation, *Biotechnology Progress,* 1:81-94 (1985).
5. L.J. Nugent and R.K. Jain, Monitoring transport in the rabbit ear chamber, *Microvascular Research,* 24:204-209 (1982).
6. L.J. Nugent and R.K. Jain, Plasma pharmacokinetics and interstitial diffusion of macromolecules in a normal capillary bed, *American Journal of Physiology,* 246:H129-H137 (1984).
7. L.E. Gerlowski and R.K. Jain, Microvascular permeability of normal and neoplastic tissues, *Microvascular Research,* 31:288-305 (1986).
8. L.J. Nugent and R.K. Jain, Extravascular diffusion in normal and neoplastic tissues, *Cancer Research,* 44:238-244 (1984).
9. L.J. Nugent and R.K. Jain, Pore and fiber-matrix models for diffusive transport in normal and neoplastic tissues, *Microvascular Research,* 28:270-274 (1984).
10. R.K. Jain and K.A. Ward-Hartley, Dynamics of cancer cell interactions with microvasculature and interstitium, *Biorheology,* 24:117-125 (1987).
11. L.E. Gerlowski and R.K. Jain, Effect of hyperthermia on microvascular permeability of normal and neoplastic tissues, *International Journal of Microcirculation: Clinical and Experimental,* 4:336-372 (1985).
12, H. Sezaki and M. Hashida, Macromolecule — drug conjugates in targeted cancer chemotherapy, *CRC Critical Reviews on Therapeutic Drug Systems,* 1:1-38 (1984).
13. G. Poste, Drug targeting in cancer therapy *In*: "Receptor-Mediated Targeting of Drugs," G. Gregoriadis, G. Poste, J. Senior and A. Trouet, eds, Plenum, New York, pp. 427-474 (1985).
14. R.K. Jain, J. Weissbrod and J. Wei, Mass transfer in tumors: Characterization and applications in chemotherapy, *Advances in Cancer Research,* 33:251-310 (1980).
15. L.E. Gerlowski and R.K. Jain, Physiologically-based pharmacokinetics: Principles and applications, *Journal of Pharmaceutical Sciences,* 72:1103-1127 (1983).
16. R.K. Jain and K.A. Ward-Hartley, Tumor blood flow: Characterization, modifications and role in hyperthermia, *IEEE Transactions in Sonics and Ultrasonics;* Special Issue on Hyperthermia, SU-31:504-526 (1984).
17. R.K. Jain and J. Wei, Dynamics of drug transport in solid tumors: Distributed parameter model, *J. Bioengineering,* 1:313-329 (1977).
18. R.K. Jain, Intersitital transport in tumors, *Advances in Microcirculation.* 13:266-284 (1987).
19. T.B. Butler, F.H. Grantham and P.M. Gullino, Bulk transfer of fluid in the interstitial compartment of mammary tumors, *Cancer Research,* 35:512-516 (1975).
20. D.L. Taylor, A.S. Waggoner, R.F. Murphy, F. Lanni, and R.R. Birge, eds., "Applications of fluorescence in the biomedical sciences," A.R. Liss, New York (1986).
21. S.C. Chary and R.K. Jain, Analysis of diffusive and convective recovery after photobleaching — uniform flow field, *Chemical Engineering Communications.* 55:235-249 (1987).

MATRIX CONTROL OF TUMOR ANGIOGENESIS

W. Reilly and B.R. McAuslan

CSIRO Division of Molecular Biology
P.O. Box 184
North Ryde, NSW 2113, Australia

INTRODUCTION

Tumor angiogenesis is the process through which certain tumors stimulate the growth of the microvascular network in the surrounding tissue. This capillary network is remarkable in that the growth is directed towards the tumor which becomes vascularized. An important fundamental question is, what is the nature of the molecular controls responsible for the directed vascularization? As cell migration is the salient feature in neovascularization the question thus becomes, what are the molecular events that control cell migration during neovascularization? A wide variety of compounds have been shown to be inducers of angiogenesis or neovascularization *in vivo*. These include both tumor or tissue derived factors as well as a number of chemical factors.[1,2,3,4,5,6] All of these, with the exception fo angiogenin, have been shown to also induce endothelial cell migration.

Clearly cell migration *in vivo* must require the modification of a number of cellular processes together with changes in the physical environment before a cell can escape from the matrix in which it is embedded. This matrix modification occurs during angiogenesis and is reported to influence cell migration and proliferation.[7,8,9] Rifkin et al. (1983)[10] proposed that during angiogenesis endothelial cells release specific proteases to help them escape matrix constraints and penetrate the surrounding stroma. Likely candidates are plasminogen activator and collagenase. These proteases were shown to be at much higher levels after exposure of the cells to angiogenesis factors. This was in accord with the idea that extracellular matrix (ECM) disruption was a likely early event in angiogenesis. ECM has been also shown to have a profound influence on the early events in organogenesis and development and has been reported to have an effect on both cell proliferation and migration.[11,12,13] These studies and others have shown ECM to not only affect the direction of migration but also the rate at which cell migration occurs.[12,14,15]

In our attempts to focus on endothelial cell migration as the major controlling event in angiogenesis, we have examined how ECM components influence cell migration and angiogenesis. In this paper we demonstrate that (i) ECM components control cellular migration rates by inhibiting the migration inducing activity of angiogenic factors and (ii) interference with ECM synthesis or assembly stimulates cell migration which leads to angiogenesis.

MATERIALS AND METHODS

Cell Cultures

All cells were of bovine origin. Clonal lines of aortal endothelial cells (BAE), retinal capillary endothelial cells (BREC), smooth muscle cells (BSM) and corneal endothelial cells (BCE) were established and maintained as described (McAuslan et al., 1987). All cells used for experimentation were between their 6th and 12th passage.

Migration Assay

Cell migration was determined using the phagokinesis assay.[16] Migration inducers were added to the medium covering the cells and track lengths measured 24 hours later. Measurements were made using a Leitz Bioquant II image analysis system. An average of 100 individual tracks were measured and the means tabulated.

Substratum Preparation

Serial dilutions of fibronectin (FN) and collagen were prepared using serum free medium. Two millilitre aliquots of each concentration in triplicate were added to 60 mm tissue culture dishes containing clean 18 mm glass coverslips. These were then air dried. Two millilitres of colloidal gold solution were then added and incubated at 37°C for 2 hours. The excess liquid was then removed and 5 ml of migration medium containing 3% FCS and 3 × 10⁴ cells added and reincubated.

Reagents

The proline analogues cis-4-hydroxy-L-proline (cisOHPro), 3,4 dehydro-L-proline (dHPRo), cis-4-hydroxy-D-proline (cisDPro) and L-azetidine—Z-carboxylic acid (Azet) were obtained from Sigma Chemical Co., USA. Fibronectin was isolated from fresh bovine plasma using the method of Hannan et al. (1984).[17] Collagen as Vitrogen 100 was purchased from The Collagen Corporation, Palo Alto, CA and is a purified form of type I collagen from calf skin. EGF was prepared from acid extracts of mouse submaxillary glands and was further purified by reverse phase HPLC.[18] ESF was prepared according to McAuslan and Hoffman (1979).[19]

In vivo Angiogenesis Assay

Slow release Elvax polymer was impregnated with saturating amounts of test material. These were sterilized and embedded in an atelo-collagen gel in a shallow silicon tube. These were then implanted subcutaneously into rabbits and examined 10 days later.[20] The implants were then surgically removed, fixed in normal saline and processed for light microscopy.

RESULTS

Changes in the Rate of Migration of Endothelial Cells in Response to Angiogenic Factors: Inhibition by ECM Components

The migratory response of endothelial cells to angiogenic factors has been well documented.[1,21,22] Two of these factors, EGF and ESF, were used to examine the possible inhibition of endothelial cell migration by the ECM components fibronectin (FN) and collagen. Bade and Nitzgen (1985)[15] have shown that FN, when bound to the substratum, inhibited the migration of Buffalo rat liver epithelial cells in response to a combination of EGF and insulin. This inhibition was shown to be FN specific and they suggested that it may be an additional control mechanism to contact inhibition.

Our approach was to examine endothelial cells for similar mechanisms by using angiogenic factors that are known to produce large increases in endothelial cell migration. The two factors, EGF and ESF, gave consistently 3-fold increases in the migration rate of the different endothelial cells tested, using BSA as the substratum for the attachment of the colloidal gold particles, and were active over a large concentration range (Table 1). However, when either of the two factors were used at optimal concentrations normally producing maximal migration, inhibition of the migration occurred if FN was used as a substratum.

A series of concentrations of FN were then tested to determine the concentration at which total inhibition occurred. Table 2 presents these results. It was found that both EGF- and ESF-induced migration was inhibited linearly as the FN concentration increased. Complete inhibition occurred at concentrations above 30 μg/cm². To ensure that the observed migration inhibition was substratum dependent a similar series of concentrations of FN were added to the medium in a set of experiments where BSA was used as the substratum. No inhibition of the EGF- or ESF-induced migration was observed under these conditions.

We next examined collagen type I substratum for its ability to inhibit migration as did the FN substratum. Bade and Nitzgen (1985)[15] had tested collagen type IV at a concentration simi-

Table 1. Stimulation of BREC migration by EGF or ESF on BSA substratum

BSA conc. μ/cm^2	EGF conc. ng/ml	Area $10^{-3}\mu m^2$	ESF conc. $\mu g/ml$	Area $10^{-3}\mu m^2$
3000	100	96.2	50	122.3
3000	50	75.4	25	65.8
3000	25	58.8	10	36.5
3000	10	42.7	0	26.8
3000	0	29.4	–	–

BREC were seeded onto BSA coated coverslips in Medium 199 plus 3% FCS and incubated at 37°C in 5% CO_2 for 24 hours. The migration trails were then measured using a BIOQUANT image analysis system. Each measurement represents the mean of 100 individual migration trails.

Table 2. The effect of fibronectin substratum on the stimulation of BREC migration by EGF or ESF

FN conc. $\mu g/cm^2$	EGF conc. ng/ml	Area $10^{-3}\mu m^2$	ESF conc. $\mu g/ml$	Area $10^{-3}\mu m^2$
0.0	100	86.9	50	97.3
0.3	100	88.7	50	92.8
3.0	100	47.8	50	48.5
30	100	29.9	50	30.8
60	100	25.7	50	26.8

BREC were seeded onto FN coated coverslips in Medium 199 plus 3% FCS and incubated at 37°C in 5% CO_2 for 24 hours. The migration trails were then measured using a BIOQUANT image analysis system. Each measurement represents the mean of 100 individual migration trails.

Table 3. The effect of collagen substratum on the stimulation of BREC migration by EGF or ESF

Collagen $\mu g/cm^2$	EGF conc. ng/ml	Area $10^{-3}\mu m^2$	ESF conc. $\mu g/ml$	Area $10^{-3}\mu m^2$
0.0	100	89.9	50	99.7
3.0	100	86.7	50	96.8
30	100	75.5	50	78.5
60	100	62.9	50	65.1
100	100	24.4	50	23.4

BREC were seeded onto collagen coated coverslips in Medium 199 plus 3% FCS and incubated at 37°C in 5% CO_2 for 24 hours. The migration trails were then measured using a BIOQUANT image analysis system. Each measurement represents the mean of 100 individual migration trails.

lar to that of FN used in these experiments and found it to have no effect. We found that collagen type I did inhibit EGF- and ESF-induced migration but at a concentration an order of magnitude greater than that required by FN (Table 3). The high concentration of collagen needed for inhibition to occur could explain why it was missed by Bade and Nitzgen. Alternatively, it is conceivable that collagen type IV does not have any effect. It will be necessary to repeat this work with collagen type IV to resolve this.

We attempted to demonstrate further that the ECM components already shown to inhibit

Table 4

Cell type	Conc. of analogue	Area			
		cisOHPro	cisDPro	Azet	dHPro
BREC	5×10^{-4}M	20.0	23.2	19.9	21.0
	1×10^{-4}M	29.2	25.2	30.1	30.5
	1×10^{-5}M	46.4	24.2	37.9	48.1
	1×10^{-5}M	24.2	24.7	25.0	25.0
BCE	5×10^{-4}M	30.0	29.8	29.5	30.5
	1×10^{-5}M	115.8	36.8	43.4	45.1
	1×10^{-6}M	36.4	38.6	43.4	45.1
BASM	1×10^{-5}M	89.4	33.6	110.6	90.8

Cell migration rates in response to proline analogues. Each measurement represents the mean of 100 cell trails. The measurements were made with a BIOQUANT II analysis system.

the migration of endothelial cells was not just a response to high concentrations of proteins on the substratum. A similar series of experiments using ovalbumin or BSA as the substratum protein were carried out. It was found that neither ovalbumin nor BSA also had any effect on induced migration over the concentration range tested. This suggests that specific ECM components may act as molecular modulators regulating cell migration. The ECM must therefore be degraded or modified for endothelial cell migration to occur during neovascularization.

Stimulation of Endothelial Cell Migration via Interference with ECM Synthesis

It has been shown that tumor angiogenic factor (TAF) activates a latent collagen type IV collagenase.[23] Further, it has been demonstrated that endothelial cells migrating in response to the angiogenic stimulus of retinal extracts actively degrade basement membrane collagens.[24] Angiogenic factors therefore may stimulate ECM degradation by either (1) activating collagenases produced by endothelial cells which in turn degrade the ECM to which they are adhering, or (2) cause some change in the synthesis or export of ECM components which in turn leads to increased enzymatic degradation and migration occurs.

In either case, and in the light of the previously reported ECM inhibition results, it should be possible to induce endothelial cell migration by modifying synthesis of certain ECM components, in particular the collagens, by the use of proline analogues. A range of concentrations of cisOHPro, cisDPro, Azet and dHPro were tested using the previously described assay with BSA as the substratum. All the analogues interfere with the synthesis and secretion of collagens. The results presented in Table 4 show cisOHPro, Azet and dHPro all produce a 2-3 fold increase in migration rate; cisDPro, which is not incorporated into collagen, was inactive. The optimal concentration was 10^{-5}M; concentrations above this produced a relative decrease in migration rate. This later finding agrees with the work of Madri and Stenn (1982).[14] They found that marked inhibition of collagen synthesis with proline analogues inhibited migration, suggesting that ECM turnover by migrating endothelial cells is necessary for continued migration.

Proline Analogues as Angiogenic Factors in vivo

It has become evident that any factor that induces endothelial cells to migrate *in vitro* is invariably angiogenic *in vivo*. We demonstrated this by implanting slow release polymers subcutaneously in rabbits.[20] These implants were removed after 10 days, fixed, processed histologically and examined microscopically. A typical field is presented in Figure 1.

Control implants showed responses that were consistent with those of a foreign body. There was an increase in granulocytes at the edge of the silicon ring with an increase in fibroblasts and the appearance of dense collagen bundles. On the other hand, implants containing the proline analogues were markedly different. These were highly vascularized with numerous large and small vessels.

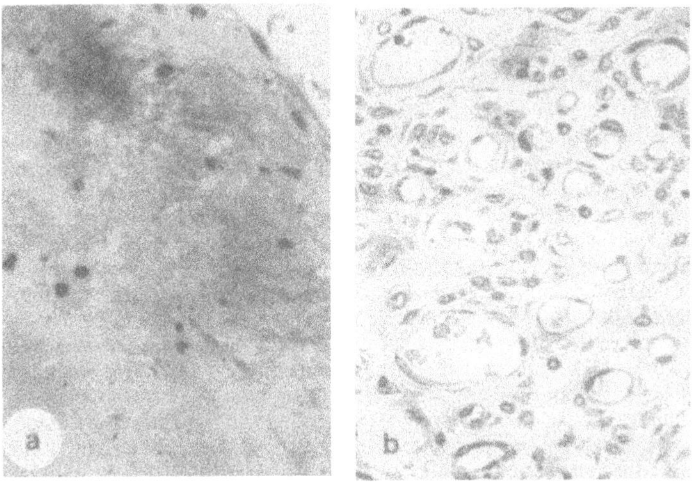

Fig. 1. (a) Control implant in collagen gel at 10 days, (b) cisOHPro implant in collagen gel at 10 days.

DISCUSSION

Extracellular matrix (ECM) has been shown to influence profoundly the behaviour of vascular cells; it plays a role in directing cell migration during development and wound healing and affects the action of soluble growth regulators.[12] The endothelial cell in turn also influences the ECM during migration, continually modifying it through the action of proteases.[25] The experiments reported above attempt to further examine these ECM-endothelial cell interactions during migration by (1) demonstrating that the ECM components fibronectin and collagen I inhibit the migration response to the angiogenic factors EGF and ESF, and (2) modulation of the synthesis of ECM collagen is sufficient to induce endothelial cell migration *in vitro* and set angiogenesis en train *in vivo*. The ability of ECM to inhibit the action of angiogenic factors is of general interest. Bade and Nitzgen (1985)[15] proposed the inhibition they observed had relevance to liver physiology as the cells used were liver epithelial cells, but these results would indicate that this control mechanism is yet another general function of the ECM.

We found that the inhibition of endothelial cell migration was proportional to the concentration of the ECM component. The maximal inhibition occurred at 30 μg/cm^2 and 100 μg/cm^2 for FN and collagen respectively. As the concentration on the substratum decreased the induction of migration by EGF or ESF increased, indicating a linear relationship for the effect. Addition of FN at a concentration of 60 μg/cm^2 to the medium in soluble form rather than as a substratum did not inhibit migration to EGF or ESF (data not presented). It is conceivable that if this effect operated *in vivo* that a factor like TAF which has been reported to activate a latent protease[23] could produce a concentration gradient which would directionally control the migration of endothelial cells during angiogenesis.

Further, our finding that the modification of ECM through the modulation of synthesis of cellular collagens leads to migration and angiogenesis supports the hypothesis that the early event in angiogenesis is matrix modification which in turn controls endothelial cell migration and directional movement. The proline analogues used to interfere with collagen secretion and synthesis, cisOHPro, Azet and dHPro, all produced an increase in the cell migration rate when used at their optimal concentrations 10^{-5}M. This produced a 2-3 fold increase over the control. Since cisDPro was inactive this suggests a structural specificity. Continuous collagen synthesis has been shown to be an obligatory requirement for cell migration.[14] Our findings suggest that small changes in the collagen structure due to the incorporation of low levels of proline analogues is sufficient to impair the assembly of collagen in the ECM. This may destabilize cell anchorage, interfere with some other step critical for cell migration or perhaps make the ECM more susceptible to degradation, with the result being an increased migration rate.

The finding that modulation of collagen synthesis or secretion can lead to altered controls on the microvascular system offers a useful model system to understand the cellular events in tumor angiogenesis in particular and organogenesis in general.

SUMMARY AND CONCLUSION

Endothelial cell migration is a key feature of angiogenesis. Epidermal Growth Factor (EGF) or Tumor Angiogenesis Factor (TAF) induce cell migration and angiogenesis. When the matrix components, collagen or fibronectin, were used as a substratum in the phagokinesis assays, EGF- or TAF-induced cell migration was inhibited. It has been proposed that TAF activates cellular protease causing the matrix degradation that is evident during neovascularization *in vitro*. If such degradation leads to cell migration and angiogenesis, then other agents that interfere with the synthesis or assembly of matrix components should stimulate cell migration and angiogenesis. The proline analogues cis hydroxyproline, azetidine and dehydroproline are known modulators of cellular collagen synthesis. At optimal concentration (10^{-5}M) these analogues caused 3-fold increases in endothelial cell migration rates *in vivo* as tested by a subcutaneous implant assay. We conclude from these studies that: (i) matrix components control cellular migration rates; high concentration of collagen or fibronectin inhibit angiogenically active inducers of endothelial cell migration. (ii) Intracellular modulation of synthesis of collagens leads to angiogenesis by stimulating cell migration.

These findings relate to tumor angiogenesis and that TAF might trigger angiogenesis either by activation of latent proteases or by some modification of matrix assembly during synthesis that affects cell adhesion and migration.

REFERENCES

1. B.R. McAuslan, W. Reilly, G.N. Hannan and G.A. Gole, Angiogenic factors and their assay: activity of formyl methionyl leucyl phenylalanine, adenosine diphosphate, heparin, copper and bovine endothelium stimulating factor, *Microvasc. Res.* **26**:323 (1983).
2. J. Folkman, E. Merler, C. Abernathy and G. Williams, Isolation of a tumor factor responsible for angiogenesis, *J. Exp. Med.* **133**:275 (1971).
3. R.D. Kissun, C.R. Hill, A. Garner, P. Phillips, S. Kumar and J.B. Weiss, A low molecular weight angiogenic factor in cat retina, *Brit. J. Ophthal.* **66**:165 (1982).
4. M.J. Banda, D.R. Knighton, T.K. Hunt and Z. Webb, Isolation of a nonmitogenic angiogenesis factor from wound fluid, *Proc. Natl. Acad. Sci. USA* **79**:7773 (1982).
5. M. Ziche, J. Jones and P.M. Gullino, Role of prostaglandin El and copper in angiogenesis, *J. Natl. Cancer Inst.* **69**:475 (1982).
6. J.W. Fett, D.J. Strydom, B.R. Lobb, E.M. Alderman, J.L. Bethune, J.F. Riordan and B.L. Vallee, Isolation and characterization of angiogenin and angiogenic protein from human carcinoma cells, *Biochemistry* **24**:5480 (1985).
7. D.M. Form, B.M. Pratt and J.A. Madri, Endothelial cell proliferation during angiogenesis, *Lab. Invest.* **55**:521 (1986).
8. K. Nabeshima, H. Kataoka and M. Koono, Enhanced migration of tumor cells in response to collagen degradation products and tumor cell collagenolytic activity, *Invasion and Metastasis*, **6**:270 (1986).
9. B.R. McAuslan and G.A. Gole, Cellular and molecular mechanisms in angiogenesis, *Trans. Ophthal. Soc. UK* **100**:354 (1980).
10. D.B. Rifkin, J.L. Gross, D. Moscatelli and E. Jaffe, Proteases, angiogenesis and invasion, *Symp. Fundam. Cancer Res.* **36**:187 (1983).
11 J.H. Greenberg, S. Seppa, H. Seppa and A.T. Hewitt, Role of collagen and fibronectin in neural crest cell adhesion and migration, *Devel. Biol.* **87**:259 (1981).
12. I.M. Herman, Extracellular matrix-cytoskeletal interactions in vascular cells, *Tissue and Cell* **19**:1 (1987).
13. D. Gospodarowicz and C.R. Ill, Extracellular matrix and control of proliferation of vascular endothelial cells, *J. Clin, Invest.* **65**:1351 (1980).
14. J.A. Madri and K.S. Stenn, Aortic endothelial cell migration. I. Matrix requirements and composition, *Am. J. Pathol.* **106**:180 (1982).
15. E.G. Bade and G. Nitzgen, Extracellular matrix (ECM) modulates the EGF induced migration of liver cells in serum free, hormone supplemented medium, *In Vitro* **21**:245 (1985).
16. B.R. McAuslan and W. Reilly, Endothelial cell phagokinesis in response to specific metal ions, *Exp. Cell Res.* **130**:147 (1980).
17. G.N. Hannan, J.W. Redman and B.R. McAuslan, Similarity of carbohydrate moieties of fibronectin derived from blood plasma and synthesized by cultured endothelial cells, *Biochim. Biophys. Acta* **801**:396 (1984).
18. J. Koch, T. Fifis, V. Bender and B.A. Moss, Molecular species of epidermal growth factor carrying immuno-suppressive activity, *J. Cell Biochem.* **25**:45 (1984).

19. B.R. McAuslan and H. Hoffman, Endothelium stimulating factor from Walker carcinoma cells: relation to tumor angiogenic factor, *Exp. Cell Res.* **119**:181 (1979).

20. B.R. McAuslan, W. Reilly, G.N. Hannan, K. Schindhelm, B. Milthorpe and B.A. Saur, Induction or endothelial cell migration by proine analogues and its relevance to angiogenesis, *Exp. Cell Res.* in press (1988).

21. B.R. McAuslan, V. Bender, W. Reilly and B.A. Moss, New functions of epidermal growth factor: stimulation of capillary endothelial cell migration and matrix dependent proliferation, *Cell Biol. Int. Reps.* **9**:175 (1985).

22. R.G. Azizkhan, J.C. Azizkhan, B.R. Zetter and J. Folkman, Mast cell heparin stimulates migration of capillary endothelial cells *in vitro*, *J. Exp. Med.* **152**:931 (1980).

23. J.B. Weiss, C.R. Hill, R.J. Davis and B. McLaughlin, Activation of mammalian procollagenase and basement membrane — degrading enzymes by a low molecular weight angiogenesis factor, *Agents and Actions,* **15**:107 (1984).

24. T. Kalebic, S. Garbisa, B. Glaser and L.A. Liotta, Basement membrane collagen: degradation by migrating endothelial cells, *Science* **July**:283 (1983).

25. J.L. Gross, D. Moscatelli and D.B. Rifkin, Increased capillary endothelial cell protease activity in response to angiogenic stimuli *in vitro*, *Proc. Natl. Acad. Sci. USA,* **80**:2623 (1983).

INDEX

Cell velocity   18-20, 24, 85, 86, 96, 206, 211, 212
Cell volume   40, 100, 102, 103, 106
Chemiluminescence (ChL)   136, 137, 139-141
Chemotaxis   109, 185, 189
Chief Cell   154, 157, 166, 171, 173
Cholecystokinin (CCK)   165
Choline acetyltransferase (ChA)   165
Cholinergic neuron   165, 169, 172
Cimetidine   146, 151-154, 157
Circle of Willis   51, 52, 57
Cisternae   7, 8
Cleft depth   3, 14
Cleft length   3, 14
Collagen   222-227
  type I   222
Collagenase   108, 165, 179, 195, 221, 224
Colloidal gold   222
Complement C5   95
Computer-assisted analysis video image   35
Computerized reconstruction   35, 40
Contact area   88, 89
Contact inhibition   43, 222
Contact length   88, 89
Convection   24, 30 147, 215
Convective coupling   30.
Convective transport   215
Convective velocity   218, 219
Cortical layer   107
Cremaster muscle   18, 21
Cushing ulcer   161, 174
Cycloheximide   130
Cyclooxygenase   115, 129, 130
Cytochalasin B (CB)   166, 195, 196, 198, 199
Cytokine   129-131, 190
Cytosolic free Ca^{2+} 7, 192
Cytotoxic T-cell   129, 132

D

Darcy's law   12
Debye length   11
Deformation index   88, 89
Degranulation   101, 107, 173
Density index (DI)   136-138
Dextran   15, 95, 98, 114, 216, 219
Diabetes   113, 117, 180
Diapedesis   84, 208
Dielectric constant   11
Diet, high cholesterol   53
Diffusion   5, 6, 15, 20, 24, 25, 29, 30, 60, 67, 73, 166, 174, 215, 216, 219, 220
  coefficient   4, 67, 215, 217, 219
Diffusive transport   215, 220
Disseminated Intravascular Coagulation (DIC)   135, 140
Dorsal skin fold chamber   78, 95, 97

E

Edema   77
EDTA   101-104

Effective molecular diameter   67
Electron microscopy   3-7, 9, 11, 16, 35, 37, 42, 57, 73, 96, 152, 165, 166, 169, 175, 195, 201
Electrical polarity   156
Electrostatic replusion   9, 10
Endarteriole   38
Endocytosis   179-183
Endoplasmic reticulum   106
Endothelial activation   185
Endothelial cell (*see* Endothelium)
Endothelium   3-17, 36, 38, 40, 42, 43, 47, 49, 56, 62, 68, 70, 71, 73, 77, 80, 82, 84-86, 89, 91, 114, 116, 123, 125, 128-130, 132, 137, 140, 145, 150, 152, 155-159, 161, 165, 169-172, 175, 179, 180-183, 185, 186, 189, 192, 193, 196, 199-201, 207-211, 213, 214, 226, 227
  bovine aorta (BAECS)   113, 130, 131
  bovine retinal capillary (BREC)   221, 223, 224
  corneal   131
  cultured   141, 166, 175, 195-199
  cytoplasm   7, 77, 80, 81
  damage   127, 135, 137, 140
  dying   70
  fenestra 175, 179
  flap   80
  gap   81, 84
  glomerular   182
  growth   186
  human umbilical vein (HUVEC)   130, 132
  junction   9, 14, 15, 70, 72, 77, 79, 81-83 150, 179, 208, 216
  lifetime   70
  migration   185, 190, 192, 221, 222, 224, 225-227
  mitosis   59-62, 70, 73, 148
  monolayer   70, 71, 185
  perforation   80
  proliferation   206
  sheath   81-83
  surface area   61
  turnover   43, 59, 70, 71
  turnover rate   70, 209
Endothelium-derived relaxing factor (EDRF)   36, 156
Endothelium-neutrophil interaction (*see* Leukocyte-endothelium adhesion)
Endotoxin   59, 81, 84, 128, 135-140
Enkephalin   165
Eosinophil   99, 100, 102, 105, 108
Epidermal growth factor (EGF)   222, 223, 225-227
Epididymal fat pad   179, 200
Epithelial cell   151, 153, 155, 156, 158, 159, 165, 166, 205, 222
Equivalent pore radius   15
Ergotamine compound   119, 124
Erythrocyte (*or* Red blood cell)   4, 15, 17-20, 24, 25, 85-87, 93, 96, 97, 100, 169-172, 175, 207

J

L

M

N

Non-Newtonian fluid 44-46
Norepinephrine (*or* Noradrenaline) 19, 164
Nuclear envelope 106
Nuclear to cytoplasmic volume ratio 36, 40
Nucleus 40, 42, 83

O

OKM-5 antibody 152
Opsonized zymosan 136
Organelle 78-80, 83, 99, 104, 106, 107, 132, 211
Osmolality 101
Osmotic pressure gradient 24
Oxygen-dervied free radicals 95, 98, 139

P

Paracellular macromolecular leakage 148
Paracellular pathway 3, 6, 7
Parasympathetic nervous system 163
Parietal cell 152, 153, 157-159, 166, 167, 173, 175
Peclet number 25, 219
Perfusion 17, 19, 21, 22, 24, 26, 27, 29, 30, 36, 41, 42, 52, 65, 87, 91, 165, 212-214, 218, 219
Periendothelial cell 208
Peripheral arterial occlusive disease (PAOD) 95
Peripheral vascular resistance 23, 214
Permeability 3, 5, 8, 12, 15-17, 23, 24, 29-31, 36, 59, 60-62, 67-72, 84, 98, 148-150, 155, 159, 160, 166, 175, 179, 182, 200, 207, 215-217, 220, 221
$PGF_{1\alpha}$, 6-keto 114-116, 119-124, 130
Phagocytosis 99, 102, 106, 141, 130, 192
Phagokinesis assay 222
Phagosome 106
Phase angle 45
Phosphoinositide 192
Phospholipid 128
Pinocytosis 102
Pinocytotic vesicle 168
Pirenzepine, ^3H- 166
Plasma derived serum (PDS) 113-116
Plasma volume 23, 30, 31, 146, 147
Plasmalemma 72, 80
Plasmalemmal vesicle 7, 8
Plasmin 128, 141, 173
Plasminogen 128, 221
  activator (PA) 120, 127-129
Platelet 35, 56, 81, 83, 101, 117, 124, 128, 132, 192
  aggregation 96, 115, 117, 124, 128-130, 132, 139
Platelet-derived growth factor (PDGF) 56
Poiseuille flow 11
Pressure gradient 13, 24, 30, 87, 91, 93, 215, 216, 218
Procoagulant 127, 131, 132

Procollagen 128
Proline analogue 222, 224, 225
Prostacyclin (PGI_2) 42, 113-117, 119, 123, 124, 125, 128-130, 132, 133, 192
  synthase 116, 117, 119-125, 129
  stimulatory activity (PSA) 113, 114, 116
Prostaglandin 42, 117, 119, 120, 124, 132, 133, 226
Protease inhibitor 135, 136, 139
Protein C 127, 131
Protein kinase C 8, 192
Protein permeability 23, 24, 29, 30, 73
Protein S 127, 131
Protein strand 9-11, 14, 15
Prothrombin 187, 189
Pseudopod 36, 79, 81, 99-105, 107
Psychogenic stress 162
Pulsatile flow 47, 52-56
Pyrilamine 151-156

Q

Quinuclidinyl benzilate 156
  ^3H- 159, 166, 175

R

Rabbit ear chamber 216
Radioautography (*or* Autoradiography) 151, 158, 160
Random walk theory 189
Reattachment point 45
Recirculation flow 53, 54, 56
Reconstruction 5, 6, 7, 35
  solid mode 38
  transparent mode 38
Red blood cell (RBC, *see* Erythrocyte)
Red cell velocity 85, 96
Reflection coefficient 24, 25, 30, 215
Refractive index 44, 52
Reilly phenomenon 163
Renovascular hypertension 36
Reperfusion 79, 95-98
  failure 95-98
Reynolds number 45, 54
Rouleau 15

S

S Phase 68, 70
Sarcoma 207
Sarcoplasmic reticulum 7, 8
Secondary flow 54-56
Serial section electron microscopy 5, 7, 16
Serine protease 128, 129, 139, 140
Serotonin 8, 160, 172, 173
Shape index 47
Shear rate 45, 85-89, 91
Shear stress 43, 45, 52, 53, 56, 57, 86-93, 98
Shock 139
Signal-transducing system 7